AT A GLANCE
YOU WILL DISCOVER IMPORTANT
DIFFERENCES BETWEEN SIMILAR FOODS:

Food and Description	Measure or Quantity	Calories	Carbo-hydrates (grams)
*Diet Pepsi Cola	6 fl. oz.	35	8.8
Tab	6 fl. oz.	<1	<.1
*Swanson Frozen Beef Dinner	11 oz.	414	32.5
Morton Frozen Beef Dinner	11 oz.	350	20.3

Here is the largest, most complete listing ever published of *precise* calorie counts, *exact* carbohydrate gram counts for practically everything edible—thousands and thousands of BRAND NAMES, BASIC FOODS, including ALCOHOLIC BEVERAGES.

No matter which diet you're following—whether you wish to maintain, gain, or lose weight—CALORIES AND CARBOHYDRATES will revolutionize your whole approach to dieting by taking the guesswork out of every mouthful you eat!

SIGNET Books of Related Interest

CALORIES AND CARBOHYDRATES

REVISED AND UPDATED

by
BARBARA KRAUS

Foreword by
Edward B. Greenspan, M.D.

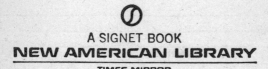

A SIGNET BOOK
NEW AMERICAN LIBRARY
TIMES MIRROR

For Rebecca K. Pecot

Library of Congress Catalog Card Number: 70–119037

SIGNET TRADEMARK REG. U.S. PAT. OFF. AND FOREIGN COUNTRIES
REGISTERED TRADEMARK—MARCA REGISTRADA
HECHO EN CHICAGO, U.S.A.

SIGNET, SIGNET CLASSICS, SIGNETTE,
MENTOR and PLUME BOOKS
are published by The New American Library, Inc.,
1301 Avenue of the Americas, New York, New York 10019

First Printing, August, 1973

1 2 3 4 5 6 7 8 9

PRINTED IN THE UNITED STATES OF AMERICA

FOREWORD

Well-documented actuarial statistics indicate that one out of every five adult Americans is overweight. (If we include overweight children in the figure, the number of Americans suffering from obesity is staggering.)

Why is this statistic so important? Because obesity has come to be regarded by the medical profession as a forerunner of some diseases. Quite simply, your chances of being afflicted with a serious ailment, such as heart disease, are greater if you are overweight.

Scientific study of the metabolisms of obese patients reveals two important facts about the way fat accumulates: 1) the ingestion of more calories than energy expended will lead to an increase in weight. 2) an excess of carbohydrates or other calorie-yielding nutrients (such as protein or fat) causes the formation of fat in the body. Clearly, it is important for each one of us to keep a close watch on the foods we eat—especially in a society so fond of rich foods, desserts, alcoholic beverages and soft drinks.

This extraordinary compilation by Barbara Kraus reveals the caloric and carbohydrate content of foods, both natural and processed, and should prove an invaluable aid not only to dietitians and physicians, but also to all individuals who wish to maintain, gain or lose weight.

Edward B. Greenspan, M.D.
Mount Sinai Hospital

CONTENTS

INTRODUCTION

This dictionary of foods lists several thousand brand-name products and basic foods with their caloric and carbohydrate content. The calorie yield of your diet versus the amount of energy you expend is the key to whether you maintain your ideal weight, gain too many pounds or lose weight.

Because of the relationship of weight to health, many individuals are "counting calories" at every meal. Interest has also been directed to the carbohydrate content of the diet in relation to weight control. Comprehensive information on these values in basic foods and brand-name products is not readily available in any one source. Nor is the information regularly reported in portions that are usually eaten or bought at the grocery store. To compound the problem, hundreds of new food items appear in our stores every year.

Arrangement of This Book

Foods are listed alphabetically by brand name or by the name of the food. The singular form is used for the entries, that is, blackberry instead of blackberries. Most items are listed individually though a few are grouped (see p. xii), for example, all candies are listed together so that if you are looking for *Mars* bar, you look first under Candy, then under *M* in alphabetical order. But, if you are looking for a breakfast food such as Oatmeal, you will find it under *O* in the main alphabet. Many cross references are included to assist in finding items called by different names.

Under the main headings, it was often not possible nor even desirable to follow an alphabetical arrangement. For basic foods such as apricots, for example, the first entries are for the fresh product weighed with seeds as it is purchased in the store, then the fruit in small portions as they may be eaten or measured. These entries are followed by the processed products, canned (although it may actually be a bottle or jar), dehydrated, dried and frozen. This basic plan, with adaptations where necessary, was followed for fruits, vegetables and meats.

In almost all entries where data were available the U.S. Department of Agriculture figures are shown first. The Department values represent averages from several manufacturers and are shown for comparison with the values from individual companies or for use where particular brands are not available.

All brand-name products have been italicized and company names appear in parentheses.

Portions Used

The portion column is a most important one to read and note. Common household measures are used insofar as possible. For some items, the amounts given are those commonly purchased in the store, such as 1 pound of meat, or a 15-ounce package of cake mix. These quantities can be divided into the number of servings used in the home and the nutritive values available to each person served can then be readily determined. Of course, any ingredients added in preparing such products must also be taken into account.

The smaller portions given are for foods as served or measured in moderate amounts, such as ½ cup of juice reconstituted, or 4 ounces of meat. Be sure to adjust the calories and carbohydrates to the actual portions you use. For example, if you serve 1 cup of juice instead of ½ cup, multiply the calories and carbohydrates shown for the smaller amount by 2.

Don't fool yourself about the size of portions you use. If you are serious about controlling the calories and carbohydrates in your diet, weigh your foods until you can accurately gauge the weight visually. Remember, the calories and carbohydrates go up with any increase in the weight of foods. Remember, too, that 4 ounces by weight may be very different from ½ cup or 4 fluid ounces. Ounces in the table are always ounces by weight unless specified as fluid ounces, or fractions of a cup or other volumetric measure. Foods that are fluffy in texture, such as flaked coconut and bean sprouts, vary greatly in weight per cup depending on how tightly they are packed into the cup. Such foods as canned green beans also vary when weighed with and without liquid, for example, canned green beans with liquid weigh 4.2 ounces for ½ cup, but drained beans weigh 2.5 ounces for the same ½ cup. Check the weights of your serving portions regularly. Bear in mind that you can cut calories and carbohydrates by cutting the serving size.

It was impossible to convert all the portions to a uniform basis. Some sources were only able to report data in terms of weights with no information on cup or other volumetric measures. We have shown small portions in quantities that might reasonably be expected to be served or measured in the home or institution. Package sizes are useful to show the composition of products as they are purchased and may be divided into the number of serving portions prepared from the entire product, taking into account any added ingredients.

You will find in the portion column the phrases "weighed with bone," or "weighed with skin and seeds" or other inedible parts. These descriptions apply to the products as you purchase them in the markets but the caloric values and the carbohydrate content as shown are for the amount of edible food after you discard the bone, skin, seed or other inedible part. The weight given in the "measure or quantity" column is to the nearest gram or fraction of an ounce.

Data on the composition of foods are constantly changing for many reasons. Better sampling and analytical methods, improvements in marketing procedures and changes in formulas of mixed products, all may alter values for carbohydrates and other nutrients as well as caloric values. Weights of packaged foods are frequently changed. It is essential to read label information to be informed about these matters and to make intelligent use of food tables.

Calories

What is a calorie? It is not a nutrient nor is it a good guide to the nutritive value of a food. It is more like a yardstick to measure the energy that a food will yield in the body. You need energy for your body functions as well as for exercise. If your diet contains more calories than your body uses for these purposes, the extra "energy" will be stored as fat. One pound of fat is equal to 3500 calories. Add this number of calories to those you need to balance your energy requirements and you will gain one pound; subtract it, and you will lose a pound.

Carbohydrates

The carbohydrate column shows the amount of this nutrient in grams for the quantities of foods indicated in the portion column. Some dietitians are giving special attention to this nutrient at present in connection with weight control. Carbohydrates include sugars, starches, acids and other nutrients. The values in this book are total carbohydrates, by difference, the basis on which calories from carbohydrates are calculated in the U.S. diet.

Other Nutrients

Do not forget that other nutrients are extremely important in diet planning—protein, fat, minerals and vitamins. Calories yielded by alcohol must also be considered in diet planning. From a nutrition viewpoint, perhaps the best advice that can be given to the dieter is to eat a varied diet with all classes of foods represented. Meat, fish, chicken, fats and oils, milk, vegetables, fruits and grain products are all important sources of essential nutrients and some foods from each of these classes of foods should be included in the diet every day. With the great abundance and variety of foods on the grocer's shelves, there is no reason why the dieter should not enjoy a tasty, nutritious and attractive diet. Just eat in moderation and there is no need to eliminate any one food altogether, except in special conditions under a doctor's directions. Choose wisely and eat well.

Sources of Data

Values in this dictionary are based on publications issued by the U.S. Department of Agriculture and on data submitted by manufacturers and processors. The U.S. Department of Agriculture issues basic tables on food composition for use in the United States. The commercial products from U.S.D.A. publications represent average values obtained on products of more than one company. The figures designated "home recipe" are based on recipes on file with the Department of Agriculture. Data on commercial products listed by brand name in this publication are based on values supplied by manufacturers and processors for their own individual products. Supermarket brand names, such as A & P's *Ann Page,* or private labels could not be included in this book inasmuch as they are not usually analyzed under these trade names. Every care has been taken to interpret the data and the descriptions supplied by the companies as fully and accurately as possible. Many values have been recalculated to different portions from those submitted in order to bring about greater uniformity among similar items.

Calories in these different sources are not always on a strictly uniform basis. In the Department of Agriculture, calories are calculated using specific factors, which make allowances for losses in digestion and metabolism. The technical explanation of these factors is given in Handbook 74 of the United States Department of Agriculture. Most manufacturers use average factors of 4, 9 and 4 for calories yielded by each gram of protein, fat and carbohydrates respectively; a factor of 7 is used as an average value to calculate the calories from one gram of alcohol. These differences in procedure will give somewhat different results for products of similar composition. Some manufacturers have adopted the values from U.S. Department of Agriculture publications as representative of their own products. In these cases, it will be apparent in the table that the data from the companies match exactly those from U.S.D.A. publications.

Analyses of foods to provide information on nutritive values are extremely expensive to conduct. Many small companies have not been able to afford to have their products analyzed and thus were unable to provide data for this book or were able to provide only the calories or only the carbohydrates. Other companies have simply never gotten around to having the analysis done. New requirements for labeling nutritive values of products may provide information on additional items in the future.

Bear in mind that small differences in calorie values on similar products of the same weight are not important in diet planning. They may be due to different methods of calculating the calories or to small differences in the nutritive values of the samples analyzed because no two foods ever have exactly the same composition. Some differences may also be due to the way the food was measured as noted in the case of green beans earlier.

Carbohydrates in this book are usually total carbohydrates by difference. A few manufacturers reported only "available carbohydrates." These values were omitted.

Foods Listed by Groups

Foods in the following classes are reported together rather than as individual items in the main alphabet: Baby Food; Bread; Cake Icing; Cake Icing Mix; Candy; Cheese; Cookie; Cookie Mix; Cracker; Gravy; Salad Dressing; and Sauce.

Barbara Kraus

ABBREVIATIONS AND SYMBOLS

(USDA) = United States Department of Agriculture
* = Prepared as package directs[1]
< = less than
& = and
" = inch
D.N.A. = Data not available
dia. = diameter
fl. = fluid
liq. = liquid
lb. = pound

med. = medium
neg. = negligible
oz. = ounce
pkg. = package
pt. = pint
qt. = quart
sq. = square
T. = tablespoon
Tr. = trace
tsp. = teaspoon
wt. = weight

italics or name in parentheses = registered trademark, ®

EQUIVALENTS

By Weight

1 pound = 16 ounces
1 ounce = 28.35 grams
3.52 ounces = 100 grams

By Volume

1 quart = 4 cups
1 cup = 8 fluid ounces
1 cup = ½ pint
1 cup = 16 tablespoons
2 tablespoons = 1 fluid ounce
1 tablespoon = 3 teaspoons
1 pound butter = 4 sticks or 2 cups

[1]If the package directions call for whole or skim milk, the data given here is for whole milk, unless otherwise stated.

Food and Description	Measure or Quantity	Calories	Carbohydrates (grams)

A

ABALONE (USDA):
Raw, meat only	4 oz.	111	3.9
Canned	4 oz.	91	2.6

ABISANTE LIQUEUR (Leroux):
100 proof	1 fl. oz.	87	1.0
120 proof	1 fl. oz.	104	1.0

AC'CENT
	¼ tsp. (1 gram)	3	0.

ACEROLA, fresh (USDA):
Fruit	½ lb. (weighed with seeds)	52	12.6
Juice	½ cup (4.3 oz.)	28	5.8

ALBACORE, raw, meat only (USDA)
	4 oz.	201	0.

ALCOHOLIC BEVERAGES
(See individual listings)

ALEWIFE (USDA):
Raw, meat only	4 oz.	144	0.
Canned, solids & liq.	4 oz.	160	0.

ALMOND:
In shell:
(USDA)	4 oz. (weighed in shell)	347	11.3
(USDA)	1 cup (2.8 oz.)	239	7.8

Shelled:
Plain:
Whole (USDA)	½ cup (2.5 oz.)	425	13.8
Whole (USDA)	1 oz.	170	5.5

(USDA): United States Department of Agriculture
DNA: Data Not Available
* Prepared as Package Directs

Food and Description	Measure or Quantity	Calories	Carbo-hydrates (grams)
Whole (USDA)	13–15 almonds (.6 oz.)	105	3.4
Chopped (USDA)	1 cup (4.5 oz.)	759	24.8
(Blue Diamond)	1 oz.	176	5.5
Blanched (Blue Diamond) salted or slivered	1 oz.	176	5.5
Chocolate-covered (See CANDY)			
Flavored (Blue Diamond) barbecue, cheese, French-fried, onion-garlic or smokehouse-style	1 oz.	180	9.5
Roasted:			
Diced (Blue Diamond)	1 oz.	176	5.5
Dry (Planters)	1 oz.	191	5.5
Salted (USDA)	1 cup (5.5 oz.)	984	30.6
Salted (USDA)	1 oz.	178	5.5
ALMOND EXTRACT (Ehlers)	1 tsp.	5	D.N.A.
ALMOND MEAL, partially defatted (USDA)	1 oz.	116	8.2
ALPHABET SOUP MIX:			
*(Golden Grain)	1 cup	54	9.0
(Lipton) vegetable	1 pkg. (2 oz.)	205	36.6
ALPHA-BITS, oat cereal (Post)	1 cup (1 oz.)	113	23.0
AMARANTH, raw (USDA):			
Untrimmed	1 lb. (weighed untrimmed)	103	18.6
Trimmed	4 oz.	41	7.4
AMBROSIA, chilled bottled (Kraft)	4 oz.	85	14.7
ANCHOVY PASTE, canned (Crosse & Blackwell)	1 T.	20	1.0
ANCHOVY, PICKLED, canned, with & without added oil (USDA)	1 oz.	50	<.1

Food and Description	Measure or Quantity	Calories	Carbo-hydrates (grams)
ANESONE LIQUEUR			
(Leroux) 90 proof	1 fl. oz.	86	2.8
ANGEL FOOD CAKE:			
Home recipe (USDA)	½2 of 8" cake		
	(1.4 oz.)	108	24.1
Loaf (Van de Kamp's)	10-oz. loaf	1006	D.N.A.
Ring, chocolate iced (Van de Kamp's)	7½" cake	2528	D.N.A.
ANGEL FOOD CAKE MIX:			
(USDA)	4 oz.	437	100.4
*(USDA)	½2 of 10" cake		
	(1.9 oz.)	137	31.5
(Betty Crocker):			
*1 step	⅟16 of cake	111	26.2
*2 step	⅟16 of cake	100	22.8
*Confetti	⅟16 of cake	114	26.8
*Lemon custard	⅟16 of cake	111	26.0
*Strawberry	⅟16 of cake	115	27.1
*(Duncan Hines)	½2 of cake		
	(2 oz.)	131	29.6
(Pillsbury) raspberry swirl	1 oz.	102	23.6
(Pillsbury) white	1 oz.	102	23.3
*(Swans Down)	½2 of cake		
	(1.8 oz.)	132	29.7
ANISE EXTRACT (Ehlers)	1 tsp.	12	D.N.A.
ANISETTE LIQUEUR:			
(Bols) 50 proof	1 fl. oz.	111	13.9
(Garnier) 54 proof	1 fl. oz.	82	9.3
(Hiram Walker) 60 proof, red or white	1 fl. oz.	92	10.8
(Leroux) 60 proof, red or white	1 fl. oz.	89	9.9
(Old Mr. Boston) 42 proof	1 fl. oz.	64	8.0
(Old Mr. Boston) 60 proof	1 fl. oz.	90	7.5

(USDA): United States Department of Agriculture
DNA: Data Not Available
* Prepared as Package Directs

Food and Description	Measure or Quantity	Calories	Carbo-hydrates (grams)
APPLE, any variety:			
Fresh (USDA):			
Eaten with skin	1 lb. (weighed with skin & core)	242	60.5
Eaten with skin	1 med., 2½″ dia. (about 3 per lb.)	80	20.0
Eaten without skin	1 lb. (weighed without skin & core)	211	55.0
Eaten without skin	1 med., 2½″ dia. (about 3 per lb.)	70	18.2
Pared, diced	1 cup (3.8 oz.)	59	15.4
Pared, quartered	1 cup (4.3 oz.)	66	17.2
Dehydrated:			
Uncooked (USDA)	1 oz.	100	26.1
Cooked, sweetened (USDA)	½ cup (4.2 oz.)	91	23.5
Dried (USDA):			
Uncooked	4 oz.	312	81.4
Uncooked (Del Monte)	1 cup (3 oz.)	238	56.7
Cooked, unsweetened	½ cup (4.3 oz.)	94	24.6
Cooked, sweetened	½ cup (4.9 oz.)	157	40.9
Frozen, sweetened, slices, not thawed (USDA)	4 oz.	105	27.6
APPLE BROWN BETTY, home recipe (USDA)	1 cup (8.1 oz.)	347	68.3
APPLE BUTTER:			
(USDA)	½ cup (5 oz.)	262	66.0
(USDA)	1 T. (.6 oz.)	33	8.4
(Musselman's)	1 T.	33	D.N.A.
(White House)	1 T.	28	7.6
APPLE CAKE MIX:			
*Cinnamon (Duncan Hines)	1⁄12 of cake (2.7 oz.)	202	35.0
*Cinnamon, pudding cake (Betty Crocker)	1⁄8 of cake	223	44.5
*Cinnamon, upside down (Betty Crocker)	1⁄9 of cake	269	44.2
APPLE CIDER (Indian Summer)	6 fl. oz.	78	19.5

Food and Description	Measure or Quantity	Calories	Carbo- hydrates (grams)
APPLE DRINK, canned:			
(Hi-C)	6 fl. oz.	87	22.2
(Del Monte)	6 fl. oz.	81	14.9
APPLE DUMPLING, frozen (Pepperidge Farm)	1 dumpling (3.3 oz.)	276	30.7
APPLE FRITTERS, frozen (Mrs. Paul's)	12-oz. pkg.	712	95.4
APPLE FRUIT ROLL, frozen (Chun King)	1 oz.	64	10.1
APPLE JACKS, cereal (Kellogg's)	1 cup (1 oz.)	112	25.8
APPLE JELLY:			
Sweetened (White House)	1 T.	46	13.0
Dietetic or low calorie:			
(Dia-Mel) fresh pressed, old fashioned, or mint	1 T.	22	5.4
(Diet Delight)	1 T. (.6 oz.)	22	5.4
(Kraft)	1 oz.	34	8.5
(Slenderella)	1 T. (.6 oz.)	22	5.6
(Tillie Lewis)	1 T.	9	2.1
APPLE JUICE:			
Canned: (USDA)	½ cup (4.4 oz.)	58	14.8
(Heinz)	5½-fl.-oz. can	88	21.7
(Musselman's)	½ cup	62	D.N.A.
(Seneca)	½ (4.4 oz.)	61	14.8
(White House)	½ cup	58	15.0
*Frozen (Seneca)	½ cup (4.4 oz.)	61	14.8
APPLE-PAPAYA FRUIT SPREAD, low calorie (Vita)	1 T.	9	D.N.A.
APPLE PIE:			
Home recipe, 2 crusts (USDA)	⅛ of 9" pie (5.6 oz.)	404	60.2

(USDA): United States Department of Agriculture
DNA: Data Not Available
* Prepared as Package Directs

Food and Description	*Measure or Quantity*	*Calories*	*Carbo-hydrates (grams)*
(Tastykake)	4-oz. pie	380	58.6
French apple (Tastykake)	4½-oz. pie	451	64.3
Frozen:			
Unbaked (USDA)	5 oz.	298	47.1
Baked (USDA)	5 oz.	361	56.8
(Banquet)	5 oz.	351	49.5
(Morton)	⅙ of 20-oz. pie	240	33.7
(Mrs. Smith's)	⅙ of 8″ pie (4.2 oz.)	303	42.0
(Mrs. Smith's) Dutch apple	⅙ of 8″ pie (4.2 oz.)	326	47.2
(Mrs. Smith's) tart	⅙ of 8″ pie (4.2 oz.)	266	44.0
APPLE PIE FILLING:			
(Comstock)	1 cup (10¾ oz.)	356	91.3
(Lucky Leaf)	8 oz.	248	60.8
APPLESAUCE, canned:			
Sweetened:			
(USDA)	½ cup (4.5 oz.)	116	30.5
(Del Monte)	½ cup (4.6 oz.)	119	32.6
(Seneca) cinnamon	½ cup (4.5 oz.)	134	30.2
(Seneca) 100% McIntosh	½ cup (4.5 oz.)	116	30.2
(Stokely-Van Camp)	½ cup(4.2 oz.)	109	28.5
(White House)	½ cup (4.5 oz.)	110	28.2
Unsweetened, dietetic or low calorie:			
(USDA)	½ cup (4.3 oz.)	50	13.2
(Blue Boy)	4 oz.	43	10.4
(Diet Delight)	½ cup (4.4 oz.)	58	14.2
(Lucky Leaf)	4 oz.	49	11.6
(S and W) *Nutradiet,* low calorie	4 oz.	54	13.7
(Tillie Lewis)	½ cup (4.2 oz.)	51	12.2
(White House)	½ cup (4.3 oz.)	48	12.2
APPLESAUCE CAKE MIX:			
*Raisin (Duncan Hines)	⅑ of cake (2.7 oz.)	200	37.2
Spice (Pillsbury)	1 oz.	117	22.7
APPLE TURNOVER, frozen			
(Pepperidge Farm)	1 turnover (3.3 oz.)	315	30.2

Food and Description	Measure or Quantity	Calories	Carbo-hydrates (grams)
APRICOT:			
Fresh (USDA):			
Whole	1 lb. (weighed with pits)	217	54.6
Whole	3 apricots (about 12 per lb.)	55	13.7
Halves	1 cup (5.5 oz.)	80	20.0
Canned:			
Juice pack, solids & liq. (USDA)	4 oz.	61	15.4
Light syrup, solids & liq. (USDA)	4 oz.	75	19.1
Heavy syrup:			
Halves & syrup (USDA)	½ cup (4.4 oz.)	108	27.7
Halves & syrup (USDA)	4 med. halves with 2 T. syrup (4.3 oz.)	105	26.8
(Hunt's)	½ cup (4.5 oz.)	103	26.9
Unsweetened or low calorie:			
Water pack, halves & liq. (USDA)	4 oz.	43	10.9
Water pack, halves & liq. (USDA)	½ cup (4.3 oz.)	46	11.7
(Diet Delight) solids & liq.	½ cup (4.4 oz.)	60	14.9
(Libby's)	4 oz.	40	10.9
(S and W) *Nutradiet,* low calorie	4 halves (3.5 oz.)	40	9.6
(Tillie Lewis) solids & liq.	½ cup (4.3 oz.)	49	11.2
Dehydrated:			
Uncooked (USDA)	4 oz.	376	95.9
Cooked, solids & liq., sugar added (USDA)	4 oz.	135	34.6
Slices (Vacu-Dry)	1 oz.	94	24.0
Dried:			
Uncooked:			
(USDA)	1 lb.	1179	301.6
(USDA)	14 large halves (½ cup or 2.8 oz.)	211	53.9

(USDA): United States Department of Agriculture
DNA: Data Not Available
* Prepared as Package Directs

Food and Description	Measure or Quantity	Calories	Carbo-hydrates (grams)
(USDA)	10 small halves (¼ cup or 1.3 oz.)	99	25.3
(Del Monte)	½ cup (2.3 oz.)	163	41.6
Cooked (USDA):			
Sweetened	½ cup with liq. (12–13 halves, 5.7 oz.)	198	50.9
Unsweetened	½ cup with liq. (4.3 oz.)	104	26.4
Frozen, sweetened, not thawed (USDA)	4 oz.	111	28.5
APRICOT-APPLE JUICE DRINK, canned (BC)	6 fl. oz.	96	D.N.A.
APRICOT, CANDIED (USDA)	1 oz.	96	24.5
APRICOT JELLY, low calorie (Tillie Lewis)	1 T. (.5 oz.)	10	2.4
APRICOT LIQUEUR:			
(Bols) 60 proof	1 fl. oz.	96	8.9
(Hiram Walker) 60 proof	1 fl. oz.	82	8.2
(Leroux) 60 proof	1 fl. oz.	85	8.9
APRICOT NECTAR, canned			
Sweetened:			
(USDA)	½ cup (4.2 oz.)	68	17.5
(Del Monte)	½ cup (4.3 oz.)	68	18.0
(Dewco)	½ cup	68	D.N.A.
(Heinz)	5½-fl.-oz. can	90	21.0
Low calorie (S and W) *Nutradiet*	4 oz. by weight	35	8.2
APRICOT-ORANGE PIE (Tastykake)	4-oz. pie	377	54.8
APRICOT PIE FILLING:			
(Comstock)	1 cup (10¾ oz.)	314	78.5
(Lucky Leaf)	8 oz.	316	77.6
APRICOT & PINEAPPLE NECTAR, unsweetened (S and W) *Nutradiet*	4 oz. (by wt.)	35	8.5

Food and Description	Measure or Quantity	Calories	Carbo-hydrates (grams)
APRICOT & PINEAPPLE PRESERVE:			
Sweetened (Bama)	1 T. (.7 oz.)	54	13.5
Dietetic or low calorie:			
(Dia-Mel)	1 T.	22	5.4
(Diet Delight)	1 T. (.6 oz.)	21	5.1
(S and W) *Nutradiet*	1 T. (.5 oz.)	10	2.5
(Tillie Lewis)	1 T. (.5 oz.)	10	2.4
APRICOT PRESERVE:			
Sweetened (Bama)	1 T. (.7 oz.)	51	12.7
Dietetic or low calorie:			
(Dia-Mel)	1 T.	22	5.4
(Polaner)	1 T.	6	.3
AQUAVIT (Leroux) 90 Proof	1 fl. oz.	75	Tr.
ARTICHOKE, Globe or French (See also **JERUSALEM ARTICHOKE**):			
Raw, whole (USDA)	1 lb. (weighed untrimmed)	85	19.2
Boiled, drained (USDA)	4 oz.	50	11.2
Frozen, hearts (Birds Eye)	5–6 hearts (3 oz.)	22	4.8
ASPARAGUS:			
Raw, whole spears (USDA)	1 lb. (weighed untrimmed)	66	12.7
Boiled, whole spears (USDA)	4 spears (½″ at base, 2.1 oz.)	12	2.2
Boiled, cut spears, 1½″–2″ pieces, drained (USDA)	1 cup (5.1 oz.)	29	5.2
Canned, regular pack:			
Green:			
Spears & liq. (USDA)	1 cup (8.6 oz.)	44	7.1
Spears only (USDA)	1 cup (7.6 oz.)	45	7.3
Spears only (USDA)	6 med. spears (3.4 oz.)	20	3.3
Liq. only (USDA)	2 T.	3	.7

(USDA): United States Department of Agriculture
DNA: Data Not Available
* Prepared as Package Directs

Food and Description	Measure or Quantity	Calories	Carbohydrates (grams)
Spears & liq. (Del Monte)	1 cup (8 oz.)	25	3.0
Spears & liq. (Green Giant)	⅓ of 15-oz. can	23	3.4
Spears & liq. (Stokely-Van Camp)	½ cup (3.9 oz.)	20	3.3
Cut, drained solids (Cannon)	4 oz.	24	3.9
White:			
Spears & liq. (USDA)	1 cup (8.4 oz.)	43	7.9
Spears only (USDA)	1 cup (7.6 oz.)	47	7.7
Spears only (USDA)	6 med. spears (3.4 oz.)	21	3.5
Liq. only (USDA)	2 T.	3	.8
Canned, dietetic pack:			
Green:			
Spears & liq. (USDA)	4 oz.	18	3.1
Drained solids (USDA)	4 oz.	23	3.5
Spears & liq. (Blue Boy)	4 oz.	20	3.2
Spears & liq. (Diet Delight)	4 oz.	19	2.9
(S and W) Nutradiet	5 whole spears (3.5 oz.)	16	2.4
(Tillie Lewis)	½ cup (4.2 oz.)	22	2.6
White, spears & liq. (USDA)	4 oz.	18	3.4
Frozen:			
Cuts & tips, not thawed (USDA)	4 oz.	26	4.1
Cuts & tips, boiled, drained (USDA)	½ cup (3.2 oz.)	20	3.2
Cuts & tips, boiled, drained (USDA)	4 oz.	25	4.0
Cuts (Birds Eye)	½ cup (3.3 oz.)	20	3.3
Cut spears in butter sauce (Green Giant)	⅓ of 9-oz. pkg.	47	4.0
Spears, not thawed (USDA)	4 oz.	27	4.4
Spears, boiled, drained (USDA)	4 oz.	26	4.3
Spears (Birds Eye)	⅓ pkg. (3.3 oz.)	22	3.6
Spears with Hollandaise sauce (Birds Eye)	⅓ pkg. (3.3 oz.)	97	3.2

Food and Description	Measure or Quantity	Calories	Carbo-hydrates (grams)
ASPARAGUS CRISPS, dehydrated snack (Epicure)	1 oz.	78	12.2
ASPARAGUS SOUP, Cream of, canned:			
Condensed (USDA)	8 oz. (by wt.)	123	19.1
*Prepared with equal volume water (USDA)	1 cup (8.5 oz.)	65	10.1
*Prepared with equal volume milk (USDA)	1 cup (8.5 oz.)	144	16.3
*(Campbell)	1 cup (8 fl. oz.)	80	10.7
ASTI WINE (Gancia) 9% alcohol	3 fl. oz.	126	18.0
AUNT JEMIMA SYRUP	¼ cup	212	54.0
AVOCADO, peeled, pitted (USDA):			
All commercial varieties:			
Whole	1 lb. (weighed with seed & skin)	568	21.4
Diced	½ cup (2.6 oz.)	124	4.7
Mashed	½ cup (4.1 oz.)	194	7.3
California varieties, mainly Fuerte:			
Whole	½ avocado (3⅛" dia.)	185	6.5
½-inch cubes	½ cup (2.7 oz.)	130	4.6
Florida varieties:			
Whole	½ avocado (3⅝" dia.)	195	13.4
½-inch cubes	½ cup (2.7 oz.)	97	6.7
***AWAKE** (Birds Eye)	½ cup (4 oz.)	55	12.6
AYDS, vanilla or chocolate	1 piece	26	4.9

(USDA): United States Department of Agriculture
DNA: Data Not Available
* Prepared as Package Directs

Food and Description	Measure or Quantity	Calories	Carbo-hydrates (grams)

B

BABY FOOD:

Apple:

& apricot, junior (Beech-Nut)	7¾ oz.	204	50.4
& apricot, strained (Beech-Nut)	4¾ oz.	121	29.1
& cranberry, junior (Heinz)	7¾ oz.	191	46.6
& cranberry, strained (Heinz)	4¾ oz.	124	30.7
& pear, junior (Heinz)	7¾ oz.	180	43.7
& pear, strained (Heinz)	4½ oz.	108	26.4
Dutch, dessert, junior (Gerber)	7⁸⁄₁₀ oz.	204	47.8
Dutch, dessert, strained (Gerber)	4⁷⁄₁₀ oz.	124	28.5
Apple-apricot juice, strained (Heinz)	4½ fl. oz.	92	22.4
Apple Betty (Beech-Nut)			
Junior	7¾ oz.	234	55.2
Strained	4¾ oz.	146	34.6
Apple-cherry juice:			
Strained (Beech-Nut)	4⅕ fl. oz.	74	18.4
Strained (Gerber)	4⅕ fl. oz.	59	14.2
Strained (Heinz)	4½ fl. oz.	86	21.1
Apple gel, strained (Beech-Nut)	4½ oz.	85	21.0
Apple-grape juice:			
Strained (Beech-Nut)	4⅕ fl. oz.	81	20.1
Strained (Heinz)	4½ fl. oz.	89	22.3
Apple juice:			
Strained (Beech-Nut)	4⅕ fl. oz.	57	14.4
Strained (Gerber)	4⅕ fl. oz.	65	16.0
Strained (Heinz)	4½ fl. oz.	88	21.7
Apple-pineapple juice, strained (Heinz)	4½ fl. oz.	92	22.5
Apple-prune & honey, junior (Heinz)	7½ oz.	181	43.8
Apple-prune & honey with tapioca, strained (Heinz)	4½ oz.	107	25.4

Food and Description	Measure or Quantity	Calories	Carbo-hydrates (grams)
Apple-prune juice, strained (Heinz)	4½ fl. oz.	89	22.0
Applesauce:			
Junior (Beech-Nut)	7¾ oz.	195	46.9
Junior (Gerber)	7⁸⁄₁₀ oz.	179	44.6
Junior (Heinz)	7¾ oz.	182	44.7
Strained (Beech-Nut)	4¾ oz.	119	28.9
Strained (Gerber)	4⁷⁄₁₀ oz.	109	27.4
Strained (Heinz)	4½ oz.	98	24.0
& apricots, junior (Gerber)	7⁸⁄₁₀ oz.	192	47.0
& apricots, junior (Heinz)	7¾ oz.	174	41.6
& apricots, strained (Gerber)	4⁷⁄₁₀ oz.	116	29.2
& apricots, strained (Heinz)	4¾ oz.	98	23.8
& cherries, junior (Beech-Nut)	7¾ oz.	204	48.6
& cherries, strained (Beech-Nut)	4¾ oz.	125	28.8
& cranberries, junior (Beech-Nut)	7¾ oz.	208	51.2
& cranberries, strained (Beech-Nut)	4¾ oz.	127	31.4
& pineapple, junior (Beech-Nut)	7¾ oz.	195	48.0
& pineapple, junior (Gerber)	7⁸⁄₁₀ oz.	162	41.7
& pineapple, strained (Beech-Nut)	4¾ oz.	119	29.3
& pineapple, strained (Gerber)	4⁷⁄₁₀ oz.	106	26.4
& raspberries, junior (Beech-Nut)	7¾ oz.	239	56.7
& raspberries, strained (Beech-Nut)	4¾ oz.	142	34.0
Apricot with tapioca:			
Junior (Beech-Nut)	7¾ oz.	186	44.9
Junior (Gerber)	7⁸⁄₁₀ oz.	178	44.1
Junior (Heinz)	7¾ oz.	224	55.0
Strained (Beech-Nut)	4¾ oz.	102	24.8

(USDA): United States Department of Agriculture
DNA: Data Not Available
* Prepared as Package Directs

Food and Description	Measure or Quantity	Calories	Carbo-hydrates (grams)
Strained (Gerber)	4⁷⁄₁₀ oz.	107	26.4
Strained (Heinz)	4¾ oz.	141	33.3
Banana:			
Strained (Heinz)	4½ oz.	105	25.0
& pineapple, junior (Heinz)	7¾ oz.	167	40.6
& pineapple with tapioca, junior (Beech-Nut)	7¾ oz.	204	49.7
& pineapple with tapioca, junior (Gerber)	7¾ oz.	185	44.4
& pineapple with tapioca, strained (Beech-Nut)	4¾ oz.	127	30.0
& pineapple with tapioca, strained (Gerber)	4⁷⁄₁₀ oz.	113	27.4
Dessert, junior (Beech-Nut)	7¾ oz.	204	49.5
Pie, junior (Heinz)	7¾ oz.	207	45.0
Pie, strained (Heinz)	4¾ oz.	116	25.0
Pudding, junior (Gerber)	7⁸⁄₁₀ oz.	210	48.2
With tapioca, strained (Beech-Nut)	4¾ oz.	119	28.8
With tapioca, strained (Gerber)	4⁷⁄₁₀ oz.	113	27.4
Bean, green:			
Junior (Beech-Nut)	7¼ oz.	55	10.9
Strained (Beech-Nut)	4½ oz.	36	6.9
Strained (Gerber)	4½ oz.	36	8.5
Strained (Heinz)	4½ oz.	37	6.4
Creamed with bacon, junior (Gerber)	7½ oz.	141	19.0
In butter sauce (Beech-Nut):			
Junior	7¼ oz.	88	15.4
Strained	4½ oz.	55	9.3
With potatoes & ham, casserole, toddler (Gerber)	6⅕ oz.	139	17.8
Beef:			
Junior (Beech-Nut)	3½ oz.	87	.3
Junior (Gerber)	3½ oz.	95	0.
Junior (Heinz)	3½ oz.	99	0.
Strained (Beech-Nut)	3½ oz.	101	0.
Strained (Gerber)	3½ oz.	90	0.
Strained (Heinz)	3½ oz.	92	0.
Beef & beef heart, strained (Gerber)	3½ oz.	85	.7

Food and Description	*Measure or Quantity*	*Calories*	*Carbo-hydrates (grams)*
Beef dinner:			
Junior (Beech-Nut)	4½ oz.	119	6.9
Strained (Beech-Nut)	4½ oz.	132	7.3
& noodles, junior (Beech-Nut)	7½ oz.	136	15.8
& noodles, junior (Gerber)	7½ oz.	107	13.1
& noodles, strained (Beech-Nut)	4½ oz.	78	11.7
& noodles, strained (Gerber)	4½ oz.	61	9.1
With vegetables, junior (Gerber)	4½ oz.	105	7.6
With vegetables, strained (Gerber)	3½ oz.	104	6.9
With vegetables & cereal, junior (Heinz)	4¾ oz.	110	6.2
With vegetables, strained (Heinz)	4¾ oz.	109	6.3
Beef lasagna, toddler (Gerber)	6½ oz.	135	16.8
Beef liver, strained (Gerber)	3½ oz.	92	2.0
Beef liver soup, strained (Heinz)	4½ oz.	57	8.1
Beef stew, toddler (Gerber)	6⅕ oz.	120	15.2
Beet:			
Strained (Gerber)	4½ oz.	48	11.0
Strained (Heinz)	4½ oz.	60	12.7
Butterscotch pudding, strained (Gerber)	4½ oz.	129	23.3
Caramel pudding (Beech-Nut):			
Junior	7¾ oz.	215	48.8
Strained	4¾ oz.	131	29.6
Carrot:			
Junior (Beech-Nut)	7½ oz.	76	16.5
Junior (Gerber)	7½ oz.	63	14.9
Junior (Heinz)	7¾ oz.	86	19.0
Strained (Beech-Nut)	4½ oz.	45	9.7
Strained (Gerber)	4½ oz.	37	9.0
Strained (Heinz)	4½ oz.	52	11.6

(USDA): United States Department of Agriculture
DNA: Data Not Available
* Prepared as Package Directs

Food and Description	Measure or Quantity	Calories	Carbo-hydrates (grams)
In butter sauce (Beech-Nut)			
Junior	7½ oz.	114	23.1
Strained	4½ oz.	69	14.2
Cereal, dry:			
Barley (Gerber)	3 T. (¼ oz.)	27	4.9
Barley, instant (Heinz)	2 T	19	3.9
High protein (Gerber)	3 T. (7 grams)	26	3.3
High protein, instant (Heinz)	2 T.	29	3.7
Hi-protein (Beech-Nut)	1 oz.	101	12.2
Mixed (Beech-Nut)	1 oz.	105	19.3
Mixed, honey (Beech-Nut)	1 oz.	106	19.9
Mixed (Gerber)	3 T. (7 grams)	27	5.3
Mixed (Heinz)	2 T.	21	4.0
Oatmeal (Beech-Nut)	1 oz.	108	18.8
Oatmeal, honey (Beech-Nut)	1 oz.	109	19.8
Oatmeal (Gerber)	3 T. (7 grams)	28	4.7
Oatmeal, instant (Heinz)	2 T.	18	3.2
Rice (Beech-Nut)	1 oz.	105	21.2
Rice, honey (Beech-Nut)	1 oz.	106	22.5
Rice (Gerber)	3 T. (7 grams)	26	5.5
Rice, instant (Heinz)	2 T.	20	4.2
Cereal, or mixed cereal:			
With applesauce & banana, strained (Gerber)	4⁷⁄₁₀ oz.	111	24.4
With egg yolks & bacon, junior (Beech-Nut)	7½ oz.	201	17.2
With egg yolks & bacon, junior (Gerber)	7½ oz.	158	15.1
With egg yolks & bacon, junior (Heinz)	7½ oz.	164	15.5
With egg yolks & bacon, strained (Beech-Nut)	4½ oz.	120	10.2
With egg yolks & bacon, strained (Gerber)	4½ oz.	92	9.0
With egg yolks & bacon, strained (Heinz)	4½ oz.	112	10.0
With fruit, strained (Beech-Nut)	4¾ oz.	111	25.7
Oatmeal with fruit, strained (Beech-Nut)	4¾ oz.	98	20.4
Oatmeal with applesauce			

Food and Description	Measure or Quantity	Calories	Carbo- hydrates (grams)
& banana, strained (Gerber)	4⁷⁄₁₀ oz.	99	20.7
Rice, with applesauce & banana, strained (Gerber)	4⁷⁄₁₀ oz.	93	21.3
Cheese:			
Cottage, with banana, junior (Heinz)	7¾ oz.	169	36.3
Cottage, with banana, strained (Heinz)	4½ oz.	97	20.9
Cottage, creamed, with pineapple, junior (Beech-Nut)	7¾ oz.	184	35.5
Cottage, creamed, with pineapple, strained (Gerber)	4½ oz.	174	23.3
Cottage, creamed, with pineapple juice, strained (Beech-Nut)	4¾ oz.	119	23.2
Cherry vanilla pudding (Gerber):			
Junior	7⁸⁄₁₀ oz.	190	43.3
Strained	4⁷⁄₁₀ oz.	115	29.8
Chicken:			
Junior (Beech-Nut)	3½ oz.	97	0.
Junior (Gerber)	3½ oz.	133	.5
Junior (Heinz)	3½ oz.	103	0.
Strained (Beech-Nut)	3½ oz.	96	0.
Strained (Gerber)	3½ oz.	131	.1
Strained (Heinz)	3½ oz.	114	0.
Chicken dinner:			
Junior (Beech-Nut)	4½ oz.	104	8.8
Strained (Beech-Nut)	4½ oz.	109	9.1
Noodle, junior (Beech-Nut)	7½ oz.	93	15.3
Noodle, junior (Gerber)	7½ oz.	93	17.0
Noodle, junior (Heinz)	7½ oz.	123	15.7
Noodle, strained (Beech-Nut)	4½ oz.	56	9.5
Noodle, strained (Gerber)	4½ oz.	60	10.4
Noodle, strained (Heinz)	4½ oz.	70	9.2

(USDA): United States Department of Agriculture
DNA: Data Not Available
* Prepared as Package Directs

Food and Description	Measure or Quantity	Calories	Carbo-hydrates (grams)
With vegetables, junior (Gerber)	4½ oz.	113	7.9
With vegetables, junior (Heinz)	4¾ oz.	128	5.3
With vegetables, strained (Gerber)	4½ oz.	110	7.7
With vegetables, strained (Heinz)	4¾ oz.	124	5.8
Chicken soup:			
Junior (Heinz)	7½ oz.	113	17.6
Strained (Beech-Nut)	4½ oz.	54	10.5
Strained (Heinz)	4½ oz.	65	8.9
Cream of, junior (Gerber)	7½ oz.	116	19.6
Cream of, strained (Gerber)	4½ oz.	73	12.4
Chicken stew, toddler (Gerber)	6 oz.	128	15.0
Chicken sticks:			
Junior (Beech-Nut)	2½ oz.	145	1.4
Junior (Gerber)	2½ oz.	134	.8
Cookie, animal-shaped (Gerber)	1 cookie (6 grams)	29	4.3
Cookie, assorted (Beech-Nut)	½ oz.	61	9.5
Corn, creamed:			
Junior (Gerber)	7½ oz.	133	29.4
Junior (Heinz)	7½ oz.	153	34.0
Strained (Beech-Nut)	4½ oz.	120	26.1
Strained (Gerber)	4½ oz.	82	18.1
Strained (Heinz)	4½ oz.	92	20.4
Custard:			
Junior (Beech-Nut)	7¾ oz.	210	40.3
Junior (Heinz)	7¾ oz.	213	36.4
Strained (Beech-Nut)	4½ oz.	125	24.6
Strained (Heinz)	4½ oz.	122	21.6
Chocolate, junior (Gerber)	7⁸⁄₁₀ oz.	208	41.1
Chocolate, strained (Beech-Nut)	4½ oz.	137	27.6
Chocolate, strained (Gerber)	4½ oz.	122	24.4
Vanilla, junior (Gerber)	7½ oz.	202	39.7
Vanilla, strained (Gerber)	4½ oz.	112	23.4
Dutch apple dessert (See Apple, Dutch, dessert)			

Food and Description	Measure or Quantity	Calories	Carbohydrates (grams)
Egg yolk:			
Strained (Beech-Nut)	3⅓ oz.	181	1.2
Strained (Gerber)	3⅓ oz.	187	0.
Strained (Heinz)	3¼ oz.	189	2.0
& bacon, strained			
(Beech-Nut)	3⅓ oz.	196	.1
& ham, strained (Gerber)	3⅓ oz.	182	0.
Fruit dessert:			
Junior (Gerber)	7¾ oz.	185	44.9
Junior (Heinz)	7¾ oz.	207	50.9
Strained (Heinz)	4½ oz.	124	30.4
Tropical, junior			
(Beech-Nut)	7¾ oz.	208	50.8
With tapioca, junior			
(Beech-Nut)	7¾ oz.	219	53.0
With tapioca, strained			
(Beech-Nut)	4¾ oz.	133	32.8
With tapioca, strained			
(Gerber)	4⁷⁄₁₀ oz.	120	29.0
Fruit juice:			
Mixed, strained			
(Beech-Nut)	4⅕ fl. oz.	79	19.0
Mixed, strained (Gerber)	4⅕ fl. oz.	77	18.3
Ham:			
Strained (Beech-Nut)	3½ oz.	115	2.2
Strained (Gerber)	3½ oz.	113	.7
Ham dinner:			
Junior (Beech-Nut)	4½ oz.	120	6.1
Strained (Beech-Nut)	4½ oz.	136	7.7
With vegetables, junior			
(Gerber)	4½ oz.	100	8.3
With vegetables, strained			
(Gerber)	4½ oz.	101	8.5
With vegetables, junior			
(Heinz)	4¾ oz.	148	12.5
With vegetables, strained			
(Heinz)	4¾ oz.	124	6.7
Lamb:			
Junior (Beech-Nut)	3½ oz.	98	0.
Junior (Gerber)	3½ oz.	96	0.

(USDA): United States Department of Agriculture
DNA: Data Not Available
* Prepared as Package Directs

Food and Description	*Measure or Quantity*	*Calories*	*Carbo-hydrates (grams)*
Junior (Heinz)	3½ oz.	97	0.
Strained (Beech-Nut)	3½ oz.	116	0.
Strained (Gerber)	3½ oz.	96	0.
Strained (Heinz)	3½ oz.	86	0.
& noodles, junior (Beech-Nut)	7½ oz.	148	17.8
Liver, strained (Heinz)	3½ oz.	79	0.
Macaroni:			
Alphabets & beef casserole, toddler (Gerber)	6⅕ oz.	146	18.6
& bacon with vegetables, junior (Beech-Nut)	7½ oz.	197	19.7
& beef with vegetables, junior (Beech-Nut)	7½ oz.	136	15.3
With tomato, beef & bacon, junior (Gerber)	7½ oz.	132	21.9
With tomato, beef & bacon, junior (Heinz)	7½ oz.	140	20.6
With tomato, beef & bacon, strained (Gerber)	4½ oz.	78	11.9
With tomato, beef & bacon, strained (Heinz)	4½ oz.	89	11.6
With tomato sauce, beef & bacon dinner, strained (Beech-Nut)	4½ oz.	106	10.8
Meat sticks, junior (Beech-Nut)	2½ oz.	135	.9
Meat sticks, junior (Gerber)	2½ oz.	115	1.0
Noodles & beef, junior (Heinz)	7½ oz.	111	16.4
Orange-apple juice, strained:			
(Beech-Nut)	4⅕ fl. oz.	98	23.2
(Gerber)	4⅕ fl. oz.	71	16.3
Orange-apple-banana juice, strained:			
(Gerber)	4⅕ fl. oz.	86	20.2
(Heinz)	4½ fl. oz.	89	21.8
Orange-apricot juice, strained:			
(Beech-Nut)	4⅕ fl. oz.	117	27.3
(Gerber)	4⅕ fl. oz.	79	18.8
Orange-apricot juice drink, strained (Heinz)	4½ fl. oz.	73	17.5
Orange-banana juice, strained (Beech-Nut)	4⅕ fl. oz.	122	28.3

Food and Description	Measure or Quantity	Calories	Carbo-hydrates (grams)
Orange juice, strained:			
(Beech-Nut)	4⅕ fl. oz.	64	14.4
(Gerber)	4⅕ fl. oz.	65	14.5
(Heinz)	4½ fl. oz.	69	16.2
Orange-pineapple dessert, strained (Beech-Nut)	4¾ oz.	154	36.6
Orange-pineapple juice, strained:			
(Beech-Nut)	4⅕ fl. oz.	104	24.7
(Gerber)	4⅕ fl. oz.	78	18.6
(Heinz)	4½ fl. oz.	72	17.5
Orange pudding, strained:			
(Gerber)	4⁷⁄₁₀ oz.	133	29.4
(Heinz)	4½ oz.	119	28.0
Pablum cereal (Drackett):			
Barley	1 oz.	100	21.7
High-protein	1 oz.	105	13.0
Mixed	1 oz.	105	19.7
Oatmeal	1 oz.	105	18.1
Rice	1 oz.	100	22.9
Pea, creamed:			
Junior (Heinz)	7¾ oz.	158	24.9
Strained (Heinz)	4½ oz.	82	12.8
Pea, split (See Split pea)			
Pea, strained:			
(Beech-Nut)	4½ oz.	81	14.1
(Gerber)	4½ oz.	56	10.1
Peach:			
Junior (Beech-Nut)	7¾ oz.	195	46.0
Junior (Gerber)	7⁸⁄₁₀ oz.	181	44.4
Junior (Heinz) freestone	7½ oz.	247	60.1
Strained (Beech-Nut)	4¾ oz.	117	27.7
Strained (Gerber)	4⁷⁄₁₀ oz.	107	26.9
Strained (Heinz)	4½ oz.	160	37.9
Peach cobbler, strained (Gerber)	4⁷⁄₁₀ oz.	116	28.5
Pear:			
Junior (Beech-Nut)	7½ oz.	148	36.5
Junior (Gerber)	7⁸⁄₁₀ oz.	152	39.4
Junior (Heinz)	7¾ oz.	167	40.0

(USDA): United States Department of Agriculture
DNA: Data Not Available
* Prepared as Package Directs

Food and Description	*Measure or Quantity*	*Calories*	*Carbo-hydrates (grams)*
Strained (Beech-Nut)	4½ oz.	91	21.6
Strained (Gerber)	4⁷⁄₁₀ oz.	92	24.3
Strained (Heinz)	4½ oz.	98	23.2
Pear & pineapple:			
Junior (Beech-Nut)	7½ oz.	159	38.6
Junior (Gerber)	7⁸⁄₁₀ oz.	156	39.5
Junior (Heinz)	7¾ oz.	158	38.0
Strained (Beech-Nut)	4½ oz.	96	23.3
Strained (Gerber)	4⁷⁄₁₀ oz.	95	24.6
Pineapple dessert, strained (Beech-Nut)	4¾ oz.	142	34.6
Pineapple-grapefruit juice drink, strained (Gerber)	4⅕ fl. oz.	76	18.6
Pineapple juice, strained (Heinz)	4½ fl. oz.	72	16.6
Pineapple-orange:			
Junior (Heinz)	7¾ oz.	152	34.1
Strained (Heinz)	4½ oz.	109	26.4
(Heinz)	4½ oz.	115	27.7
Plum with tapioca:			
Junior (Beech-Nut)	7¾ oz.	217	52.6
Junior (Gerber)	7⁸⁄₁₀ oz.	218	53.8
Strained (Beech-Nut)	4¾ oz.	141	34.2
Strained (Gerber)	4⁷⁄₁₀ oz.	132	32.7
Strained (Heinz)	4½ oz.	129	31.7
Pork:			
Junior (Beech-Nut)	3½ oz.	110	1.1
Junior (Gerber)	3½ oz.	113	0.
Strained (Beech-Nut)	3½ oz.	112	.3
Strained (Gerber)	3½ oz.	109	0.
Strained (Heinz)	3½ oz.	93	0.
Potatoes, creamed, with ham & bacon, toddler (Gerber)	6 oz.	181	18.4
Pretzel (Gerber)	1 pretzel (5 grams)	19	3.9
Prune-orange juice, strained:			
(Beech-Nut)	4⅕ fl. oz.	95	22.8
(Gerber)	4⅕ fl. oz.	99	23.6
Prune-orange juice drink, strained (Heinz)	4½ fl. oz.	73	17.5
Prune with tapioca:			
Junior (Beech-Nut)	7¾ oz.	201	48.6
Junior (Gerber)	7⁸⁄₁₀ oz.	201	49.4
Strained (Beech-Nut)	4¾ oz.	127	30.7

Food and Description	Measure or Quantity	Calories	Carbohydrates (grams)
Strained (Gerber)	4⁷⁄₁₀ oz.	118	29.3
Strained (Heinz)	4¾ oz.	142	33.8
Spaghetti & meat balls, toddler (Gerber)	6⅕ oz.	135	21.5
Spaghetti, tomato sauce & beef:			
Junior (Beech-Nut)	7½ oz.	157	19.7
Junior (Gerber)	7½ oz.	145	27.2
Junior (Heinz)	7½ oz.	168	26.8
Strained (Heinz)	4½ oz.	96	14.6
Spinach, creamed:			
Junior (Gerber)	7½ oz.	95	14.1
Strained (Gerber)	4½ oz.	53	8.3
Strained (Heinz)	4½ oz.	56	8.3
Split pea with bacon, junior (Gerber)	7½ oz.	179	26.6
Split pea, vegetables & bacon:			
Junior (Beech-Nut)	7½ oz.	142	22.5
Junior (Heinz)	7½ oz.	213	23.6
Strained (Heinz)	4½ oz.	120	13.4
Split pea, vegetables & ham, junior (Beech-Nut)	7½ oz.	134	25.0
Squash:			
Junior (Beech-Nut)	7½ oz.	70	15.1
Junior (Gerber)	7½ oz.	57	13.4
Strained (Beech-Nut)	4½ oz.	44	9.0
Strained (Gerber)	4½ oz.	35	8.5
Strained (Heinz)	4½ oz.	50	10.5
In butter sauce (Beech-Nut):			
Junior	7½ oz.	106	20.8
Strained	4½ oz.	60	11.9
Sweet potato:			
Junior (Beech-Nut)	7¾ oz.	131	30.2
Junior (Gerber)	7⁸⁄₁₀ oz.	153	35.9
Strained (Beech-Nut)	4¾ oz.	72	16.4
Strained (Gerber)	4⁷⁄₁₀ oz.	92	21.7
Strained (Heinz)	4½ oz.	84	18.8
In butter sauce, junior (Beech-Nut)	7¾ oz.	153	32.4

(USDA): United States Department of Agriculture
DNA: Data Not Available
* Prepared as Package Directs

Food and Description	Measure or Quantity	Calories	Carbo-hydrates (grams)
In butter sauce, strained (Beech-Nut)	4½ oz.	88	18.8
Teething biscuit (Gerber)	1 piece (.4 oz.)	43	8.2
Teething ring, honey (Beech-Nut)	½ oz.	56	10.7
Tuna with noodles, strained (Heinz)	4½ oz.	55	9.3
Turkey:			
Junior (Beech-Nut)	3½ oz.	100	.7
Strained (Beech-Nut)	3½ oz.	103	.9
Strained (Gerber)	3½ oz.	129	.3
Turkey dinner:			
Junior (Beech-Nut)	4½ oz.	88	8.3
Strained (Beech-Nut)	4½ oz.	106	10.6
With rice & vegetables, junior (Beech-Nut)	7½ oz.	85	16.7
With rice, strained (Beech-Nut)	4½ oz.	64	12.5
With vegetables, junior (Gerber)	4½ oz.	93	8.1
With vegetables, strained (Gerber)	4½ oz.	96	7.8
With vegetables, strained (Heinz)	4¾ oz.	94	7.9
Tutti frutti dessert (Heinz):			
Junior	7¾ oz.	187	44.6
Strained	4½ oz.	108	25.1
Veal:			
Junior (Beech-Nut)	3½ oz.	88	0.
Junior (Gerber)	3½ oz.	99	0.
Junior (Heinz)	3½ oz.	93	0.
Strained (Beech-Nut)	3½ oz.	110	0.
Strained (Gerber)	3½ oz.	89	0.
Strained (Heinz)	3½ oz.	90	0.
Veal dinner:			
Junior (Beech-Nut)	4½ oz.	129	6.7
Strained (Beech-Nut)	4¼ oz.	119	7.4
With vegetables, junior (Gerber)	4½ oz.	83	9.4
With vegetables, strained (Gerber)	4½ oz.	82	8.6
With vegetables, strained (Heinz)	4¾ oz.	84	6.3
Vegetables:			

Food and Description	Measure or Quantity	Calories	Carbo-hydrates (grams)
Garden, strained (Beech-Nut)	4½ oz.	55	10.4
Garden, strained (Gerber)	4½ oz.	41	7.9
Mixed, junior (Gerber)	7½ oz.	85	18.4
Mixed, junior (Heinz)	7½ oz.	100	20.8
Mixed, strained (Gerber)	4½ oz.	49	10.9
Vegetables & bacon:			
Junior (Beech-Nut)	7½ oz.	155	17.6
Junior (Gerber)	7½ oz.	137	18.7
Junior (Heinz)	7½ oz.	153	16.3
Strained (Beech-Nut)	4½ oz.	91	9.5
Strained (Gerber)	4½ oz.	94	13.0
Strained (Heinz)	4½ oz.	65	9.0
Vegetables & beef:			
Junior (Beech-Nut)	7½ oz.	134	14.8
Junior (Gerber)	7½ oz.	108	14.7
Junior (Heinz)	7½ oz.	106	17.1
Strained (Beech-Nut)	4½ oz.	87	9.7
Strained (Gerber)	4½ oz.	67	8.6
Strained (Heinz)	4½ oz.	70	8.5
Vegetables & chicken (Gerber):			
Junior	7½ oz.	105	21.2
Strained	4½ oz.	53	9.0
Vegetables, dumplings, beef & bacon:			
Junior (Heinz)	7½ oz.	145	16.9
Strained (Heinz)	4½ oz.	79	10.3
Vegetables, egg noodles & chicken:			
Junior (Heinz)	7½ oz.	134	17.6
Strained (Heinz)	4½ oz.	80	11.2
Vegetables, egg noodles & turkey:			
Junior (Heinz)	7½ oz.	113	16.6
Strained (Heinz)	4½ oz.	54	7.4
Vegetables & ham:			
Strained (Beech-Nut)	4½ oz.	79	10.1
Junior (Heinz)	7½ oz.	132	15.4

(USDA): United States Department of Agriculture
DNA: Data Not Available
* Prepared as Package Directs

Food and Description	Measure or Quantity	Calories	Carbohydrates (grams)
With bacon, junior (Gerber)	7½ oz.	122	18.5
With bacon, strained (Gerber)	4½ oz.	70	9.8
With bacon, strained (Heinz)	4½ oz.	79	7.3
Vegetables & lamb:			
Junior (Beech-Nut)	7½ oz.	123	14.8
Junior (Gerber)	7½ oz.	106	16.2
Junior (Heinz)	7½ oz.	117	17.4
Strained (Beech-Nut)	4½ oz.	69	9.9
Strained (Gerber)	4½ oz.	64	9.9
Strained (Heinz)	4½ oz.	56	8.1
Vegetables & liver:			
Junior (Beech-Nut)	7½ oz.	95	16.3
Strained (Beech-Nut)	4½ oz.	55	9.7
With bacon, junior (Gerber)	7½ oz.	104	17.9
With bacon, strained (Gerber)	4½ oz.	76	8.4
Vegetable soup:			
Junior (Beech-Nut)	7½ oz.	83	17.6
Junior (Heinz)	7½ oz.	106	20.4
Strained (Beech-Nut)	4½ oz.	50	10.9
Strained (Heinz)	4½ oz.	55	10.2
Vegetables & turkey (Gerber):			
Junior	7½ oz.	89	17.7
Strained	4½ oz.	57	11.0
Toddler	6⅛ oz.	158	18.0
BACO NOIR BURGUNDY WINE (Great Western) 12% alcohol	3 fl. oz.	78	2.1
BAC*O CHIPS (General Mills)	1 oz.	129	8.1
BAC*O'S (General Mills)	1 T.	29	1.0
BACON, cured: Raw: (USDA) sliced	1 lb.	3016	4.5

Food and Description	Measure or Quantity	Calories	Carbo-hydrates (grams)
(USDA) sliced	1 oz.	189	.3
(Wilson)	1 oz.	169	.3
Broiled or fried crisp (USDA):			
Thin slice, drained	1 slice (5 grams)	31	.2
Medium slice, drained	1 slice (8 grams)	46	.2
Thick slice, drained	1 slice (12 grams)	73	.4
Canned (USDA)	3 oz.	582	.9
BACON BITS, imitation:			
(Durkee)	1 tsp. (2 grams)	8	.5
(McCormick)	1 oz.	113	7.7
BACON, CANADIAN:			
Unheated:			
(USDA)	1 oz.	61	Tr.
(Wilson)	1 oz.	42	<.1
Broiled or fried (USDA)	1 oz.	79	Tr.
BAGEL (USDA):			
Egg	3″ dia. (1.9 oz.)	165	28.0
Water	3″ dia. (1.9 oz.)	165	30.0
BAKING POWDER:			
Phosphate (USDA)	1 tsp. (5 grams)	6	1.4
SAS (USDA)	1 tsp. (4 grams)	5	1.2
Tartrate (USDA)	1 tsp. (4 grams)	3	.7
(Royal)	1 tsp. (4 grams)	5	1.3
BAKON DELITES (Wise):			
Regular	½ oz. bag	72	0.
Barbecue flavored	½ oz. bag	70	.3
BALI HAI WINE (Italian Swiss Colony—Gold Medal)			
11% alcohol	3 fl. oz.	89	9.2
BAMBOO SHOOT, raw, whole (USDA)	½ lb. (weighed untrimmed)	18	3.4

(USDA): United States Department of Agriculture
DNA: Data Not Available
* Prepared as Package Directs

Food and Description	Measure or Quantity	Calories	Carbo-hydrates (grams)
BANANA (USDA):			
Common			
Fresh:			
Whole	1 lb. (weighed with skin)	262	68.5
Small size	4.9-oz. banana (7¾" x 1¹¹⁄₃₂")	81	21.1
Medium size	6.2-oz. banana (8¾" x 1¹³⁄₃₂")	101	26.4
Large size	7-oz. banana (9¾" x 1⁷⁄₁₆")	116	30.2
Mashed	1 cup (about 2 med.)	189	49.3
Sliced	1 cup (1¼ med.)	124	32.4
Dehydrated or powder (USDA)	1 oz.	96	25.1
Red, fresh, whole (USDA)	1 lb. (weighed with skin)	278	72.2
BANANA, BAKING (See PLANTAIN)			
BANANA CAKE MIX:			
*(Betty Crocker) Layer	¹⁄₁₂ of cake	205	36.6
*(Duncan Hines)	¹⁄₁₂ of cake (2.7 oz.)	203	35.0
(Pillsbury)	1 oz.	120	22.7
(Pillsbury) loaf cake	1 oz.	117	22.6
BANANA CREAM PIE:			
(Tastykake)	4-oz. pie	485	82.4
Frozen (Banquet)	2½ oz.	185	25.0
Frozen (Morton)	⅛ of 14.4-oz. pie	171	23.3
Frozen (Mrs. Smith's)	⅙ of 8" pie (2.3 oz.)	203	23.2
BANANA CREAM PUDDING or PIE FILLING MIX:			
*Instant (Jell-O)	½ cup (5.3 oz.)	178	30.5
*Instant (Royal)	½ cup (5.1 oz.)	177	30.5
*Regular (Jell-O)	½ cup (5.2 oz.)	173	29.3
*Regular (My-T-Fine)	½ cup (5 oz.)	175	32.6
*Regular (Royal)	½ cup (5.1 oz.)	168	27.6

Food and Description	Measure or Quantity	Calories	Carbo-hydrates (grams)
BANANA CUSTARD PIE, home recipe (USDA)	⅛ of 9" pie (5.4 oz.)	336	46.7
BANANA LIQUEUR (Leroux):			
56 proof	1 fl. oz.	92	11.4
100 proof	1 fl. oz.	116	9.2
BANANA PUDDING, canned (Del Monte)	5-oz. container	187	31.7
BANANA SOFT DRINK (Yoo-Hoo):			
Regular	6 fl. oz.	90	18.0
High-protein	6 fl. oz.	114	24.6
BARBADOS CHERRY (See ACEROLA)			
BARBECUE DINNER MIX (Hunt's) *Skillet*	2-lb. 1-oz. pkg.	1404	247.1
BARBECUE SAUCE (See SAUCE, Barbecue)			
BARBECUE SEASONING (Lawry's):			
Bar-B-Q	1 pkg. (4½ oz.)	408	97.8
Sweet 'N Sour	1 pkg. (4½ oz.)	394	88.4
BARBERA WINE (Louis M. Martini) 12½% alcohol	3 fl. oz.	90	.2
BARDOLINO WINE, Italian red (Antinori) 12% alcohol	3 fl. oz.	84	6.3
BARLEY: Pearled, dry, light:			
(USDA)	¼ cup (1.8 oz.)	174	39.4

(USDA): United States Department of Agriculture
DNA: Data Not Available
* Prepared as Package Directs

Food and Description	Measure or Quantity	Calories	Carbo-hydrates (grams)
(Albers)	¼ cup	177	40.0
(Quaker-Scotch)	¼ cup (1.7 oz.)	174	37.3
Pot or Scotch, dry (USDA)	2 oz.	197	43.8
BARRACUDA, raw, meat only (USDA)	4 oz.	128	0.
BASS (USDA):			
Black sea:			
Raw, whole	1 lb. (weighed whole)	165	0.
Baked, stuffed, home recipe	4 oz.	294	12.9
Smallmouth & largemouth, raw:			
Whole	1 lb. (weighed whole)	146	0.
Meat only	4 oz.	118	0.
Striped:			
Raw, whole	1 lb. (weighed whole)	205	0.
Raw, meat only	4 oz.	119	0.
Oven-fried	4 oz.	222	7.6
White, raw, meat only	4 oz.	111	0.
B & B LIQUEUR (Julius Wile) 86 proof	1 fl. oz.	94	5.7
BAVARIAN PIE FILLING (Lucky Leaf)	8 oz.	306	51.8
BAVARIAN PIE or PUDDING MIX:			
*Cream (My-T-Fine)	½ cup (5 oz.)	175	32.5
*Custard, *Rice-A-Roni*	4 oz.	143	24.6
BAVARIAN-STYLE VEGE-TABLES (Birds Eye) frozen	⅓ pkg. (3⅓ oz.)	135	11.8
BEAN, BAKED:			
Canned:			
(B & M) New England-style sauce	1 cup (7.9 oz.)	336	50.8
(Heinz) in molasses sauce	1 cup (9¼ oz.)	283	52.8

Food and Description	Measure or Quantity	Calories	Carbohydrates (grams)
Canned with pork:			
(Campbell) home style	1 cup	302	52.0
(Hunt's)	5-oz. can	169	35.3
(Van Camp)	1 cup (7.7 oz.)	286	41.8
Canned with pork & molasses sauce:			
(USDA)	1 cup (9 oz.)	382	53.8
(Heinz) Boston-style	1 cup (8¾ oz.)	303	50.8
Canned with pork & tomato sauce:			
(USDA)	1 cup (9 oz.)	311	48.4
(Campbell)	1 cup	262	42.7
(Heinz)	1 cup (9¼ oz.)	293	48.5
Canned with tomato sauce:			
(USDA)	1 cup (9 oz.)	306	58.6
(Heinz) *Campside,* smoky beans	1 cup (9½ oz.)	350	51.1
(Heinz) vegetarian	1 cup (9¼ oz.)	267	48.9
(Van Camp)	1 cup (8.1 oz.)	276	52.0
BEAN, BARBECUE (Campbell)	1 cup	287	51.1
BEAN, BAYO, dry (USDA)	4 oz.	384	69.4
BEAN, BLACK, dry (USDA)	4 oz.	384	69.4
BEAN, BROWN, dry (USDA)	4 oz.	384	69.4
BEAN, CALICO, dry (USDA)	4 oz.	396	72.2
BEAN, CHILI (See **CHILI**)			
BEAN & FRANKFURTER, canned:			
(Campbell) in tomato & molasses sauce	1 cup	364	35.7
(Heinz)	8¾-oz. can	399	38.0

(USDA): United States Department of Agriculture
DNA: Data Not Available
* Prepared as Package Directs

Food and Description	Measure or Quantity	Calories	Carbo-hydrates (grams)
BEAN & FRANKFURTER			
DINNER, frozen:			
(Banquet)	10¾-oz. dinner	687	70.5
(Morton)	12-oz. dinner	554	81.3
(Swanson)	11½-oz. dinner	610	70.1
BEAN, GREEN or SNAP:			
Fresh (USDA):			
Whole	1 lb. (weighed untrimmed)	128	28.3
1½″ to 2″ pieces	½ cup (1.8 oz.)	17	3.7
French-style	½ cup (1.4 oz.)	13	2.8
Boiled, drained, whole (USDA)	½ cup (2.2 oz.)	16	3.3
Boiled, drained, 1½″ to 2″ pieces (USDA)	½ cup (2.4 oz.)	17	3.7
Canned, regular pack:			
Solids & liq. (USDA)	½ cup (4.2 oz.)	22	5.0
Drained solids, whole (USDA)	4 oz.	27	5.9
Drained solids, cut (USDA)	½ cup (2.5 oz.)	17	3.6
Drained liq. (USDA)	4 oz.	11	2.7
Drained solids (Butter Kernel)	½ cup (3.9 oz.)	20	4.6
Blue Lake, drained solids (Cannon)	4 oz.	27	5.9
(Fall River)	½ cup	20	4.6
Solids & liq., ½″ cut (Green Giant)	½ of 8.5-oz. can	22	5.1
Canned, dietetic pack:			
Solids & liq. (USDA)	4 oz.	18	4.1
Drained solids (USDA)	4 oz.	25	5.4
Drained liq. (USDA)	4 oz.	9	2.0
Cut, solids & liq. (Blue Boy)	4 oz.	26	5.3
Solids & liq. (Diet Delight)	½ cup (4.2 oz.)	20	3.8
Cut (S and W) *Nutradiet*	4 oz.	18	3.6
Solids & liq. (Tillie Lewis)	½ cup (4.2 oz.)	20	3.6
Frozen:			
Cut or french-style, not thawed (USDA)	10-oz. pkg.	74	17.0

Food and Description	Measure or Quantity	Calories	Carbohydrates (grams)
Cut or french-style, boiled, drained (USDA)	½ cup (2.8 oz.)	20	4.6
Cut (Birds Eye)	⅓ pkg. (3 oz.)	22	5.1
Whole (Birds Eye)	½ cup (3 oz.)	23	5.2
(Blue Goose)	4 oz.	35	6.4
French-style (Birds Eye)	⅓ pkg. (3 oz.)	22	5.1
French-style, with sliced mushrooms (Birds Eye)	⅓ pkg. (3 oz.)	26	5.5
French-style, with toasted almonds (Birds Eye)	½ cup (3 oz.)	52	6.0
In butter sauce (Birds Eye)	½ cup (3 oz.)	48	4.5
In butter sauce, kitchen-sliced (Green Giant)	⅓ of 9-oz. pkg.	31	4.0
In mushroom sauce (Green Giant)	⅓ of 10-oz. pkg.	47	4.0

BEAN & GROUND BEEF, canned (Campbell)

	1 cup	259	34.8

BEAN, ITALIAN, frozen:

(Birds Eye)	⅓ pkg. (3 oz.)	23	4.1
In butter sauce (Green Giant) boil-in-the-bag	4 oz.	70	5.3

BEAN, KIDNEY or RED:
Dry:

(USDA)	1 lb.	1556	280.8
(USDA)	½ cup (3.3 oz.)	319	57.6
(Sinsheimer)	1 oz.	99	17.6
Cooked (USDA)	½ cup (3.3 oz.)	109	19.8
Canned:			
Solids & liq. (USDA)	½ cup (4.5 oz.)	115	21.0
Drained solids (Butter Kernel)	½ cup	108	19.7
Red kidney & chili gravy (Nalley's)	4 oz.	113	18.5

BEAN, LIMA, young:
Raw, whole (USDA)

	1 lb. (weighed in pod)	223	40.1

(USDA): United States Department of Agriculture
DNA: Data Not Available
* Prepared as Package Directs

Food and Description	Measure or Quantity	Calories	Carbo- hydrates (grams)
Raw, without shell (USDA)	1 lb. (weighed shelled)	558	100.2
Boiled, drained (USDA)	½ cup (3 oz.)	94	16.8
Canned, regular pack:			
Solids & liq. (USDA)	½ cup (4.4 oz.)	88	16.6
Drained solids (USDA)	½ cup (3 oz.)	84	15.9
Drained liq. (USDA)	4 oz.	23	4.4
Drained solids (Del Monte)	½ cup (3.1 oz.)	84	15.9
With ham (Nalley's)	4 oz.	125	14.3
Canned, dietetic pack:			
Solids & liq., low sodium (USDA)	4 oz.	79	14.6
Drained solids, low sodium (USDA)	4 oz.	108	20.1
Solids & liq., unseasoned (Blue Boy)	4 oz.	79	12.6
Frozen:			
Baby butter beans (Birds Eye)	⅓ pkg. (3.3 oz.)	123	23.6
Baby limas:			
Not thawed (USDA)	4 oz.	138	26.1
Boiled, drained solids (USDA)	4 oz.	134	25.3
Boiled, drained solids (USDA)	½ cup (3 oz.)	101	19.2
(Birds Eye)	½ cup (3.3 oz.)	111	21.0
In butter sauce (Green Giant)	⅓ of 10-oz. pkg.	110	17.5
Tiny (Birds Eye)	½ cup (2.5 oz.)	83	16.2
Fordhooks:			
Not thawed (USDA)	4 oz.	116	22.1
Boiled, drained (USDA)	½ cup (3 oz.)	83	16.0
(Birds Eye)	⅓ pkg. (3.3 oz.)	94	17.9
BEAN, LIMA, MATURE:			
Dry:			
Baby (USDA)	½ cup (3.4 oz.)	331	61.4
Large (USDA)	½ cup (3.1 oz.)	304	56.3
(Sinsheimer)	1 oz.	92	17.5
Boiled, drained (USDA)	½ cup (3.4 oz.)	131	24.3
BEAN, MUNG, dry (USDA)	½ cup (3.7 oz.)	357	63.3

Food and Description	Measure or Quantity	Calories	Carbo-hydrates (grams)
BEAN, PINTO:			
Dry (USDA)	4 oz.	396	72.2
Dry (USDA)	½ cup (3.4 oz.)	335	61.2
Dry (Sinsheimer)	1 oz.	99	17.6
*(Uncle Ben's) quick-cooked, including broth	¾ cup (6 oz.)	148	25.9
BEAN, RED (See BEAN, KIDNEY or BEAN, RED MEXICAN)			
BEAN, RED MEXICAN, dry (USDA)	4 oz.	396	72.2
BEAN, REFRIED, canned (Rosarita)	4 oz.	120	17.2
BEAN SALAD, MIXED:			
Solids & liq. (Comstock-Greenwood)	4 oz.	81	7.5
(Hunt's) Snack Pack	5-oz. can	111	23.7
BEAN SOUP, canned:			
*(Manischewitz)	8 fl. oz.	111	17.6
*With bacon (Campbell)	1 cup (8 oz.)	152	19.4
With pork, condensed (USDA)	8 oz. (by wt.)	304	39.3
*With pork, prepared with equal volume water (USDA)	1 cup (8.8 oz.)	168	21.8
With smoked ham (Heinz) *Great American*	1 cup (8¾ oz.)	201	24.5
*With smoked pork (Heinz)	1 cup (8½ oz.)	157	20.1
BEAN SOUP, BLACK, canned:			
*(Campbell)	1 cup	91	13.9
(Crosse & Blackwell)	6½ oz. (½ can)	96	15.5

(USDA): United States Department of Agriculture
DNA: Data Not Available
* Prepared as Package Directs

Food and Description	Measure or Quantity	Calories	Carbo-hydrates (grams)
*BEAN SOUP, LIMA, canned (Manischewitz)	8 oz. (by wt.)	93	15.3
BEAN SOUP, NAVY, dehydrated (USDA)	1 oz.	93	17.8
BEAN SPROUT:			
Mung:			
Raw (USDA)	½ lb.	80	15.0
Raw (USDA)	½ cup (1.6 oz.)	16	3.0
Boiled, drained (USDA)	½ cup (2.2 oz.)	17	3.2
Soy:			
Raw (USDA)	½ lb.	104	12.0
Raw (USDA)	½ cup (1.9 oz.)	25	2.9
Boiled, drained (USDA)	4 oz.	43	4.2
Canned (Chun King)	1 cup	39	2.5
BEAN, WAX (See BEAN, YELLOW)			
BEAN, WHITE, dry:			
Raw:			
Great Northern (USDA)	½ cup (3.1 oz.)	303	54.6
Navy or pea (USDA)	½ cup (3.7 oz.)	354	63.8
Navy or pea (Sinsheimer)	1 oz.	99	17.6
White (USDA)	1 oz.	96	17.4
Cooked:			
Great Northern (USDA)	½ cup (3 oz.)	100	18.0
Navy or pea (USDA)	½ cup (3.4 oz.)	113	20.4
All other white (USDA)	4 oz.	134	24.0
(Uncle Ben's) quick-cooked, including broth	¾ cup (6.3 oz.)	132	23.5
BEAN, YELLOW or WAX:			
Raw, whole (USDA)	1 lb. (weighed untrimmed)	108	24.0
Boiled, drained 1" pieces (USDA)	½ cup (2.9 oz.)	18	3.7
Canned, regular pack:			
Solids & liq. (USDA)	½ cup (4.2 oz.)	23	5.0
Drained solids (USDA)	½ cup (2.2 oz.)	15	3.2
Drained liq. (USDA)	4 oz.	12	2.8
Drained solids (Butter Kernel)	½ cup (3.9 oz.)	20	4.6

Food and Description	Measure or Quantity	Calories	Carbo-hydrates (grams)
Golden, ½″ cut, solids & liq. (Green Giant)	½ of 8.5-oz. can	20	5.1
Canned, dietetic pack:			
Solids & liq. (USDA)	4 oz.	17	3.9
Drained solids (USDA)	4 oz.	24	5.3
Drained liq. (USDA)	4 oz.	8	1.6
Solids & liq. (Blue Boy)	4 oz.	24	5.0
Frozen:			
Cut, not thawed (USDA)	4 oz.	32	7.4
Boiled, drained (USDA)	4 oz.	31	7.0
Cut (Birds Eye)	⅓ pkg. (3 oz.)	24	5.4
BEAUJOLAIS WINE, French Burgundy:			
(Barton & Guestier) St. Louis, 11% alcohol	3 fl. oz.	60	.1
(Chanson) St. Vincent, 11% alcohol	3 fl. oz.	78	6.3
(Cruse) 12% alcohol	3 fl. oz.	72	D.N.A.
BEAUNE WINE:			
Clos de Feves, French Burgundy (Chanson) 12% alcohol	3 fl. oz.	84	6.3
St. Vincent, French Burgundy (Chanson) 12% alcohol	3 fl. oz.	84	6.3
BEAVER, roasted (USDA)	4 oz.	281	0.
BEECHNUT:			
Whole (USDA)	4 oz. (weighed in shell)	393	14.0
Shelled (USDA)	4 oz. (weighed shelled)	644	23.0

BEEF. Values for beef cuts are given below for "lean and fat" and for "lean only." Beef purchased by the consumer at the retail store usually is

(USDA): United States Department of Agriculture
DNA: Data Not Available
* Prepared as Package Directs

Food and Description	Measure or Quantity	Calories	Carbohydrates (grams)
trimmed to about one-half inch layer of fat. This is the meat described as "lean and fat." If all the fat that can be cut off with a knife is removed, the remainder is the "lean only." These cuts still contain flecks of fat known as "marbling" distributed through the meat. Cooked meats are medium done. Choice grade cuts (USDA):			
Brisket:			
Raw	1 lb. (weighed with bone)	1284	0.
Braised:			
Lean & fat	4 oz.	467	0.
Lean only	4 oz.	252	0.
Chuck:			
Raw	1 lb. (weighed with bone)	984	0.
Briaised or pot-roasted:			
Lean & fat	4 oz.	371	0.
Lean only	4 oz.	243	0.
Dried (See BEEF, CHIPPED)			
Fat, separable, cooked	1 oz.	207	0.
Filet mignon. There are no data available on its composition. For dietary estimates, the data for sirloin steak, lean only, afford the closest approximation.			
Flank:			
Raw	1 lb.	653	0.
Braised	4 oz.	222	0.
Foreshank:			
Raw	1 lb. (weighed with bone)	531	0.
Simmered:			
Lean & fat	4 oz.	310	0.

Food and Description	Measure or Quantity	Calories	Carbo-hydrates (grams)
Lean only	4 oz.	209	0.
Ground:			
Lean:			
Raw	1 lb.	812	0.
Raw	1 cup (8 oz.)	405	0.
Broiled	4 oz.	248	0.
Regular:			
Raw	1 lb.	1216	0.
Raw	1 cup (8 oz.)	606	0.
Broiled	4 oz.	324	0.
Heel of round:			
Raw	1 lb.	966	0.
Roasted:			
Lean & fat	4 oz.	296	0.
Lean only	4 oz.	204	0.
Hindshank:			
Raw	1 lb. (weighed with bone)	604	0.
Braised:			
Lean & fat	4 oz.	409	0.
Lean only	4 oz.	209	0.
Neck:			
Raw	1 lb. (weighed with bone)	820	0.
Pot-roasted:			
Lean & fat	4 oz.	332	0.
Lean only	4 oz.	222	0.
Plate:			
Raw	1 lb. (weighed with bone)	1615	0.
Simmered:			
Lean & fat	4 oz.	538	0.
Lean only	4 oz.	252	0.
Rib roast:			
Raw	1 lb. (weighed with bone)	1673	0.
Roasted:			
Lean & fat	4 oz.	499	0.
Lean only	4 oz.	273	0.

(USDA): United States Department of Agriculture
DNA: Data Not Available
* Prepared as Package Directs

Food and Description	Measure or Quantity	Calories	Carbo-hydrates (grams)
Round:			
Raw	1 lb. (weighed with bone)	863	0.
Broiled:			
Lean & fat	4 oz.	296	0.
Lean only	4 oz.	214	0.
Rump:			
Raw	1 lb. (weighed with bone)	1167	0.
Roasted:			
Lean & fat	4 oz.	393	0.
Lean only	4 oz.	236	0.
Steak, club:			
Raw	1 lb. (weighed without bone)	1724	0.
Broiled:			
Lean & fat	4 oz.	515	0.
Lean only	4 oz.	277	0.
One 8-oz. steak (weighed without bone before cooking) will give you:			
Lean & fat	5.9 oz.	754	0.
Lean only	3.4 oz.	234	0.
Steak, porterhouse:			
Raw	1 lb. (weighed with bone)	1603	0.
Broiled:			
Lean & fat	4 oz.	527	0.
Lean only	4 oz.	254	0.
One 16-oz. steak (weighed with bone before cooking) will give you:			
Lean & fat	10.2 oz.	1339	0.
Lean only	5.9 oz.	372	0.
Steak, ribeye, broiled:			
One 10-oz. steak (weighed before cooking without bone) will give you:			
Lean & fat	7.3 oz.	911	0.
Lean only	3.8 oz.	258	0.

Food and Description	Measure or Quantity	Calories	Carbo-hydrates (grams)
Steak, sirloin, double-bone:			
Raw	1 lb. (weighed with bone)	1240	0.
Broiled:			
Lean & fat	4 oz.	463	0.
Lean only	4 oz.	245	0.
One 16-oz. steak (weighed before cooking with bone) will give you:			
Lean & fat	8.9 oz.	1028	0.
Lean only	5.9 oz.	359	0.
One 12-oz. steak (weighed before cooking with bone) will give you:			
Lean & fat	6.6 oz.	767	0.
Lean only	4.4 oz.	268	0.
Steak, sirloin, hipbone:			
Raw	1 lb. (weighed with bone)	1585	0.
Broiled:	4 oz.	552	0.
Lean & fat	4 oz.	272	0.
Lean only			
Steak, sirloin, wedge & round-bone:	1 lb. (weighed		
Raw	with bone)	1316	0.
Broiled:	4 oz.	439	0.
Lean & fat	4 oz.	235	0.
Lean only			
Steak, T-bone:			
Raw	1 lb. (weighed with bone)	1596	0.
Broiled:			
Lean & fat	4 oz.	536	0.
Lean only	4 oz.	253	0.
One 16-oz. steak (weighed before			

Food and Description	Measure or Quantity	Calories	Carbo-hydrates (grams)
cooking with bone) will give you:			
Lean & fat	9.8 oz.	1315	0.
Lean only	5.5 oz.	348	0.
BEEFARONI, canned (Chef Boy-Ar-Dee)	8 oz. (⅕ of 40-oz. can	206	27.9
BEEF & BEEF STOCK (Bunker Hill)	15-oz. can	920	0.
BEEF BOUILLON, cubes or powder:			
(Croyden House)	1 tsp. (5 grams)	12	2.2
(Herb-Ox)	1 cube (4 grams)	6	.5
(Herb-Ox) instant	1 packet (4 grams)	8	.8
(Knorr Swiss)	1 cube	13	D.N.A.
(Knorr Swiss)	1 tsp.	11	D.N.A.
(Maggi)	1 cube	7	.5
(Maggi) instant	1 tsp.	7	.5
(Wyler's)	1 cube	7	.4
(Wyler's) instant	1 tsp.	7	.4
BEEF, CHIPPED Uncooked:			
(USDA)	½ cup (2.9 oz.)	166	0.
(USDA)	2 oz. (about ⅓ cup)	116	0.
(Armour Star)	1 oz.	48	0.
(Eckrich) *Slender Sliced*	1 oz.	40	D.N.A.
Cooked, creamed, home recipe (USDA)	1 cup (8.6 oz.)	377	17.4
Canned, creamed (Swanson)	½ cup	96	5.8
Frozen, creamed (Banquet)	5 oz.	126	9.2
BEEF, CHOPPED, canned (Hormel)	12-oz. can	867	2.0
BEEF, CORNED (See **CORNED BEEF**)			
BEEF DINNER, frozen:			
(Banquet)	11-oz. dinner	309	24.0

Food and Description	Measure or Quantity	Calories	Carbohydrates (grams)
(Morton)	11-oz. dinner	292	22.0
(Swanson)	11½-oz. dinner	371	30.3
(Swanson) 3-course	15-oz. dinner	567	57.8
Chopped (Banquet)	9-oz. dinner	386	27.0
Chopped sirloin (Swanson)	10-oz. dinner	447	40.0
Pot roast, includes potatoes, peas and corn (USDA)	10 oz.	301	17.3
Sliced (Morton) 3-course	1-lb. 1-oz. dinner	563	60.1
Stew (Tom Thumb)	3-lb. 8-oz. tray	1375	97.3
BEEF GOULASH:			
Canned (Heinz)	8½-oz. can	253	20.1
Seasoning mix (Lawry's)	1 pkg. (1.7 oz.)	127	24.1
BEEF, GROUND (See **BEEF, ground**)			
BEEF HASH, ROAST:			
Canned (Hormel) *Mary Kitchen*	15-oz. can	701	37.8
Frozen (Stouffer's)	11½-oz. pkg.	460	21.7
BEEF JERKY	1 piece (¼ oz.)	25	.3
BEEF KABOBS, frozen (Colonial Beef)	6 oz.	540	D.N.A.
BEEF PIE:			
Baked, home recipe (USDA)	4¼" pie (8 oz. before baking)	558	42.7
Frozen:			
Commercial, unheated (USDA)	8 oz.	435	40.8
(Banquet)	8-oz. pie	411	40.5
(Morton)	8-oz. pie	369	35.1
(Stouffer's)	10-oz. pie	572	42.9
(Swanson)	8-oz. pie	434	38.6
(Swanson) deep dish	1-lb. pie	703	56.8

(USDA): United States Department of Agriculture
DNA: Data Not Available
* Prepared as Package Directs

Food and Description	Measure or Quantity	Calories	Carbo- hydrates (grams)
BEEF PUFFS, hors d'oeuvres, frozen (Durkee)	1 piece (½ oz.)	47	3.1
BEEF RAGOUT, frozen (Swanson)	8.5-oz. pkg.	177	13.7
BEEF, ROAST, canned (USDA)	4 oz.	254	0.
BEEF, SLICED, with barbecue sauce:			
Buffet (Banquet)	2 lb.	1115	81.8
Cookin' bag (Banquet)	5 oz.	152	13.0
BEEF SOUP, canned:			
*(Campbell) *Chunky*	1 cup	185	18.8
*Barley (Manischewitz)	1 cup	83	11.2
Bouillon, condensed (USDA)	8 oz. (by wt.)	59	5.0
*Bouillon, prepared with equal volume water (USDA)	1 cup (8.5 oz.)	31	2.6
Broth:			
Condensed (USDA)	8 oz. (by wt.)	59	5.0
*Prepared with equal volume water (USDA)	1 cup (8.5 oz.)	31	2.6
*(Campbell)	1 cup	25	2.2
*Cabbage (Manischewitz)	1 cup	62	9.0
Consommé, condensed (USDA)	8 oz. (by wt.)	59	5.0
*Consommé, prepared with equal volume water (USDA)	1 cup (8.5 oz.)	31	2.6
Noodle:			
Condensed (USDA)	8 oz. (by wt.)	129	13.2
*Prepared with equal volume water (USDA)	1 cup (8.5 oz.)	67	7.0
*(Campbell)	1 cup	67	8.2
*(Heinz)	1 cup (8½ oz.)	74	6.7
*(Manischewitz)	8 oz. (by wt.)	64	8.0
With dumplings (Heinz) *Great American*	1 cup (8¾ oz.)	109	11.1
*Vegetable (Manischewitz)	8 oz. (by wt.)	59	8.9
BEEF SOUP MIX, noodle: (USDA)	1 oz.	110	18.5

Food and Description	Measure or Quantity	Calories	Carbo-hydrates (grams)
*(USDA)	1 cup (8.1 oz.)	64	11.0
(Lipton) *Cup-A-Soup*	1 pkg. (.4 oz.)	36	6.6
*(Wyler's)	6 fl. oz.	37	7.0
BEEF STEW:			
Home recipe (USDA)	1 cup (8.6 oz.)	218	15.2
Canned:			
(USDA)	1 cup (8.6 oz.)	194	17.4
(Armour Star)	24-oz. can	590	38.8
(Austex)	15½-oz. can	347	31.2
(B&M)	1 cup (7.9 oz.)	152	15.2
(Bounty)	1 cup	181	15.9
(Bunker Hill)	15-oz. can	422	18.0
(Dinty Moore)	15-oz. can	306	21.2
(Heinz)	8½-oz. can	253	24.2
(Morton House)	15-oz. can	570	D.N.A.
(Nalley's)	8 oz.	204	18.8
(Wilson)	15½-oz.	343	30.8
Dietetic (Claybourne)	8-oz. can	365	18.4
Meatball (Hormel)	1-lb. 8-oz. can	631	27.9
Frozen, buffet (Banquet)	2-lb. pkg.	720	82.2
BEEF STEW SEASONING MIX:			
(French's)	1⅞-oz. pkg.	133	28.5
(Lawry's)	1⅜-oz. pkg.	131	24.2
BEEF STROGANOFF (See STROGANOFF)			
BEER, canned:			
Regular:			
(USDA) 4.5% alcohol	12 fl. oz.	151	13.7
Andeker	12 fl. oz.	165	D.N.A.
Buckeye, 4.6% alcohol	12 fl. oz.	144	11.0
Budweiser, 4.9% alcohol	12 fl. oz.	156	12.3
Budweiser, 3.9% alcohol	12 fl. oz.	137	11.9
Busch Bavarian, 4.9% alcohol	12 fl. oz.	156	12.3
Busch Bavarian, 3.9% alcohol	12 fl. oz.	137	11.9

(USDA): United States Department of Agriculture
DNA: Data Not Available
* Prepared as Package Directs

Food and Description	Measure or Quantity	Calories	Carbo-hydrates (grams)
Eastside Lager	12 fl. oz.	145	D.N.A.
Gold Medal	12 fl. oz.	160	9.6
Hamm's	12 fl. oz.	151	13.3
Knickerbocker, 4.6% alcohol	12 fl. oz.	160	13.7
Meister Brau Premium, 4.6% alcohol	12 fl. oz.	144	11.0
Meister Brau Premium Draft, 4.6% alcohol	12 fl. oz.	144	11.0
Michelob, 4.9% alcohol	12 fl. oz.	160	12.8
Narragansett, 4.7% alcohol	12 fl. oz	155	14.4
North Star, regular, 4.8% alcohol	12 fl oz	165	14.9
North Star, 3.2 low gravity	12 fl. oz.	142	13.6
Pabst Blue Ribbon	12 fl. oz.	150	D.N.A.
Pfeifer, regular, 4.8% alcohol	12 fl. oz.	165	14.9
Pfeifer, 3.2 low gravity	12 fl. oz.	142	13.6
Rheingold, 4.6% alcohol	12 fl. oz.	160	13.7
Schlitz	12 fl. oz.	155	D.N.A.
Schmidt, regular, 4.8% alcohol	12 fl. oz.	165	14.9
Schmidt, extra special, regular	12 fl. oz.	165	14.9
Schmidt, 3.2 low gravity	12 fl. oz.	142	13.6
Utica Club	12 fl. oz.	150	D.N.A.
Yuengling Premium	12 fl. oz.	144	15.1
Low carbohydrate:			
Dia-beer	12 fl. oz.	145	4.2
Dia-beer	7 fl. oz.	85	2.8
Gablinger's 4.5% alcohol	12 fl. oz.	99	.2
Meister Brau Lite, 4.6% alcohol	12 fl. oz.	96	1.4
BEER, NEAR, Select (Schmidt)	12 fl. oz.	78	D.N.A.
BEET:			
Raw (USDA)	1 lb. (weighed with skins, without tops)	137	31.4

Food and Description	Measure or Quantity	Calories	Carbo-hydrates (grams)
Raw, diced (USDA)	½ cup (2.4 oz.)	29	6.6
Boiled, drained (USDA):			
Whole	2 beets (2″ dia. 3.5 oz.)	32	7.2
Diced	½ cup (3 oz.)	27	6.1
Slices	½ cup (3.6 oz.)	33	7.3
Canned, regular pack:			
Solids & liq. (USDA)	½ cup (4.3 oz.)	42	9.7
Drained solids, whole (USDA)	½ cup (2.8 oz.)	30	7.0
Drained solids, diced (USDA)	½ cup (2.9 oz.)	30	7.2
Drained solids, sliced (USDA)	½ cup (3.1 oz.)	33	7.7
Drained liq. (USDA)	4 oz.	29	7.0
Drained solids (Butter Kernel)	½ cup (4.1 oz.)	38	9.1
Harvard, solids & liq. (Comstock-Greenwood)	4 oz.	54	12.9
Pickled, solids & liq. (Comstock-Greenwood)	4 oz.	60	14.1
Canned, dietetic pack:			
Solids & liq. (USDA)	4 oz.	36	8.8
Drained solids (USDA)	4 oz.	42	9.9
Drained liq. (USDA)	4 oz.	28	6.7
Whole (Blue Boy)	10 small (3.5 oz.)	43	9.3
Pickled, solids & liq. (Del Monte)	½ cup (4 oz.)	75	18.8
Diced, solids & liq. (Blue Boy)	4 oz.	25	5.1
Sliced (Blue Boy)	10 slices (3.5 oz.)	32	7.0
Sliced (S and W) Nutradiet	4 oz.	32	7.3
(Tillie Lewis)	½ cup (4.3 oz.)	46	9.0
Frozen, sliced, in orange flavor glaze (Birds Eye)	½ cup (3.3 oz.)	54	14.9
BEET GREENS (USDA):			
Raw, whole	1 lb. (weighed untrimmed)	61	11.7

(USDA): United States Department of Agriculture
DNA: Data Not Available
* Prepared as Package Directs

Food and Description	Measure or Quantity	Calories	Carbo-hydrates (grams)
Boiled, leaves & stems, drained	½ cup (2.6 oz.)	13	2.4
BENEDICTINE LIQUEUR (Julius Wile) 86 proof	1 fl. oz.	112	10.3
BERNKASTELER, German Moselle wine (Deinhard) 11% alcohol	3 fl. oz.	60	1.0
BERNKASTELER DOKTOR, 1966 German Moselle wine (Deinhard) 11% alcohol	3 fl. oz.	60	1.0
BEVERAGE (See individual listings.)			
BIANCA DELLA COSTA TOSCANA, Italian white wine (Antinori) 12½% alcohol	3 fl. oz.	87	6.3
BIF (Wilson) canned luncheon meat	3 oz.	272	1.5
BIRCH BEER, soft drink:			
(Pennsylvania Dutch)	6 fl. oz.	84	19.7
(Yukon Club)	6 fl. oz.	89	22.3
BISCUIT:			
Baking powder, home recipe (USDA)	1 oz. biscuit (2″ dia.)	103	12.8
Egg (Stella D'oro):			
Dietetic	1 piece (.4 oz.)	42	6.6
Regular	1 piece (.4 oz.)	42	6.9
Roman	1 piece (1.1 oz.)	135	19.2
Sugared	1 piece (.5 oz.)	59	11.0
BISCUIT DOUGH:			
Frozen, commercial (USDA)	1 oz.	93	13.9
Refrigerated:			
Commercial (USDA)	1 oz.	79	13.2
(Pillsbury) *Ballard,* ovenready	1 oz.	72	12.8

Food and Description	Measure or Quantity	Calories	Carbo-hydrates (grams)
(Pillsbury) baking powder, Tenderflake:			
Regular	1 oz.	92	11.1
Buttermilk	1 oz.	94	11.1
(Pillsbury) buttermilk:			
Regular	1 oz.	72	12.8
Extra light	1 oz.	75	12.0
Hungry Jack, regular	1 oz.	77	12.2
Hungry Jack, flaky	1 oz.	97	10.9
Tenderflake	1 oz.	94	11.1
(Pillsbury) country style	1 oz.	72	12.8
(Pillsbury) Hungry Jack:			
Butter tastin'	1 oz.	101	10.4
Flaky	1 oz.	97	10.6
(Pillsbury) Tenderburst	1 oz.	95	11.0
BISCUIT MIX:			
Dry, with enriched flour (USDA)	1 oz.	120	19.5
*Baked from mix, with added milk (USDA)	1-oz. biscuit	92	14.8
Bisquick (Betty Crocker)	1 cup	503	79.4
BI-SICLE (Popsicle Industries)	3 fl. oz.	116	D.N.A.
BITTER LEMON, soft drink:			
(Hoffman)	6 fl. oz.	85	21.3
(Schweppes)	6 fl. oz.	96	23.6
BITTER ORANGE, soft drink (Schweppes)	6 fl. oz.	92	22.6
BITTERS (Angostura)	½ tsp.	7	1.0
BLACKBERRY (USDA):			
Fresh (includes boysenberry, dewberry, youngberry):			
With hulls	1 lb. (weighed untrimmed)	250	55.6
Hulled	4 oz. (weighed hulled)	66	14.6
Hulled	½ cup (2.6 oz.)	42	9.4

(USDA): United States Department of Agriculture
DNA: Data Not Available
* Prepared as Package Directs

Food and Description	Measure or Quantity	Calories	Carbo-hydrates (grams)
Canned, regular, solids & liq.:			
Juice pack	4 oz.	61	13.7
Light syrup	4 oz.	82	19.6
Heavy syrup	½ cup (4.6 oz.)	118	28.9
Extra heavy syrup	4 oz.	125	30.7
Canned, water pack:			
Solids & liq.	4 oz.	45	10.2
Solids & liq.	½ cup (4.3 oz.)	49	11.0
Frozen:			
Sweetened, not thawed	4 oz.	109	27.7
Unsweetened, not thawed	4 oz.	55	12.9
BLACKBERRY CRISPS,			
dehydrated snack (Epicure)	1 oz.	90	21.2
BLACKBERRY JAM,			
dietetic:			
(Dia-Mel)	1 T.	22	5.4
(Diet Delight)	1 T. (.6 oz.)	22	5.5
BLACKBERRY JELLY, low			
calorie (Slenderella)	1 T. (.6 oz.)	22	5.6
BLACKBERRY JUICE,			
canned, unsweetened (USDA)	½ cup (4.3 oz.)	45	9.5
BLACKBERRY LIQUEUR:			
(Bols) 60 proof	1 fl. oz.	96	8.9
(Hiram Walker) 60 proof	1 fl. oz.	100	12.8
BLACKBERRY PIE:			
Home recipe (USDA)	⅛ of 9″ pie (5.6 oz.)	384	54.4
(Tastykake)	4-oz. pie	386	60.1
Frozen (Banquet)	5-oz. serving	376	55.5
BLACKBERRY PIE FILLING			
(Lucky Leaf)	8 oz.	258	62.4
BLACKBERRY WINE (Mogen David) 12% alcohol	3 fl. oz.	135	18.7

Food and Description	Measure or Quantity	Calories	Carbo-hydrates (grams)
BLACK-EYED PEA, frozen (See also **COWPEA**):			
Not thawed (USDA)	10-oz. pkg.	371	66.9
Cooked, drained (USDA)	½ cup	111	20.1
(Birds Eye)	½ cup (2.5 oz.)	92	15.7
BLANCMANGE (See **VANILLA PUDDING**)			
BLINTZE, frozen (Aunt Leah's):			
Apple, blueberry or cherry	1 blintze (2.5 oz.)	80	D.N.A.
Cheese	1 blintze (2.5 oz.)	70	D.N.A.
BLOOD PUDDING or SAUSAGE (USDA)	1 oz.	112	.1
BLOODY MARY MIX (Bar-Tender's)	1 serving (.3 oz.)	26	5.7
BLUEBERRY:			
Fresh, whole (USDA)	1 lb. (weighed untrimmed)	259	63.8
Fresh, trimmed (USDA)	½ cup (2.6 oz.)	45	11.2
Canned, solids & liq. (USDA):			
Syrup pack, extra heavy	½ cup (4.4 oz.)	126	32.5
Water pack	½ cup (4.3 oz.)	47	11.9
Frozen:			
Sweetened, solids & liq. (USDA)	½ cup (4 oz.)	120	30.2
Quick thaw (Birds Eye)	½ cup (5 oz.)	114	28.7
Unsweetened, solids & liq. (USDA)	4 oz.	62	15.4
Unsweetened, solids & liq. (USDA)	½ cup (2.9 oz.)	45	11.2
BLUEBERRY PIE:			
Home recipe (USDA)	⅙ of 9″ pie (5.6 oz.)	382	55.1
(Tastykake)	4-oz. pie	376	57.8

(USDA): United States Department of Agriculture
DNA: Data Not Available
* Prepared as Package Directs

Food and Description	Measure or Quantity	Calories	Carbo-hydrates (grams)
Frozen:			
(Banquet)	5-oz. serving	366	55.8
(Mrs. Smith's)	⅛ of 8″ pie		
	(4.2 oz.)	288	39.2
BLUEBERRY PIE FILLING:			
(Comstock)	1 cup (10¾ oz.)	332	82.8
(Lucky Leaf)	8 oz.	256	61.4
BLUEBERRY PRESERVE, dietetic (Dia-Mel)	1 T.	22	5.4
BLUEBERRY SYRUP, dietetic (Dia-Mel)	1 T.	22	5.5
BLUEBERRY TURNOVER, frozen (Pepperidge Farm)	1 turnover		
	(3.3 oz.)	321	32.0
BLUEFISH (USDA):			
Raw, whole	1 lb. (weighed whole)	271	0.
Raw, meat only	4 oz.	133	0.
Baked or broiled	4.4-oz. piece (3½″ x 3″ x ½″)	199	0.
Fried	5.3-oz. piece (3½″ x 3″ x ½″)	308	7.0
BOCKWURST (USDA)	1 oz.	75	.2
BOLOGNA:			
All meat, very thin slice (USDA)	3″ x ⅛″ slice (.5 oz.)	36	.5
With cereal, very thin slice (USDA)	1 oz.	74	1.1
(Armour Star)	1 oz.	99	0.
(Eckrich):			
All meat	1 oz.	92	D.N.A.
All meat sandwich	1 oz.	84	D.N.A.
German brand	1 oz.	79	D.N.A.
Pure beef	1 oz.	64	D.N.A.
(Vienna)	1 oz.	67	.7
(Wilson)	1 oz.	87	.5

Food and Description	Measure or Quantity	Calories	Carbohydrates (grams)
BONITO, raw (USDA):			
Whole	1 lb. (weighed whole)	442	0.
Meat only	4 oz.	191	0.
BORDEAUX, rouge (Cruse) 10½% alcohol	3 fl. oz.	63	D.N.A.
BORDEAUX WINE (See also individual regional, vineyard or brand names or **CLARET WINE**)			
BORSCHT:			
(Manischewitz)	8 oz. (by wt.)	72	17.5
*Concentrate, frozen (Aunt Leah's)	8 fl. oz.	46	D.N.A.
*Concentrate, frozen, diet (Aunt Leah's)	8 fl. oz.	25	D.N.A.
Low calorie (Gold's)	8 oz.	24	D.N.A.
BOSCO (Best Foods)	1 T. (.6 oz.)	45	10.4
BOSTON BROWN BREAD (See **BREAD**)			
BOSTON CREAM PIE:			
Home recipe (USDA)	½₁₂ of 8" pie (2.4 oz.)	208	34.4
*Mix (Betty Crocker)	⅛ of pie	265	47.9
BOUILLON CUBE (See also individual flavors):			
(USDA) flavor not indicated	1 cube (½", 4 grams)	5	Tr.
(Steero) flavor not indicated	1 cube	7	D.N.A.
(Steero) instant, flavor not indicated	1 tsp.	7	D.N.A.

(USDA): United States Department of Agriculture
DNA: Data Not Available
* Prepared as Package Directs

Food and Description	Measure or Quantity	Calories	Carbo-hydrates (grams)
BOURBON WHISKEY, Unflavored (See **DISTILLED LIQUOR**)			
BOURBON WHISKEY, PEACH FLAVORED (Old Mr. Boston) 70 proof	1 fl. oz.	100	8.0
BOYSENBERRY, fresh (See **BLACKBERRY,** fresh)			
BOYSENBERRY PIE, frozen (Banquet)	5-oz. serving	374	55.8
BOYSENBERRY PRE-SERVE, low calorie:			
(Tillie Lewis)	1 T. (.5 oz.)	10	2.4
(S and W) *Nutradiet*	1 T. (.5 oz.)	11	2.5
BRAINS, all animals, raw (USDA)	4 oz.	142	.9
BRAN BREAKFAST CEREAL: Plain:			
All-Bran (Kellogg's)	½ cup (1 oz.)	107	21.8
Bran-Buds (Kellogg's)	½ cup (1 oz.)	106	21.9
40% bran flakes (USDA)	1 cup (1.2 oz.)	106	28.2
40% bran flakes (Kellogg's)	¾ cup (1 oz.)	109	22.9
40% bran flakes (Post)	⅔ cup (1 oz.)	97	21.0
100% bran (Nabisco)	½ cup (1 oz.)	97	18.6
Raisin bran flakes:			
(USDA)	1 cup (1.8 oz.)	144	39.7
(Kellogg's)	½ cup (1 oz.)	104	22.7
(Post)	½ cup (1 oz.)	92	21.0
Cinnamon (Post)	½ cup (1 oz.)	92	21.0
BRANDY, Unflavored (See **DISTILLED LIQUOR**)			
BRANDY EXTRACT (Ehlers)	1 tsp.	7	D.N.A.

Food and Description	Measure or Quantity	Calories	Carbo-hydrates (grams)
BRANDY, FLAVORED:			
Apricot:			
(Bols) 70 proof	1 fl. oz.	100	7.4
(Garnier) 70 proof	1 fl. oz.	86	7.1
(Hiram Walker) 70 proof	1 fl. oz.	88	7.5
(Leroux) 70 proof	1 fl. oz.	92	8.6
(Old Mr. Boston) 70 proof	1 fl. oz.	100	8.0
(Mr. Boston's) apricot & brandy, 42 proof	1 fl. oz.	75	8.0
Blackberry:			
(Bols) 70 proof	1 fl. oz.	100	7.4
(Garnier) 70 proof	1 fl. oz.	86	7.1
(Hiram Walker) 70 proof	1 fl. oz.	86	7.0
(Leroux) 70 proof	1 fl. oz.	91	8.3
(Leroux) Polish, 70 proof	1 fl. oz.	92	8.6
(Old Mr. Boston) 70 proof	1 fl. oz.	100	8.0
(Mr. Boston's) blackberry & brandy, 42 proof	1 fl. oz.	75	8.0
Cherry:			
(Bols) 70 proof	1 fl. oz.	100	7.4
(Garnier) 70 proof	1 fl. oz.	86	7.1
(Hiram Walker) 70 proof	1 fl. oz.	86	7.0
(Leroux) 70 proof	1 fl. oz.	91	8.3
(Old Mr. Boston) wild cherry, 70 proof	1 fl. oz.	100	8.0
(Mr. Boston's) wild cherry & brandy, 42 proof	1 fl. oz.	75	8.0
Coffee:			
(Garnier) 70 proof	1 fl. oz.	86	7.1
(Old Mr. Boston) 70 proof	1 fl. oz.	74	1.0
(Leroux) coffee & brandy, 70 proof	1 fl. oz.	91	8.3
Ginger:			
(Garnier) 70 proof	1 fl. oz.	74	4.0
(Hiram Walker) 70 proof	1 fl. oz.	72	3.5
(Leroux) 70 proof	1 fl. oz.	76	4.4
(Leroux) sharp, 70 proof	1 fl. oz.	77	4.7

(USDA): United States Department of Agriculture
DNA: Data Not Available
* Prepared as Package Directs

Food and Description	Measure or Quantity	Calories	Carbohydrates (grams)
(Old Mr. Boston) 70 proof	1 fl. oz.	74	1.0
(Mr. Boston's) ginger & brandy, 42 proof	1 fl. oz.	75	8.0
Peach:			
(Garnier) 70 proof	1 fl. oz.	86	7.1
(Hiram Walker) 70 proof	1 fl. oz.	87	7.2
(Leroux) 70 proof	1 fl. oz.	93	8.9
(Old Mr. Boston) 70 proof	1 fl. oz.	100	8.0
(Mr. Boston's) peach & brandy, 42 proof	1 fl. oz.	75	8.0
BRAUNSCHWEIGER:			
(USDA)	2 slices (2" x ¼", .7 oz.)	64	.5
(Eckrich) beef	1 oz.	71	D.N.A.
(Wilson)	1 oz.	90	.7
BRAZIL NUT (USDA):			
Whole	1 lb. (weighed in shell)	1424	23.7
Shelled	½ cup (2.5 oz.)	458	7.6
Shelled	4 nuts (.6 oz.)	114	1.9
BREAD (listed by type or brand name):			
Banana nut loaf (Van de Kamp's)	14-oz. loaf	1288	D.N.A.
Boston brown (USDA)	1.7-oz. slice (3" x ¾")	101	21.9
Cheese, 1-lb. loaf (Van de Kamp's)	.8-oz. slice	61	D.N.A.
Cinnamon raisin (Thomas')	.8-oz. slice	60	12.2
Cinnamon raisin (Wonder)	.8-oz. slice	60	13.0
Corn & molasses (Pepperidge Farm)	.9-oz. slice	71	14.3
Cracked-wheat:			
(USDA) 20 slices to 1 lb.	.8-oz. slice	60	12.0
(Pepperidge Farm)	.9-oz. slice	69	13.0
Honey (Wonder)	.8-oz. slice	63	11.2
Daffodil Farm (Wonder)	.8-oz. slice	58	11.3
Date-nut loaf:			
(Thomas')	1.1-oz. slice	94	18.5

Food and Description	Measure or Quantity	Calories	Carbohydrates (grams)
(Van de Kamp's)	1-lb. 2-oz. loaf	1720	D.N.A.
Dutch Crunch, 1-lb. loaf			
(Van de Kamp's)	.8-oz. slice	63	D.N.A.
Egg sesame, 1-lb. loaf			
(Van de Kamp's)	.9-oz. slice	77	D.N.A.
English muffin loaf, 1-lb. loaf			
(Van de Kamp's)	1-oz. slice	65	D.N.A.
Finn Crisp	1 piece (6 grams)	22	4.8
Flat, Norwegian (Ideal)	1 double wafer	25	5.5
French:			
(USDA) 20 slices to 1 lb.	.8-oz. slice	67	12.7
Brown & serve (Pepperidge Farm)	1″ slice (1.1 oz.)	87	15.8
Giraffe	.8-oz. slice	70	11.2
Glutogen Gluten (Thomas')	1 slice (.5 oz.)	35	6.4
Hollywood, dark or light	1 slice	46	10.0
Honey bran, 1-lb. loaf (Van de Kamp's)	.7-oz. slice	77	D.N.A.
Italian:			
(USDA) 20 slices to 1 lb.	.8-oz. slice	63	13.0
Brown & serve (Pepperidge Farm)	1″ slice (1.2 oz.)	90	16.3
King's Bread (Wasa)	1 slice (3.5 oz.)	365	75.0
Low sodium, 1-lb. loaf (Van de Kamp's)	.8-oz. slice	66	D.N.A.
Oatmeal:			
(Arnold)	.8-oz. slice	64	10.9
(Pepperidge Farm)	.9-oz. slice	68	12.4
Irish, 1-lb. loaf (Van de Kamp's)	.9-oz. slice	69	D.N.A.
100% Milk 'n Butter, 1-lb. loaf (Van de Kamp's)	.9-oz. slice	71	D.N.A.
Orange raisin (Arnold)	.8-oz. slice	69	11.8
Panettone, wine fruit loaf (Van de Kamp's)	1½ lb.	2167	D.N.A.
Profile light (Wonder)	.8-oz. slice	57	11.2
Protogen Protein (Thomas')	.7-oz. slice	46	8.9
Pumpernickel:			
(USDA) 20 slices to 1 lb.	.8-oz. slice	57	12.2
(Levy's)	1.1-oz. slice	70	12.4

(USDA): United States Department of Agriculture
DNA: Data Not Available
* Prepared as Package Directs

Food and Description	Measure or Quantity	Calories	Carbo-hydrates (grams)
Family (Pepperidge Farm)	1.2-oz. slice	79	15.8
(Van de Kamp's) 1-lb. loaf	.6-oz. slice	48	D.N.A.
Raisin:			
(USDA) 18 slices to 1 lb.	.9-oz. slice	66	13.4
Tea (Arnold)	.8-oz. slice	76	12.2
With cinnamon (Pepperidge Farm)	.9-oz. slice	74	13.6
Rite Diet (Thomas')	.7-oz. slice	50	9.3
Roman Light	.8-oz. slice	57	10.4
Roman Meal	.8-oz. slice	58	10.9
Rye:			
Light (USDA) 18 slices to 1 lb.	.9-oz. slice	61	13.0
Family (Pepperidge Farm)	1.2-oz. slice	82	15.7
Jewish (Arnold)	1.2 oz. slice	94	16.7
Westchester, with or without caraway seeds (Levy's)	1.1-oz. slice	55	12.1
With or without caraway seeds (Levy's)	1.1-oz. slice	70	12.1
Salt rising (USDA)	.9-oz. slice	67	13.0
Salt rising (Van de Kamp's)	.9-oz. slice	67	D.N.A.
Slender Key (Arnold)	.8-oz. slice	56	10.1
Soft sandwich, 1½-lb. loaf (Arnold)	.8-oz. slice	67	10.6
Toaster cake (See **TOASTER CAKE**)			
Vienna, 20 slices to 1 lb. (USDA)	.8-oz. slice	67	12.7
Wheat germ (Pepperidge Farm)	.9-oz. slice	68	12.2
White, enriched or unenriched:			
Prepared with 1–2% nonfat dry milk (USDA)	.8-oz. slice	62	11.6
Prepared with 3–4% nonfat dry milk (USDA)	.8-oz. slice	62	11.6
Prepared with 5–6% nonfat dry milk (USDA)	.8-oz. slice	63	11.5
(Arnold) small family	.8-oz. slice	68	11.0
(Arnold) toasting	1.1-oz. slice	88	14.0
English Tea Loaf (Pepperidge Farm)	.9-oz. slice	72	12.0

Food and Description	Measure or Quantity	Calories	Carbo-hydrates (grams)
Hearthstone (Arnold) 1-lb. loaf	.9-oz. slice	71	12.0
Hearthstone (Arnold) 30-oz. loaf	1.1-oz. slice	84	13.9
Home Pride (Wonder)	.9-oz. slice	69	13.2
Large loaf (Pepperidge Farm)	1-oz. slice	77	13.1
Oven Krust (Levy's)	.8-oz. slice	73	12.0
Sandwich (Pepperidge Farm)	.8-oz. slice	70	11.5
(Thomas')	.9-oz. slice	69	13.5
(Van de Kamp's) 1-lb. loaf	.9-oz. slice	69	D.N.A.
(Wonder)	1 slice (.9 oz.)	66	12.7
Wheat, 1-lb. loaf (Van de Kamp's)	1.1-oz. slice	69	D.N.A.
Whole-wheat:			
Prepared with 2% nonfat dry milk (USDA)	.9-oz. slice	61	11.9
Prepared with 2% nonfat dry milk (USDA)	.8-oz. slice	56	11.0
Prepared with water (USDA)	.9-oz. slice	60	12.3
Brick Oven, 1-lb. loaf (Arnold)	.8-oz. slice	65	10.0
Cap Sheaf (Freund)	1 slice	45	D.N.A.
Krinko, 1-lb. loaf (Van de Kamp's)	.9-oz. slice	63	D.N.A.
(Pepperidge Farm)	.9-oz. slice	62	11.8
(Thomas')	.9-oz. slice	64	12.0
BREAD, CANNED:			
Banana nut (Dromedary)	½″ slice (1 oz.)	75	12.4
Brown with raisins (B&M)	½″ slice (1.5 oz.)	78	1.0
Chocolate nut (Crosse & Blackwell)	½″ slice (1 oz.)	65	14.8
Chocolate nut (Dromedary)	½″ slice (1 oz.)	86	14.5
Date & nut (Crosse & Blackwell)	½″ slice (1 oz.)	65	12.6
Date & nut (Dromedary)	½″ slice (1 oz.)	74	12.8

(USDA): United States Department of Agriculture
DNA: Data Not Available
* Prepared as Package Directs

Food and Description	Measure or Quantity	Calories	Carbohydrates (grams)
Fruit & nut (Crosse & Blackwell)	½″ slice (1 oz.)	76	13.6
Orange nut (Crosse & Blackwell)	½″ slice (1 oz.)	76	15.4
Orange nut (Dromedary)	½″ slice (1 oz.)	78	13.4
Spice nut (Crosse & Blackwell)	½″ slice (1 oz.)	62	13.2
BREAD CRUMBS:			
Dry, grated (USDA)	1 cup (3.5 oz.)	392	73.4
Dry, grated (USDA)	1 T. (6 grams)	25	4.7
(Wonder)	1 oz.	108	20.5
BREAD PUDDING with raisins, home recipe (USDA)	1 cup (9.3 oz.)	496	75.3
BREAD STICK:			
Cheese (Keebler)	1 piece (3 grams)	10	1.8
Garlic (Keebler)	1 piece (3 grams)	11	1.9
Onion (Keebler)	1 piece (3 grams)	10	1.9
Onion (Stella D'oro)	1 piece (.4 oz.)	42	6.8
Regular (Stella D'oro)	1 piece (10 grams)	40	6.6
Salt:			
(USDA)	1 oz.	109	21.3
Vienna type (USDA)	1 oz.	86	16.4
(Keebler)	1 piece (3 grams)	10	1.9
Salt free (Stella D'oro)	1 piece (9 grams)	39	6.3
Sesame (Stella D'oro)	1 piece (9 grams)	42	5.7
BREAD STUFFING MIX:			
Dry (USDA)	4 oz.	421	82.1
Dry (USDA)	1 cup (2½ oz.)	263	51.4
*Crumb type, prepared with water & fat (USDA)	4 oz.	406	40.4
*Crumb type, prepared with water & fat (USDA)	1 cup (5 oz.)	505	50.2
*Moist type, prepared with water, egg & fat (USDA)	4 oz.	236	22.3
*Moist type, prepared with water, egg & fat (USDA)	1 cup (7.2 oz.)	422	40.0
Corn bread (Pepperidge Farm)	8-oz. pkg.	836	167.1
Cube (Pepperidge Farm)	7-oz. pkg.	756	147.0

Food and Description	Measure or Quantity	Calories	Carbo-hydrates (grams)
Herb seasoned (Pepperidge Farm)	8-oz. pkg.	836	178.8
BREADFRUIT, fresh (USDA):			
Whole	1 lb. (weighed untrimmed)	360	91.5
Peeled & trimmed	4 oz. (weighed trimmed)	117	29.7
BROCCOLI:			
Raw, whole (USDA)	1 lb. (weighed untrimmed)	89	16.3
Raw, large leaves removed (USDA)	1 lb. (weighed partially trimmed)	113	20.9
Boiled, ½" pieces, drained (USDA)	½ cup (2.8 oz.)	20	3.5
Boiled, drained (USDA)	1 med. stalk (6.3 oz.)	47	8.1
Frozen:			
Chopped or cut:			
Not thawed (USDA)	10-oz. pkg.	82	14.7
Boiled, drained (USDA)	1⅜ cups (10-oz. pkg.)	65	11.2
(Birds Eye)	½ cup (3.3 oz.)	27	3.6
In cream sauce (Green Giant)	⅓ of 10-oz. pkg.	57	6.4
Spears:			
Not thawed (USDA)	10-oz. pkg.	79	14.4
Boiled, drained (USDA)	½ cup (3.3 oz.)	24	4.3
(Birds Eye)	⅓ of 10-oz. pkg.	26	3.6
& noodle casserole (Green Giant)	⅓ of 10-oz. pkg.	103	9.5
Baby spears (Birds Eye)	⅓ pkg. (3.3 oz.)	26	3.6
In butter sauce (Green Giant)	⅓ of 10-oz. pkg.	49	5.3

(USDA): United States Department of Agriculture
DNA: Data Not Available
* Prepared as Package Directs

Food and Description	Measure or Quantity	Calories	Carbo-hydrates (grams)
In Hollandaise sauce (Birds Eye)	⅓ of 10-oz. pkg. (3.3 oz.)	100	3.2
BROTH & SEASONING (See also individual kinds):			
Beef (Maggi)	1 T.	32	4.6
Chicken (Maggi)	1 T.	34	5.4
Golden (George Washington)	1 packet (4 grams)	5	1.0
Onion (Maggi)	1 T.	33	4.8
Rich brown (George Washington)	1 packet (4 grams)	5	1.2
Vegetable (Maggi)	1 T.	32	4.4
BROWNIE (See **COOKIE**)			
BRUSSELS SPROUT:			
Raw (USDA)	1 lb.	188	34.6
Boiled, 1¼″–1½″ dia., drained (USDA)	1 cup (7–8 sprouts, 5.5 oz.)	56	9.9
Frozen:			
(USDA)	10-oz. pkg.	102	20.7
Boiled, drained (USDA)	4 oz.	37	7.4
Baby sprouts (Birds Eye)	½ cup (3.3 oz.)	34	5.7
Au gratin, casserole (Green Giant)	⅓ of 10-oz. pkg.	68	7.9
In butter sauce (Green Giant)	⅓ of 10-oz. pkg.	54	7.1
BUCKWHEAT:			
Flour (See **FLOUR**)			
Groats:			
(Birkett)	1 oz.	109	23.1
(Pocono)	1 oz.	104	22.0
Whole-grain (USDA)	1 oz.	95	20.7
BUFFALOFISH, raw (USDA):			
Whole	1 lb. (weighed whole)	164	0.
Meat only	4 oz.	128	0.
BULGAR (from hard red winter wheat) (USDA):			
Dry	1 lb.	1605	343.4

Food and Description	Measure or Quantity	Calories	Carbo-hydrates (grams)
Canned:			
Unseasoned (USDA)	4 oz.	191	39.7
Seasoned (USDA)	4 oz.	206	37.2
BULLHEAD, raw (USDA):			
Whole	1 lb. (weighed whole)	72	0.
Meat only	4 oz.	95	0.
BULLOCK'S-HEART (See **CUSTARD APPLE**)			
BUN (See **ROLL**)			
BURBOT, raw (USDA):			
Whole	1 lb. (weighed whole)	56	0.
Meat only	4 oz.	93	0.
BURGUNDY WINE (See also individual regional, vineyard, grape, or brand names):			
(Gallo) 13% alcohol	3 fl. oz.	52	.9
(Gallo) hearty, 14% alcohol	3 fl. oz.	48	1.2
(Gold seal) 12% alcohol	3 fl. oz.	82	.4
(Italian Swiss Colony-Gold Medal) Napa-Sonoma-Medocino, 12.3% alcohol	3 fl. oz.	65	1.1
(Italian Swiss Colony-Gold Medal) 12.3% alcohol	3 fl. oz.	63	.7
(Italian Swiss Colony-Private Stock) 12% alcohol	3 fl. oz.	60	.2
(Louis M. Martini) 12½% alcohol	3 fl. oz.	90	.2
(Mogen David) American, 12% alcohol	3 fl. oz.	24	1.8
(Taylor) 12.5% alcohol	3 fl. oz.	72	Tr.

(USDA): United States Department of Agriculture
DNA: Data Not Available
* Prepared as Package Directs

Food and Description	Measure or Quantity	Calories	Carbohydrates (grams)
BURGUNDY WINE, SPARKLING:			
(Barton & Guestier) French red, 12% alcohol	3 fl. oz.	69	2.2
(Chanson) French red	3 fl. oz.	72	3.6
(Gold Seal) 12% alcohol	3 fl. oz.	87	2.6
(Great Western) 12% alcohol	3 fl. oz.	88	5.0
(Italian Swiss Colony-Private Stock) 12% alcohol	3 fl. oz.	67	2.3
(Lejon) 12% alcohol	3 fl. oz.	67	2.3
(Taylor) 12.5% alcohol	3 fl. oz.	78	1.8
BURRITOS, frozen (Rosarita):			
Bean	8-oz. pkg.	486	D.N.A.
Green or red chili	7½-oz. pkg.	444	D.N.A.
BUTTER, salted or unsalted:			
(USDA)	¼ lb. (1 stick, ½ cup)	812	.5
(USDA)	1 T. (⅛ stick, .5 oz.)	100	<.1
(Breakstone)	1 T. (.5 oz.)	102	.1
(Hotel Bar)	1 T.	100	Tr.
(Land O'Lakes)	1 T.	102	.1
(Sealtest)	1 T. (.5 oz.)	110	.2
Whipped (Breakstone)	1 T. (9 grams)	67	<.1
Whipped (Sealtest)	1 T. (9 grams)	68	.1
BUTTER BEAN (See BEAN, LIMA)			
***BUTTER BRICKLE CAKE MIX** (Betty Crocker)	¹⁄₁₂ of cake	203	35.9
BUTTER CAKE (Van de Kamp's)	1-lb. loaf	1284	D.N.A.
BUTTERFISH, raw (USDA):			
Gulf:			
Whole	1 lb. (weighed whole)	220	0.
Meat only	4 oz.	108	0.

Food and Description	Measure or Quantity	Calories	Carbohydrates (grams)
Northern:			
Whole	1 lb. (weighed whole)	391	0.
Meat only	4 oz.	192	0.
BUTTER FLAVORING, imitation (Ehlers)	1 tsp.	7	D.N.A.
BUTTERMILK (See MILK)			
BUTTERNUT (USDA):			
Whole	1 lb. (weighed in shell)	399	5.3
Shelled	4 oz.	713	9.5
BUTTER OIL or dehydrated butter (USDA)	1 cup (7.2 oz.)	1787	0.
BUTTERSCOTCH MORSELS (Nestlé's)	6 oz.	900	102.1
BUTTERSCOTCH PIE:			
Home recipe (USDA)	⅙ of 9″ pie (5.4 oz.)	406	58.2
Frozen, cream (Banquet)	2½-oz. serving	187	27.0
BUTTERSCOTCH PIE FILLING MIX:			
*With whole milk, low calorie (D-Zerta)	½ cup (4.5 oz.)	99	9.8
*With nonfat milk, low calorie (D-Zerta)	½ cup (4.5 oz.)	60	10.0
BUTTERSCOTCH PUDDING:			
Canned (Del Monte)	5-oz. can	190	32.7
Canned (Betty Crocker)	½ cup	171	29.2
Canned (Hunt's)	5-oz. can	238	30.3
Chilled (Sealtest)	4 oz.	124	20.6

(USDA): United States Department of Agriculture
DNA: Data Not Available
* Prepared as Package Directs

Food and Description	Measure or Quantity	Calories	Carbo- hydrates (grams)
BUTTERSCOTCH PUDDING MIX:			
Sweetened:			
*Instant (Jell-O)	½ cup (5.3 oz.)	178	30.6
Instant (My-T-Fine)	1 oz.	82	20.6
*Instant (Royal)	½ cup (5.1 oz.)	177	29.0
Regular (My-T-Fine)	1 oz.	122	26.8
*Regular (Royal)	½ cup (5.1 oz.)	191	31.8
*(Thank You)	½ cup	169	29.2
Low calorie:			
*With whole milk (D-Zerta)	½ cup (4.6 oz.)	107	12.2
*With nonfat milk (D-Zerta)	½ cup (4.5 oz.)	72	12.7
B-V (Wilson)	1 tsp. (¼ oz.)	11	.6

Food and Description	Measure or Quantity	Calories	Carbo-hydrates (grams)

C

CABBAGE:
White (USDA):
Raw:

Whole	1 lb. (weighed untrimmed)	86	19.3
Finely shredded or chopped	1 cup (3.2 oz.)	22	4.9
Coarsely shredded or sliced	1 cup (2.5 oz.)	17	3.8
Wedge	3½" x 4½"	24	5.4

Boiled:

Shredded, in small amount of water, short time, drained	½ cup (2.6 oz.)	15	3.1
Wedges, in large amount of water, long time, drained	½ cup (3.2 oz.)	16	3.7
Dehydrated	1 oz.	87	20.9
Red, raw, whole (USDA)	1 lb. (weighed untrimmed)	111	24.7
Red, canned (Comstock-Greenwood)	4 oz.	77	18.0
Savoy, raw, whole (USDA)	1 lb. (weighed untrimmed)	86	16.5

CABBAGE, CHINESE or CELERY, raw (USDA):

Whole	1 lb. (weighed untrimmed)	62	13.2
1" pieces, leaves with stalk	½ cup (1.3 oz.)	5	1.1

CABBAGE ROLLS, stuffed with beef, in tomato sauce, frozen (Holloway House)

	1 roll (7 oz.)	184	D.N.A.

(USDA): United States Department of Agriculture
DNA: Data Not Available
* Prepared as Package Directs

Food and Description	Measure or Quantity	Calories	Carbo-hydrates (grams)
CABBAGE, SPOON or WHITE MUSTARD (USDA):			
Raw, untrimmed	1 lb.	69	12.5
Boiled, drained	½ cup (3 oz.)	12	2.0
CABERNET SAUVIGNON WINE (Louis M. Martini) 12½% alcohol	3 fl. oz.	90	.2
CACTUS COOLER, soft drink (Canada Dry)	6 fl. oz.	85	22.2
CAKE: Most cakes are listed elsewhere by kind of cake such as **ANGEL FOOD** or **CHOCOLATE** or brand name, such as **YANKEE DOODLES** (USDA):			
Plain, home recipe:			
Without icing	⅑ of 9″ sq. (3″ x 3″ x 1″, 3 oz.)	313	48.1
With chocolate icing	3.5-oz. piece (¹⁄₁₆ of 10″ layer cake)	368	59.4
With boiled white icing	⅑ of 9″ sq. (3″ x 3″ x 1″, 3 oz.)	401	70.6
With uncooked white icing	3.5-oz. piece (¹⁄₁₆ of 10″ layer cake)	367	63.3
White, home recipe:			
Without icing	⅑ of 9″ sq. (3″ x 3″ x 1″, 3 oz.)	322	46.4
With coconut icing	¹⁄₁₆ of 10″ layer cake (3.5 oz.)	371	60.7
With uncooked white icing	¹⁄₁₆ of 10″ layer cake (3.5 oz.)	375	62.9
Yellow, home recipe:			
Without icing	⅑ of 9″ sq. (3″ x 3″ x 1″, 3 oz.)	312	50.1
With caramel icing	3.5-oz. piece	362	61.3

Food and Description	Measure or Quantity	Calories	Carbohydrates (grams)
With chocolate icing, 2-layer	1/16 of 9" cake (2.6 oz.)	274	45.3
CAKE DECORATOR, canned, any color (Pillsbury)	1 oz.	110	21.0
CAKE FROSTING (See CAKE ICING & CAKE ICING MIX)			
CAKE ICING:			
Butterscotch (Betty Crocker)	1/12 of 16.5-oz. can	164	27.8
Caramel, home recipe (USDA)	4 oz.	408	86.8
Chocolate, home recipe (USDA)	4 oz.	426	76.4
Chocolate (Betty Crocker)	1/12 of 16.5-oz. can	162	25.0
Chocolate (Q-T)	4 oz.	452	D.N.A.
Coconut, home recipe (USDA)	4 oz.	413	84.9
Dark Dutch fudge (Betty Crocker)	1/12 of 16.5-oz. can	153	24.7
Milk chocolate (Betty Crocker)	1/12 of 16.5-oz. can	164	27.2
Sunkist Lemon (Betty Crocker)	1/12 of 16.5-oz. can	166	28.0
Vanilla (Betty Crocker)	1/12 of 16.5-oz. can	166	28.0
White, boiled, home recipe (USDA)	4 oz.	358	91.1
White, uncooked, home recipe (USDA)	4 oz.	426	92.5
CAKE ICING MIX:			
*Banana, creamy (Betty Crocker)	1/12 of cake's icing	139	29.5
Butter Brickle, creamy (Betty Crocker)	1/12 of cake's icing	140	29.7
*Caramel, creamy (Betty Crocker)	1/12 of cake's icing	139	29.6
*Cherry, creamy (Betty Crocker)	1/12 of cake's icing	139	29.3

(USDA): United States Department of Agriculture
DNA: Data Not Available
* Prepared as Package Directs

Food and Description	Measure or Quantity	Calories	Carbohydrates (grams)
*Cherry fluff (Betty Crocker)	1/12 of cake's icing	59	16.6
Cherry fudge, creamy (Betty Crocker)	1/12 of cake's icing	132	28.5
*Chocolate, fluffy (Betty Crocker)	1/12 of cake's icing	70	12.8
Chocolate fudge (USDA)	1 oz.	116	24.5
*Chocolate fudge (USDA)	4 oz.	429	76.0
*Chocolate fudge, creamy (Betty Crocker)	1/12 of cake's icing	134	28.6
*Chocolate malt, creamy (Betty Crocker)	1/12 of cake's icing	136	28.7
*Chocolate, walnut, creamy (Betty Crocker)	1/12 of cake's icing	131	26.6
*Coconut-pecan, creamy (Betty Crocker)	1/12 of cake's icing	102	16.6
*Coconut, toasted, creamy (Betty Crocker)	1/12 of cake's icing	141	28.7
*Dark chocolate fudge, creamy (Betty Crocker)	1/12 of cake's icing	130	27.4
*Pineapple, creamy (Betty Crocker)	1/12 of cake's icing	134	28.4
Fudge, creamy (USDA)	1 oz.	109	24.1
*Fudge, creamy, prepared with water (USDA)	4 oz.	384	84.6
*Fudge, creamy, prepared with water & fat (USDA)	4 oz.	434	74.7
*Fudge (Dromedary)	1" x 1" x 1/2" piece (5 oz.)	55	9.9
*Fudge nugget, creamy (Betty Crocker)	1/12 of cake's icing	133	28.6
*Sour cream, chocolate fudge, creamy (Betty Crocker)	1/12 of cake's icing	129	27.5
*Sour cream, white (Betty Crocker)	1/12 of cake's icing	130	29.0
*Spice, creamy (Betty Crocker)	1/12 of cake's icing	139	29.2
*Sunkist Lemon, creamy (Betty Crocker)	1/12 of cake's icing	134	28.5
*Sunkist Lemon, fluff (Betty Crocker)	1/12 of cake's icing	134	28.3
*Sunkist Orange, creamy (Betty Crocker)	1/12 of cake's icing	58	14.9

Food and Description	Measure or Quantity	Calories	Carbo-hydrates (grams)
*White, creamy (Betty Crocker)	1/12 of cake's icing	140	29.8
*White, fluffy (Betty Crocker)	1/12 of cake's icing	58	14.9

CAKE MIX. Most cake mixes are listed by kind of cake, such as **ANGEL FOOD CAKE MIX, CHOCOLATE CAKE MIX,** etc.

White:			
*Layer (USDA)	1 oz.	123	22.2
*With chocolate icing, 2-layer (USDA)	1/16 of 9" cake (2.5 oz.)	249	44.6
*Layer (Betty Crocker)	1/12 of cake	190	35.5
*Sour cream, layer (Betty Crocker)	1/12 of cake	191	34.1
*Party White (Crutchfield's)	4 oz.	397	71.2
*(Duncan Hines)	1/12 of cake (2.5 oz.)	190	36.3
(Pillsbury)	1 oz.	121	21.4
Loaf (Pillsbury)	1 oz.	122	21.8
Whipping cream (Pillsbury)	1 oz.	127	20.8
*(Swans Down)	1/12 of cake (2.5 oz.)	177	36.2
Yellow:			
(USDA)	1 oz.	124	22.0
*With chocolate icing (USDA)	2-oz. serving	191	32.7
*(Betty Crocker)	1/12 of cake	119	23.2
Butter recipe (Betty Crocker)	1-lb. 2.5-oz. pkg.	2220	429.2
*Butter recipe (Betty Crocker)	1/12 of cake	278	37.0
*Party Yellow (Crutchfield's)	4-oz. serving	381	65.3
*(Duncan Hines)	1 cake	2424	420.0

(USDA): United States Department of Agriculture
DNA: Data Not Available
* Prepared as Package Directs

Food and Description	Measure or Quantity	Calories	Carbo-hydrates (grams)
*(Duncan Hines)	¹⁄₁₂ of cake (2.7 oz.)	202	35.0
*Golden butter (Duncan Hines)	1 cake	3396	444.0
*Golden butter (Duncan Hines)	¹⁄₁₂ of cake (3.3 oz.)	283	37.0
(Pillsbury)	1 oz.	122	21.9
Butter flavor (Pillsbury)	1 oz.	122	21.9
Loaf (Pillsbury)	1 oz.	120	21.6
*(Swans Down)	¹⁄₁₂ of cake (2.5 oz.)	187	36.2
CALYPSO COOLER, syrup, low calorie	1 oz.	<1	Tr.

CANADIAN WHISKY (See **DISTILLED LIQUOR**)

CANDIED FRUIT (See individual kinds)

CANDY. The following values of candies from the U.S. Department of Agriculture are representative of the types sold commercially. These values may be useful when individual brands or sizes are not known:

Almond:			
Chocolate-coated	1 cup (6.3 oz.)	1024	71.3
Chocolate-coated	1 oz.	161	11.2
Sugar-coated or Jordan	1 oz.	129	19.9
Butterscotch	1 oz.	113	26.9
Caramel:			
Plain	1 oz.	113	21.7
Plain with nuts	1 oz.	121	20.0
Chocolate	1 oz.	113	21.7
Chocolate with nuts	1 oz.	121	20.0
Chocolate-flavored roll	1 oz.	112	23.4
Chocolate:			
Bittersweet	1 oz.	135	13.3
Milk:			
Plain	1 oz.	147	16.1

Food and Description	Measure or Quantity	Calories	Carbohydrates (grams)
With almonds	1 oz.	151	14.5
With peanuts	1 oz.	154	12.6
Semisweet	1 oz.	144	16.2
Sweet	1 oz.	150	16.4
Chocolate discs, sugar-coated	1 oz.	132	20.6
Coconut center, chocolate-coated	1 oz.	124	20.4
Fondant, plain	1 oz.	103	25.4
Fondant, chocolate-covered	1 oz.	116	23.0
Fudge:			
Chocolate fudge	1 oz.	113	21.3
Chocolate fudge, chocolate-coated	1 oz.	122	20.7
Chocolate fudge with nuts	1 oz.	121	19.6
Chocolate fudge with nuts, chocolate-coated	1 oz.	128	19.1
Vanilla fudge	1 oz.	113	21.2
Vanilla fudge with nuts	1 oz.	120	19.5
With peanuts & caramel, chocolate-coated	1 oz.	130	16.6
Gum drops	1 oz.	98	24.8
Hard	1 oz.	109	27.6
Honeycombed hard candy, with peanut butter, chocolate-covered	1 oz.	131	20.0
Jelly beans	1 oz.	104	26.4
Marshmallows	1 oz.	90	22.8
Nougat & caramel, chocolate-covered	1 oz.	118	20.6
Peanut bar	1 oz.	146	13.4
Peanut brittle	1 oz.	119	23.0
Peanuts, chocolate-covered	1 oz.	159	11.1
Raisins, chocolate-covered	1 oz.	120	20.0
Vanilla creams, chocolate-covered	1 oz.	123	19.9

CANDY, COMMERCIAL
(See also **CANDY, DIETETIC**):

Air Bon (Whitman's)	1 piece	10	D.N.A.

(USDA): United States Department of Agriculture
DNA: Data Not Available
* Prepared as Package Directs

Food and Description	Measure or Quantity	Calories	Carbo-hydrates (grams)
Almond Cluster (Peter Paul)	1 bar (1¾₆ oz.)	171	19.8
Almond Joy (Peter Paul)	1 bar (1½ oz.)	198	24.1
Almonds, chocolate-covered:			
Candy-coated (Hershey's)	1 oz.	142	17.2
(Kraft)	1 piece (3 grams)	14	1.0
Babies, chocolate flavor			
(Heide)	1 oz.	101	D.N.A.
Baby Ruth (Curtiss)	1 oz.	135	21.0
Baffle Bar (Cardinet's)	1 bar (1¾ oz.)	189	10.9
Berries, French gum drop			
(Mason)	1 oz.	100	D.N.A.
Bit-O-Honey (Schutter)	1 oz.	116	D.N.A.
Black Crows (Mason)	1 oz.	100	D.N.A.
Brazil nuts, chocolate-covered (Kraft)	1 piece (6 grams)	32	1.7
Bridge Mix:			
Almond (Kraft)	1 piece (4 grams)	22	1.6
Caramelette (Kraft)	1 piece (3 grams)	12	1.9
Jelly (Kraft)	1 piece (3 grams)	12	1.9
Malted milk ball (Kraft)	1 piece (2 grams)	11	1.4
Mintette (Kraft)	1 piece (3 grams)	12	1.8
Peanut (Kraft)	1 piece (1 gram)	8	.5
Peanut crunch (Kraft)	1 piece (5 grams)	23	3.4
Raisin (Kraft)	1 piece (1 gram)	5	.8
(Nabisco)	1 piece (2 grams)	8	1.4
Butter Chip Bar (Hershey's)	1 oz.	144	18.7
Butterfinger (Curtiss)	1 oz.	134	21.0
Butternut (Hollywood)	1 bar (1¼ oz.)	168	20.6
Candy Corn:			
(Brach's)	1 piece (2 grams)	7	1.8
(Goelitz)	1 oz.	94	D.N.A.
(Heide)	1 oz.	101	D.N.A.
Caramel:			
(Curtiss)	1 oz.	119	24.1
Caramelette (Kraft)	1 piece (3 grams)	12	1.9
Chocolate (Kraft)	1 piece (8 grams)	33	6.2
Chocolate, bar (Kraft)	1 piece (6 grams)	26	4.9
Chocolate-covered (Brach's)	1 piece (8 grams)	33	5.9
Coconut (Kraft)	1 piece (8 grams)	32	5.5
Milk Maid (Brach's)	1 piece (.4 oz.)	45	8.4
Rum (Reed's)	1 piece	17	D.N.A.
Treats (Kraft)	1 piece (8 grams)	34	6.4
Vanilla, plain (Kraft)	1 piece (8 grams)	33	6.2

Food and Description	Measure or Quantity	Calories	Carbo-hydrates (grams)
Vanilla, chocolate-covered			
(Kraft)	1 piece (9 grams)	39	6.2
Caravelle (Peter Paul)	10¢ bar (1½ oz.)	190	28.5
Carmallow (Queen Anne)	1 piece	83	D.N.A.
Cashew crunch, canned			
(Planters)	1 oz.	134	14.4
Charleston Chew:			
Bar	5¢ bar	125	D.N.A.
Bite-size	1 piece	28	D.N.A.
Cherry, chocolate-covered:			
(Brach's)	1 piece (.6 oz.)	66	13.2
Dark (Nabisco)	1 piece (⅔ oz.)	76	14.6
Milk (Nabisco)	1 piece (⅔ oz.)	72	15.5
Cherry-A-Let (Hoffman)	1 piece	215	D.N.A.
Chewees (Curtiss)	1 oz.	116	24.1
Chocolate bar:			
Milk chocolate:			
(Ghirardelli)	1.1-oz. bar	169	18.9
(Hershey's)	10¢ bar (1¾ oz.)	266	27.8
(Hershey's)	1 oz.	152	15.9
(Nestlé's)	1 oz.	148	13.1
Plain (Nestlé's) *Gala*	1 oz.	148	13.8
Sweet (Nestlé's) *Gala*	1 oz.	152	14.6
Mint chocolate			
(Ghirardelli)	1.1-oz. bar	171	18.7
Semisweet (Hershey's)	1 oz.	147	17.5
Semisweet (Nestlés)	1 oz.	141	17.3
Chocolate with almonds:			
(Ghirardelli)	1.1-oz. bar	173	17.6
(Hershey's)	10¢ bar (1⅝ oz.)	250	22.4
(Hershey's)	1 oz.	154	13.8
(Nestlé's)	1 oz.	149	15.3
Chocolate blocks, milk:			
(Ghirardelli)	1 sq. (1 oz.)	147	16.2
(Hershey's)	1 oz.	145	17.8
Chocolate Crisp Bar			
(Ghirardelli)	1-oz. bar	161	17.6
Chocolate Crunch Bar			
(Nestlé's)	1 oz.	140	17.8
Chocolate Drops (Nabisco)	1 piece (.4 oz.)	54	10.6

(USDA): United States Department of Agriculture
DNA: Data Not Available
* Prepared as Package Directs

Food and Description	Measure or Quantity	Calories	Carbo-hydrates (grams)
Chocolate Parfait			
(Pearson's)	1 piece	34	D.N.A.
Chocolate Sponge (Schutter)	1 oz.	122	D.N.A.
Choc-Shop (Hoffman)	1 piece	241	D.N.A.
Chuckles	1 oz.	92	23.0
Chunky	1 oz.	131	D.N.A.
Circlets (Curtiss)	1 oz.	108	26.1
Circus Peanuts (Brach's)	1 piece (7 grams)	27	6.4
Cluster:			
Almond (Kraft)	1 piece (.4 oz.)	63	4.6
Cashew, chocolate-covered			
(Kraft)	1 piece (.4 oz.)	58	4.9
Crispy (Nabisco)	1 piece (.6 oz.)	64	13.6
Peanut, chocolate-covered:			
(Brach's)	1 piece (.5 oz.)	79	7.0
(Hoffman)	1 cluster	204	D.N.A.
(Kraft)	1 piece (.4 oz.)	70	5.0
Royal Clusters (Nabisco)	1 piece (.6 oz.)	96	10.4
Coconut:			
(Welch's)	1 piece (1 oz.)	132	21.1
Bar (Curtiss)	1 oz.	126	21.0
Bon Bons (Brach's)	1 piece (.6 oz.)	70	12.6
Cream egg (Hershey's)	1 oz.	142	20.4
Neapolitan (Brach's)	1 piece (.4 oz.)	48	8.0
Squares (Nabisco)	1 piece (.5 oz.)	64	12.2
Coffee-ets (Saylor's)	1 piece	13	D.N.A.
Coffee Nips (Pearson's)	1 piece	26	D.N.A.
Coffee Time (F&F)	1 piece	10	D.N.A.
Cup-O-Gold (Hoffman)	1 piece	210	D.N.A.
Dainties, semisweet chocolate			
(Hershey's)	1 oz.	147	17.5
Dots (Mason)	1 oz.	100	D.N.A.
Eagle Bar (Ghirardelli)	1 sq. (1 oz.)	151	16.7
Frappe (Welch's)	1 piece	115	21.4
5th Avenue Bar (Luden's):			
5¢ size	1 bar	71	D.N.A.
10¢ size	1 bar	129	D.N.A.
15¢ size	1 bar	179	D.N.A.
Fruit 'n Nut chocolate bar			
(Nestlé's)	1 oz.	140	16.5
Fudge:			
Bar (Nabisco)	1 piece (1.1 oz.)	130	22.8
Fudgies, regular (Kraft)	1 piece (8 grams)	33	6.1
Nut, bar (Nabisco)	1 piece (.6 oz.)	84	3.6

Food and Description	Measure or Quantity	Calories	Carbohydrates (*grams*)
Nut, square (Nabisco)	1 piece (.6 oz.)	84	3.6
Hard candy:			
(Bonomo)	1 oz.	112	D.N.A.
(H-B)	1 piece	12	2.9
(Peerless Maid)	1 piece	22	5.6
Butterscotch:			
(Reed's)	1 piece	17	D.N.A.
Disks (Brach's)	1 piece (6 grams)	23	5.7
Skimmers (Nabisco)	1 piece (6 grams)	22	5.4
Cherry, wild, drops, old fashioned (Nabisco)	1 piece (2 grams)	11	2.7
Cinnamon (Reed's)	1 piece	17	D.N.A.
Honey & horehound drops, old fashioned (Nabisco)	1 piece (2 grams)	11	2.7
Lemon drops (Brach's)	1 piece (4 grams)	15	3.8
Peppermint (Reed's)	1 piece	17	D.N.A.
Pops, assorted (Brach's)	1 piece (5 grams)	19	4.8
Root beer (Reed's)	1 piece	17	D.N.A.
Sherbit (F&F)	1 piece	9	2.2
Sour balls (Brach's)	1 piece (6 grams)	22	5.7
Spearmint (Reed's)	1 piece	17	D.N.A.
Wintergreen (Reed's)	1 piece	17	D.N.A.
Hershey-Ets, candy-coated	1 oz.	134	21.0
Hollywood	1½ oz.	185	24.1
Jelly (See also individual flavors and brand names in this section):			
Beans:			
(Brach's)	1 piece (3 grams)	11	2.8
(Heide)	1 oz.	90	D.N.A.
Big Ben Jellies (Brach's)	1 piece (8 grams)	26	6.8
Iced Jelly Cones (Brach's)	1 piece (4 grams)	15	3.4
Nougats (Brach's)	1 piece (.4 oz.)	43	10.0
Jube Jels (Brach's)	1 piece (3 grams)	11	2.7
Jujubes, assorted (Heide)	1 oz.	93	D.N.A.
Jujyfruits (Heide)	1 oz.	94	D.N.A.
Kisses, milk chocolate (Hershey's)	1 piece (5/16 oz.)	25	2.7
Krackel Bar (Hershey's)	1 oz.	148	15.0

(USDA): United States Department of Agriculture
DNA: Data Not Available
* Prepared as Package Directs

Food and Description	Measure or Quantity	Calories	Carbohydrates (grams)
Licorice:			
(Y&S)	1 oz.	100	D.N.A.
Diamond Drops (Heide)	1 oz.	94	D.N.A.
Pastilles (Heide)	1 oz.	96	D.N.A.
Twist (American Licorice Co.):			
Black	1 piece	27	6.4
Red	1 piece	33	7.3
Life Savers (Beech-Nut):			
Drop	1 piece (2 grams)	9	2.2
Mint	1 piece (2 grams)	6	1.6
Lozenges, mint or wintergreen (Brach's)	1 piece (3 grams)	11	2.9
Mallo Cup (Boyer):			
5¢ size	¾-oz. cup	104	14.8
10¢ size	1¼-oz. cup	173	24.6
15¢ size	1⅝-oz. cup	225	32.5
Malted Milk Balls, milk chocolate-covered (Brach's)	1 piece (2 grams)	9	1.6
Malted Milk Crunch (Welch's)	1 piece (1 gram)	8	.9
Maple Nut Goodies (Brach's)	1 piece (6 grams)	29	4.0
Mars Almond Bar (M&M/Mars)	1 oz.	130	16.9
Marshmallow:			
(Campfire)	1 piece (¼ oz.)	25	5.8
Royal Marshmallow (Curtiss)	1 oz.	90	22.0
Chocolate (Kraft)	1 piece (7 grams)	24	5.4
Coconut (Kraft)	1 piece (.4 oz.)	40	7.5
Plain	1 piece (6 grams)	18	4.6
Chocolate-covered	1 piece (7 grams)	32	4.7
Flavored, regular (Kraft)	1 piece (7 grams)	23	5.8
Flavored, miniature (Kraft)	1 piece (<1 gram)	2	.5
White, miniature (Kraft)	1 piece (<1 gram)	2	.5
White, regular (Kraft)	1 piece (7 grams)	23	5.8
Mary Jane (Miller):			
1¢ size	1 piece (.3 oz.)	31	5.6
5¢ size	1 piece (1.2 oz.)	125	21.8
Merrimints (Delson)	1 piece	30	D.N.A.
Milk Shake (Hollywood)	1¼ oz.	150	26.8
Milky Way, milk or dark chocolate (M&M/Mars)	1 oz.	120	17.7

Food and Description	Measure or Quantity	Calories	Carbohydrates (grams)
Mint:			
Anise, regular (Kraft)	1 piece (<1 gram)	7	1.8
Buttermint (Kraft)	1 piece (2 grams)	8	2.0
Candy-coated mint chocolate (Hershey's)	1 oz.	133	21.1
Chocolate-covered bar (Brach's)	1 piece (1 oz.)	124	23.0
Dessert (Brach's)	1 piece (<1 gram)	4	.9
Encore (Kraft)	1 piece (2 grams)	6	1.7
Jamaica Mints (Nabisco)	1 piece (5 grams)	21	5.2
Liberty Mints (Nabisco)	1 piece (5 grams)	21	5.2
Mini-mint (Kraft)	1 piece (3 grams)	12	1.9
Mint Parfait (Pearson's)	1 piece	34	D.N.A.
Party (Kraft)	1 piece (2 grams)	8	2.0
Pattie, chocolate-covered:			
(Brach's)	1 piece (.4 oz.)	50	9.2
(Hoffman)	1 piece	120	D.N.A.
Junior Mint Pattie (Nabisco)	1 piece (2 grams)	8	2.1
Mason Mints	1 oz.	200	D.N.A.
Peppermint pattie (Nabisco)	1 piece (.6 oz.)	67	13.3
Sherbit pressed mints (F&F)	1 piece	7	1.8
Starlight Mints (Brach's)	1 piece (5 grams)	19	4.8
Swedish (Brach's)	1 piece (2 grams)	8	1.9
Thin (Delson)	1 piece	45	D.N.A.
Thin (Nabisco)	1 piece (.4 oz.)	44	8.7
White, midget (Kraft)	1 piece (<1 gram)	3	.8
White, regular (Kraft)	1 piece (<1 gram)	7	1.8
Mounds (Peter Paul)	10¢ pkg. (1⅝ oz.)	202	26.6
M&M's (M&M/Mars):			
Chocolate	1 oz.	140	18.1
Peanut	1 oz.	140	16.8
Mr. Goodbar (Hershey's)	1 oz.	153	12.5
Necco:			
Canada Mints	1 piece	13	D.N.A.
Necco Wafers	1 piece	7	D.N.A.
Wintergreen	1 piece	13	D.N.A.
North Pole (F&F)	1 bar (1⅜ oz.)	150	31.0

(USDA): United States Department of Agriculture
DNA: Data Not Available
* Prepared as Package Directs

Food and Description	Measure or Quantity	Calories	Carbo-hydrates (grams)
Nutty Crunch, bar (Nabisco)	1 piece (4 grams)	20	2.8
Nutty Crunch, squares (Nabisco)	1 piece (½ oz.)	71	10.1
Old Nick (Schutter)	1 oz.	134	D.N.A.
$100,000 Bar (Nestlé's)	1 oz.	121	18.9
Orange Slices (Brach's)	1 piece (.6 oz.)	55	14.4
Payday (Hollywood)	1¼ oz.	150	22.3
Peaks (Mason)	1 oz.	175	D.N.A.
Peanut:			
Chocolate-covered:			
(BB)	1 oz.	158	6.5
(Brach's)	1 piece (2 grams)	11	1.1
(Hershey's) candy-coated	1 oz.	139	17.9
(Kraft) bite-size	1 piece (9 grams)	43	7.6
(Kraft) boxed	1 piece (2 grams)	12	.9
(Nabisco)	1 piece (4 grams)	23	1.6
French Burnt (Brach's)	1 piece (1 gram)	5	.6
Peanut Brittle:			
(Bonomo)	1 oz.	132	D.N.A.
(Kraft)	1 oz.	126	19.8
Coconut (Kraft)	1 oz.	125	21.7
Jumbo Peanut Block Bar (Planters)	1 oz.	139	14.0
Peanut Butter Cup:			
(Boyer):			
5¢ size	¾-oz. cup	130	10.8
10¢ size	1¼-oz. cup	216	17.9
15¢ size	1⅝-oz. cup	281	23.6
(Reese's)	1 oz.	143	15.4
Smoothie (Boyer):			
5¢ size	¾-oz. cup	135	10.8
10¢ size	1¼-oz. cup	224	17.9
15¢ size	1⅝-oz. cup	292	23.6
Peanut Butter Egg (Reese's)	1 oz.	135	12.4
P-Nut Butter Crunch (Pearson's)	1 piece	35	D.N.A.
Pom Poms (Nabisco)	1 piece	12	2.2
Poppycock	1 oz.	147	22.0
Raisin, chocolate-covered:			
(Brach's)	1 piece (1 gram)	4	.7
(Nabisco)	1 piece (<1 gram)	4	.6
Bar (Ghirardelli)	1.1-oz. bar	160	19.4
Raisinets (B&B)	5¢ box	140	15.4

Food and Description	Measure or Quantity	Calories	Carbo-hydrates (grams)
Red Hot Dollars (Heide)	1 oz.	94	D.N.A.
Saf-T-Pops (Curtiss)	1 oz.	108	26.1
Snickers (M&M/Mars)	1 oz.	130	15.0
Spearmint Leaves (Brach's)	1 piece (7 grams)	23	5.9
Spicettes (Brach's)	1 piece (3 grams)	10	2.5
Sprigs, sweet chocolate (Hershey's)	1 oz.	136	18.3
Sprint, chocolate wafer bar (M&M/Mars)	1 oz.	150	16.2
Stark Wafer Roll	5¢ roll (1¼ oz.)	132	32.9
Stars, chocolate:			
(Brach's)	1 piece (3 grams)	16	1.7
(Nabisco)	1 piece (2 grams)	9	1.0
Sugar Babies (Nabisco)	1 piece	4	.9
Sugar Daddy (Nabisco):			
Giant sucker	1 piece (1 lb.)	1806	398.2
Junior sucker	1 piece (.4 oz.)	42	9.3
Junior sucker, chocolate-flavored	1 piece (.4 oz.)	43	9.1
Nugget	1 piece (6 grams)	26	5.7
Sucker	1 piece (1.1 oz.)	129	28.4
Sugar Mama, pop (Nabisco)	1 piece (1 oz.)	121	22.6
Sugar Wafer (F&F)	1¼-oz. pkg.	180	26.0
Taffy:			
Salt water (Brach's)	1 piece (8 grams)	31	6.8
Turkish (Bonomo):			
Bar	1⅛ oz.	115	29.3
Bite-size	1 piece	19	4.6
Miniatures	1 piece	21	5.6
Nibbles, chocolate-covered	1 piece	9	1.7
Pop	1 piece	45	11.3
Roll	1¢ size	21	5.6
3 Musketeers Bar (M&M/Mars)	1 oz.	120	19.6
Toffee:			
Almond (Kraft)	1-oz. bar	142	7.9
Almond, chocolate-covered (Kraft)	1 piece (6 grams)	50	6.3
Assorted (Brach's)	1 piece (7 grams)	28	5.2

(USDA): United States Department of Agriculture
DNA: Data Not Available
* Prepared as Package Directs

Food and Description	Measure or Quantity	Calories	Carbo-hydrates (grams)
Chocolate (Kraft)	1 piece (7 grams)	27	5.1
Coffee (Kraft)	1 piece (7 grams)	28	5.2
Rum butter (Kraft)	1 piece (7 grams)	28	5.2
Vanilla (Kraft)	1 piece (7 grams)	28	5.2
Tootsie Roll:			
Regular:			
1¢ size or midgee	1 piece (.23 oz.)	27	5.0
2¢ size	1 piece (.37 oz.)	43	8.1
5¢ size	1 piece (1 oz.)	116	21.5
10¢ size	1 piece (1.75 oz.)	202	37.7
Vending-machine size	1 piece (.18 oz.)	21	3.9
Pop	1 piece (.5 oz.)	55	13.2
Pop-drop	1 piece (.16 oz.)	18	4.4
Triple Decker bar (Nestlé's)	1 oz.	148	16.8
U-No (Cardinet's)	1 bar (⅞ oz.)	161	9.3
Virginia Nut Roll (Queen Anne)	10¢ size	250	D.N.A.
Walnut Hill (F&F)	1 bar (1⅜ oz.)	177	29.0
Wetem & Wearem (Heide)	1 oz.	94	D.N.A.
Whirligigs (Nabisco)	1 piece (4 grams)	14	3.0
CANDY, DIETETIC:			
Almond, chocolate-covered	1 piece	22	1.6
Chocolate, assorted:			
Bittersweet (Estee)	1 piece	51	3.0
Milk (Estee)	1 piece	50	3.3
Miniatures (Dia-Mel)	1 piece (8 grams)	37	4.4
Chocolate bar with almonds:			
(Estee)	1 section of 2-oz. bar	14	1.0
(Estee)	1 section of 4-oz. bar	87	5.8
(Estee)	1 bar (¾ oz.)	127	8.7
Chocolate bar, bittersweet:			
(Estee)	1 bar (¾ oz.)	125	8.9
(Estee)	1 section of 2-oz. bar	14	1.0
(Estee)	1 section of 4-oz. bar	83	5.9
Chocolate bar, crunch:			
(Estee)	1 bar (⅝ oz.)	101	8.6
(Estee)	1 section of 3-oz. bar	61	5.1

Food and Description	Measure or Quantity	Calories	Carbo-hydrates (grams)
Chocolate bar, fruit-nut (Estee)	1 section of 4-oz. bar	81	6.6
Chocolate bar, milk: (Estee)	1 section of 2-oz. bar	14	1.0
(Estee)	1 section of 4-oz. bar	84	6.2
Chocolate bar, peppermint (Estee)	1 bar (¾ oz.)	126	9.4
Chocolate bar, white (Estee)	1 section of 4-oz. bar	79	6.1
Chocolettes, milk (Estee)	1 piece	18	1.5
Chocolettes, peppermint (Estee)	1 piece	18	1.5
Coconut chocolate bar (Estee)	1 bar (¾ oz.)	124	8.5
Creams, assorted (Estee)	1 piece	49	3.4
Cream, peppermint (Estee)	1 piece	49	3.4
Gum drops: (Dia-Mel)	1 piece (2 grams)	3	0.
Assorted & cherry (Estee)	1 piece	3	.8
Licorice (Estee)	1 piece	2	.6
Hard candy: All flavors (Estee)	1 piece	12	3.0
Assorted flavors (Barton's)	1 piece	11	2.8
Coffee (Barton's)	1 piece	8	1.7
Coffee (Estee)	1 piece	12	2.8
Licorice (Estee)	1 piece	12	3.0
Lollipops (Estee)	1 pop	12	3.0
Peppermint (Estee)	1 piece	12	3.0
Licorice (Dia-Mel)	1 piece (2 grams)	3	0.
Marshmallow (Dia-Mel)	1 piece (8 grams)	27	2.9
Mint: Butterscotch (Estee)	1 piece	4	1.0
Chocolate (Estee)	1 piece	4	1.0
Fruit flavors (Estee)	1 piece	4	1.0
Peppermint (Estee)	1 piece	4	1.0
Spearmint (Estee)	1 piece	4	1.0
Thin (Dia-Mel)	1 piece (6 grams)	22	1.5
Wintermint (Estee)	1 piece	4	1.0

(USDA): United States Department of Agriculture
DNA: Data Not Available
* Prepared as Package Directs

Food and Description	Measure or Quantity	Calories	Carbohydrates (grams)
Nut, chocolate-covered (Estee)	1 piece	48	3.2
Peanut butter cup (Estee)	1 cup	42	2.5
Petit fours (Estee)	1 piece	48	2.5
Raisin, chocolate-covered (Estee)	1 piece	4	.5
Soff Jells (Dia-Mel)	1 piece (2 grams)	3	0.
Tri-Pak, chocolate-covered assorted bars (Dia-Mel)	3-oz. pkg.	305	34.0
Truffle, chocolate (Estee)	1 piece	51	2.7
TV mix (Estee)	1 piece	11	.8
CANE SYRUP (USDA)	1 T.	53	13.6
CANTALOUPE, fresh:			
Whole, medium (USDA)	1⅔ lbs., 5″ dia. (weighed with skin & cavity contents)	115	28.8
Whole (USDA)	½ med. melon, 5″ dia. (13.6 oz.)	60	14.0
Cubed (USDA)	½ cup (2.9 oz.)	24	6.1
CAPE GOOSEBERRY (See **GROUND-CHERRY**)			
CAPERS (Crosse & Blackwell)	1 T.	6	1.0
CAPICOLA or CAPACOLA SAUSAGE (USDA)	1 oz.	141	0.
CAP'N CRUNCH, cereal (Quaker)	¾ cup (1 oz.)	123	22.8
CAPPELLA WINE (Italian Swiss Colony—Gold Medal) 12.3% alcohol	3 fl. oz.	66	1.2
CARAMBOLA, raw (USDA)			
Whole	1 lb. (weighed whole)	149	34.1
Flesh only	4 oz.	40	9.1
CARAMEL CAKE, home recipe (USDA):			
Without icing	2-oz. serving	218	30.4
With caramel icing	2-oz. serving	215	33.5

Food and Description	Measure or Quantity	Calories	Carbohydrates (grams)
CARAMEL CAKE MIX:			
*(Duncan Hines)	1/12 of cake (2.7 oz.)	202	35.0
*Pudding (Betty Crocker)	1/8 of cake	225	44.4
*CARAMEL NUT PUDDING, instant (Royal)	1/2 cup (5.1 oz.)	189	29.9
CARAWAY SEED (Information supplied by General Mills Laboratory)	1 oz.	72	12.3
CARISSA or NATAL PLUM, raw:			
Whole (USDA)	1 lb. (weighed whole)	273	62.4
Flesh only (USDA)	4 oz.	79	18.1
***CARNATION INSTANT BREAKFAST**	1 envelope with 8 fl. oz. whole milk	290	35.1
CAROB FLOUR (See **FLOUR**)			
***CAROUSEL WINE** (Gold Seal):			
Pink or white, 13–14% alcohol	3 fl oz.	125	9.8
Red, 13–14% alcohol	3 fl. oz.	104	5.2
CARP, raw (USDA):			
Whole	1 lb. (weighed whole)	156	0.
Meat only	4 oz.	130	0.
CARROT:			
Raw (USDA):			
Whole	1 lb. (weighed with full tops)	112	26.0

(USDA): United States Department of Agriculture
DNA: Data Not Available
* Prepared as Package Directs

Food and Description	Measure or Quantity	Calories	Carbo- hydrates (grams)
Partially trimmed	1 lb. (weighed without tops, with skins)	156	36.1
Trimmed	5½" x 1" carrot (1.8 oz.)	21	4.8
Trimmed	25 thin strips (1.8 oz.)	21	4.8
Chunks	½ cup (2.4 oz.)	29	6.7
Diced	½ cup (2.5 oz.)	30	7.0
Grated or shredded	½ cup (1.9 oz.)	23	5.3
Slices	½ cup (2.2 oz.)	27	6.2
Strips	½ cup (2 oz.)	24	5.6
Boiled (USDA):			
Chunks, drained	½ cup (2.8 oz.)	25	5.8
Diced, drained	½ cup (2.4 oz.)	22	5.0
Slices, drained	½ cup (2.6 oz.)	24	5.4
Canned, regular pack:			
Diced, solids & liq. (USDA)	½ cup (4.3 oz.)	34	8.0
Diced, drained (USDA)	½ cup (2.8 oz.)	24	5.4
(Butter Kernel)	½ cup	29	7.0
(Fall River)	½ cup	29	7.0
Solids & liq. (Stokely-Van Camp)	4 oz.	32	7.4
Canned, dietetic pack:			
Low sodium, solids & liq. (USDA)	4 oz.	25	5.7
Low sodium, drained solids (USDA)	½ cup (2.8 oz.)	20	4.5
Diced, solids & liq. (Blue Boy)	4 oz.	25	5.2
Slices (S and W) Nutradiet	4 oz.	25	5.7
(Tillie Lewis)	½ cup (4.3 oz.)	27	5.4
Dehydrated (USDA)	1 oz.	97	23.0
Frozen, with brown sugar glaze (Birds Eye)	½ cup (3.3 oz.)	78	15.4
CASABA MELON, fresh (USDA):			
Whole	1 lb. (weighed whole)	61	14.7
Flesh only	4 oz.	31	7.4

Food and Description	Measure or Quantity	Calories	Carbo-hydrates (grams)
CASANOVE, Italian liqueur (Leroux) 80 proof	1 fl. oz.	104	9.5
CASHEW NUT:			
(USDA)	1 oz.	159	8.3
(USDA)	½ cup (2.5 oz.)	393	20.5
(USDA)	5 large or 8 med.	60	3.1
Dry roasted (Planters)	1 oz.	171	7.9
Dry roasted (Skippy)	1 oz.	175	8.4
Oil roasted (Planters)	1 oz.	178	7.8
Oil roasted (Skippy)	1 oz.	177	8.1
CATAWBA WINE:			
(Gold Seal) 13–14% alcohol	3 fl. oz.	125	9.8
(Great Western) pink, 13% alcohol	3 fl. oz.	116	11.0
(Mogen David) pink, New York State, 12% alcohol	3 fl. oz.	75	11.6
(Mogen David) red, New York State, 12% alcohol	3 fl. oz.	75	11.6
CATFISH, freshwater, raw, fillet (USDA)	4 oz.	117	0.
CATSUP:			
Regular pack:			
(USDA)	1 T. (.6 oz.)	19	4.6
(USDA)	½ cup (5 oz.)	149	35.8
(Heinz)	1 T.	16	3.8
(Hunt's)	1 T. (.6 oz.)	25	5.7
(Nalley's)	1 oz.	28	6.9
(Smucker's)	1 oz.	52	D.N.A.
Dietetic pack:			
(Diet Delight)	1 T.	6	1.2
(Tillie Lewis)	1 T.	6	1.2
CAULIFLOWER:			
Raw (USDA):			
Whole	1 lb. (weighed untrimmed)	48	9.2

(USDA): United States Department of Agriculture
DNA: Data Not Available
* Prepared as Package Directs

Food and Description	Measure or Quantity	Calories	Carbo-hydrates (grams)
Flowerbuds	1 lb. (weighed trimmed)	122	23.6
Slices	½ cup (1.4 oz.)	11	2.2
Boiled, flowerbuds, drained (USDA)	½ cup (2.2 oz.)	14	2.5
Frozen:			
Not thawed (USDA)	10-oz. pkg.	62	12.2
Boiled, drained (USDA)	½ cup (3.2 oz.)	16	3.0
(Birds Eye)	⅓ pkg. (3.3 oz.)	21	3.2
(Stokely-Van Camp)	4 oz.	24	4.8
Au gratin (Stouffer's)	10-oz. pkg.	339	17.9
Cut, in butter sauce (Green Giant)	⅓ of 10-oz. pkg.	37	4.1
In cheese sauce (Green Giant)	4 oz.	61	6.7
CAULIFLOWER CRISPS, dehydrated snack (Epicure)	1 oz.	82	15.9
CAULIFLOWER, SWEET PICKLED (Smucker's)	1 bud (.5 oz.)	24	5.5
CAVIAR, STURGEON (USDA):			
Pressed	1 oz.	90	1.4
Whole eggs	1 oz.	74	.9
CELERIAC ROOT, raw (USDA):			
Whole	1 lb. (weighed unpared)	156	33.2
Pared	4 oz.	45	9.6
CELERY, all varieties (USDA):			
Fresh:			
Whole	1 lb. (weighed untrimmed)	58	13.3
1 large outer stalk	8″ x 1½″ at root end (1.4 oz.)	7	1.6
Diced, chopped or cut in chunks	½ cup (2.1 oz.)	10	2.3
Slices	½ cup (1.8 oz.)	9	2.1
Boiled, drained solids:			
Diced or cut in chunks	½ cup (2.7 oz.)	11	2.4
Slices	½ cup (3 oz.)	12	2.6

Food and Description	Measure or Quantity	Calories	Carbo-hydrates (grams)
CELERY CABBAGE (See **CABBAGE, CHINESE**)			
CELERY SOUP, Cream of:			
Condensed (USDA)	8 oz. (by wt.)	163	16.8
*Prepared with equal volume water (USDA)	1 cup (8.5 oz.)	86	8.9
*Prepared with equal volume milk (USDA)	1 cup (8.4 oz.)	169	15.2
*(Campbell)	1 cup	75	7.3
*(Heinz)	1 cup	101	9.0
CEREAL BREAKFAST FOODS (See kind of cereal such as **CORN FLAKES** or brand name such as **KIX**)			
CERVELAT (USDA):			
Dry	1 oz.	128	.5
Soft	1 oz.	87	.5
CERTS (Warner-Lambert)	1 piece	6	1.5
CHABLIS WINE:			
(Barton & Guestier) 12% alcohol	3 fl. oz.	60	.1
(Chanson) St. Vincent, 11½% alcohol	3 fl. oz.	81	6.3
(Cruse) 11% alcohol	3 fl. oz.	66	D.N.A.
(Gallo) 12% alcohol	3 fl. oz.	50	.9
(Gallo) pink, 13% alcohol	3 fl. oz.	61	3.0
(Gold Seal) 12% alcohol	3 fl. oz.	82	.4
(Grest Western) 12% alcohol	3 fl. oz.	76	1.7
(Italian Swiss Colony—Gold Medal) 11.6% alcohol	3 fl. oz.	59	.6
(Italian Swiss Colony—Gold Medal) Napa-Sonoma-Mendocino, 12% alcohol	3 fl. oz.	64	1.2
(Italian Swiss Colony—			

(USDA): United States Department of Agriculture
DNA: Data Not Available
* Prepared as Package Directs

Food and Description	Measure or Quantity	Calories	Carbohydrates (grams)
Private Stock) 12% alcohol	3 fl. oz.	59	<.1
(Italian Swiss Colony—Gold Medal) gold or pink, 12.3% alcohol	3 fl. oz.	69	3.0
(Louis M. Martini) 12½% alcohol	3 fl. oz.	90	.2
CHAMPAGNE:			
(Bollinger)	3 fl. oz.	72	3.6
(Gold Seal) brut, 12% alcohol	3 fl. oz.	85	1.4
(Gold Seal) brut C.F., 12% alcohol	3 fl. oz.	82	.7
(Gold Seal) pink, extra dry, 12% alcohol	3 fl. oz.	87	2.6
(Great Western) brut, 12% alcohol	3 fl. oz.	82	3.2
(Great Western) extra dry, 12% alcohol	3 fl. oz.	75	4.5
(Great Western) pink, 12% alcohol	3 fl. oz.	88	4.7
(Great Western) special reserve, 12% alcohol	3 fl. oz.	79	3.8
(Italian Swiss Colony— Private Stock) 12% alcohol	3 fl. oz.	69	2.8
(Italian Swiss Colony— Private Stock) pink, 12% alcohol	3 fl. oz.	69	2.6
(Lejon) extra dry, 12% alcohol	3 fl. oz.	68	2.4
(Lejon) pink, 12% alcohol	3 fl. oz.	69	2.6
(Mandia)	3 fl. oz.	75	D.N.A.
(Mogen David) American Concord red, 12% alcohol	3 fl. oz.	90	8.9
(Mogen David) American dry, 12% alcohol	3 fl. oz.	36	4.4
(Mumm's) Cordon Rouge brut, 12% alcohol	3 fl. oz.	65	1.4
(Mumm's) extra dry, 12% alcohol	3 fl. oz.	82	5.6
(Taylor) brut, 12.5% alcohol	3 fl. oz.	75	1.4
(Taylor) dry, 12.5% alcohol	3 fl. oz.	78	2.0

Food and Description	Measure or Quantity	Calories	Carbo-hydrates (grams)
(Taylor) pink, 12.5% alcohol	3 fl. oz.	81	2.9
(Veuve Clicquot) 12.5% alcohol	3 fl. oz.	78	.6
CHARD, Swiss (USDA)			
Raw, whole	1 lb. (weighed untrimmed)	104	19.2
Boiled, drained solids	½ cup (3.4 oz.)	17	3.2
CHARLOTTE RUSSE, with ladyfingers, whipped cream filling, home recipe (USDA)	4 oz.	324	38.0
CHATEAU LA GARDE CLARET, French red Bordeaux (Chanson) 11½% alcohol	3 fl. oz.	60	6.3
CHATEAUNEUF-DU-PAPE, French red Rhone:			
(Barton & Guestier) 13.5% alcohol	3 fl. oz.	70	.5
(Chanson) 13% alcohol	3 fl. oz.	90	6.3
(Cruse) 12% alcohol	3 fl. oz.	72	D.N.A.
CHATEAU OLIVIER BLANC, French white Graves (Chanson) 11½% alcohol	3 fl. oz.	60	6.3
CHATEAU OLIVIER ROUGE, French red Graves (Chanson) 11½% alcohol	3 fl. oz.	60	6.3
CHATEAU PONTET CANET (Cruse) 12% alcohol	3 fl. oz.	72	D.N.A.

(USDA): United States Department of Agriculture
DNA: Data Not Available
* Prepared as Package Directs

Food and Description	Measure or Quantity	Calories	Carbohydrates (grams)
CHATEAU RAUSAN SEGLA, French red Bordeaux (Chanson) 11½% alcohol	3 fl. oz.	60	6.3
CHATEAU ST. GERMAIN, French red Bordeaux (Chanson) 11½% alcohol	3 fl. oz.	60	6.3
CHATEAU VOIGNY, French Sauternes (Chanson) 13% alcohol	3 fl. oz.	96	7.5
CHAYOTE, raw (USDA):			
Whole	1 lb. (weighed unpared)	108	27.4
Pared	4 oz.	32	8.1
***CHEDDAR CHEESE SOUP**, (Campbell)	1 cup	141	9.7
CHEERIOS, cereal (General Mills)	1¼ cup (1 oz.)	112	20.2
CHEESE:			
American or cheddar:			
Natural:			
(USDA)	1" cube (.6 oz.)	68	.4
Diced (USDA)	1 cup (4.6 oz.)	521	2.8
Grated or shredded (USDA)	1 cup (3.9 oz.)	442	2.3
Grated or shredded (USDA)	1 T. (7 grams)	27	.1
(Kraft)	1 oz.	113	.6
Cheddar (Sealtest)	1 oz.	115	.6
Sharp cheddar, *Wispride*	1 T. (.5 oz.)	50	1.5
Process:			
(USDA)	1 oz.	105	.5
*(Borden)	1-oz. slice	106	.9
(Breakstone)	1 oz.	105	.5
(Kraft) loaf or slice	1 oz.	105	.5
(Sealtest)	1 oz.	105	.5
With Brick cheese (Kraft)	1 oz.	101	.5

Food and Description	Measure or Quantity	Calories	Carbo- hydrates (grams)
With Monterey (Kraft)	1 oz.	101	.5
With Muenster (Kraft)	1 oz.	100	.5
Dried, sharp cheddar (Information supplied by General Mills Laboratory)	1 oz.	171	1.7
Asiago (Frigo)	1 oz.	113	.6
Bleu or blue:			
(USDA) natural	1 oz.	104	.6
(Borden) Flora Danica	1 oz.	105	.6
(Foremost Blue Moon)	1 T.	52	Tr.
(Frigo)	1 oz.	99	.5
(Kraft) natural	1 oz.	99	.5
(Stella)	1 oz.	112	.6
Wispride	1 T. (.5 oz.)	49	1.6
Bondost, natural (Kraft)	1 oz.	103	.4
Brick:			
Natural (USDA)	1 oz.	105	.5
Natural (Kraft)	1 oz.	103	.3
Process, slices (Kraft)	1 oz.	101	.4
Camembert, domestic:			
Natural (USDA)	1 oz.	85	.5
(Borden)	1 oz.	86	.5
Natural (Kraft)	1 oz.	85	.5
Caraway, natural (Kraft)	1 oz.	111	.6
Chantelle, natural (Kraft)	1 oz.	90	.3
Cheddar (See American)			
Ched-ett, process, cold pack (Kraft)	1 oz.	85	2.1
Colby, natural (Kraft)	1 oz.	111	.6
Cottage:			
Creamed, unflavored:			
(USDA) large or small curd	1 cup (8.6 oz.)	260	7.1
(USDA) large or small curd	1 T. (.5 oz.)	16	.4
(Borden)	8-oz. container	240	6.6
Lite Line, low fat (Borden)	1 cup	189	7.0

(USDA): United States Department of Agriculture
DNA: Data Not Available
* Prepared as Package Directs

Food and Description	Measure or Quantity	Calories	Carbohydrates (grams)
California (Breakstone)	8-oz. container	216	4.8
Tangy small curd (Breakstone)	8-oz. container	216	4.8
Tiny soft curd (Breakstone)	8-oz. container	216	4.8
Tiny soft curd (Breakstone)	1 T. (.6 oz.)	15	.3
(Foremost Blue Moon)	1 oz.	30	.4
(Kraft)	1 oz.	27	.9
(Sealtest)	1 cup (7.9 oz.)	213	4.7
Light n' Lively, low fat (Sealtest)	1 cup (7.9 oz.)	155	5.6
Low fat, 2% fat (Sealtest)	1 cup (7.9 oz.)	193	7.4
Creamed, flavored:			
Chive (Breakstone)	8-oz. container	216	4.8
Chive (Sealtest)	1 cup (7.9 oz.)	211	4.7
Pineapple, low fat (Breakstone)	8-oz. container	268	34.2
Pineapple (Breakstone)	1 T. (.6 oz.)	1.9	2.4
Pineapple (Sealtest)	1 cup (7.9 oz.)	222	16.1
Spring Garden Salad (Sealtest)	1 cup (7.9 oz.)	208	6.7
Uncreamed:			
(USDA)	1 cup (7 oz.)	172	5.4
(USDA)	1 oz.	24	.8
(Borden)	1 cup	200	6.2
(Kraft)	1 oz.	26	.6
(Sealtest)	1 cup (7.9 oz.)	179	1.6
Pot style (Breakstone)	8-oz. container	172	3.9
Pot style (Breakstone)	1 T. (.6 oz.)	12	.3
Skim milk, no salt added (Breakstone)	8-oz. container	182	1.6
Skim milk, no salt added (Breakstone)	1 T. (.6 oz.)	13	.1
Cream Cheese:			
Plain, unwhipped:			
(USDA)	1 oz.	106	.6
(USDA)	1 T. (.5 oz.)	52	.3
(Borden)	1 oz.	96	.6
(Breakstone)	1 oz.	98	.6
(Breakstone)	1 T. (.5 oz.)	49	.3
(Kraft) *Hostess*	1 oz.	98	.6
(Sealtest)	1 oz.	98	.6

Food and Description	Measure or Quantity	Calories	Carbo-hydrates (grams)
Imitation *Philadelphia* (Kraft)	1 oz.	52	1.9
Plain, whipped (Breakstone):			
Temp-Tee	1 oz.	98	.6
Temp-Tee	1 T. (9 grams)	32	.2
Flavored, unwhipped (Kraft) *Hostess:*			
With bacon & horseradish	1 oz.	91	.5
With chive	1 oz.	84	.8
With olive-pimiento	1 oz.	84	.8
With pimiento	1 oz.	85	.7
With pineapple	1 oz.	86	2.5
With Roquefort	1 oz.	80	.7
Flavored, whipped (Kraft):			
Catalina	1 oz.	94	1.1
With bacon & horseradish	1 oz.	96	.7
With blue cheese	1 oz.	97	1.2
With chive	1 oz.	92	1.0
With onion	1 oz.	93	1.5
With pimiento	1 oz.	91	1.2
With Roquefort cheese	1 oz.	99	1.3
With salami	1 oz.	88	1.2
With smoked salmon	1 oz.	90	1.7
Edam (House of Gold)	1 oz.	105	.3
Edam, natural (Kraft)	1 oz.	104	.3
Farmer cheese, midget (Breakstone)	1 oz.	40	.6
Fontina (Stella)	1 oz.	112	.6
Frankenmuth, natural (Kraft)	1 oz.	113	.7
Gjetost, natural (Kraft)	1 oz.	134	13.0
Gorgonzola (Foremost Blue Moon)	1 oz.	110	Tr.
Gorgonzola, natural (Kraft)	1 oz.	111	.4
Gouda, baby (Foremost Blue Moon)	1 oz.	120	Tr.
Gouda, natural (Kraft)	1 oz.	107	.5

(USDA): United States Department of Agriculture
DNA: Data Not Available
* Prepared as Package Directs

Food and Description	Measure or Quantity	Calories	Carbo-hydrates (grams)
Gruyère (Gerber)	1 oz.	101	.5
Gruyère, natural (Kraft)	1 oz.	110	.6
Gruyère *Swiss Knight*	1 oz.	101	.5
Jack-dry, natural (Kraft)	1 oz.	101	.4
Jack-fresh, natural (Kraft)	1 oz.	95	.4
Lagerkase, natural (Kraft)	1 oz.	107	.3
Leyden, natural (Kraft)	1 oz.	80	.7
Liederkranz (Borden)	1 oz.	86	.4
Limburger, natural (USDA)	1 oz.	98	.6
Limburger, natural (Kraft)	1 oz.	98	.6
MacLaren's, process, cold pack (Kraft)	1 oz.	109	.6
Monterey Jack (Frigo)	1 oz.	103	.4
Monterey Jack, natural (Kraft)	1 oz.	102	.4
Mozzarella:			
(Frigo)	1 oz.	79	.3
Natural, low moisture, part skim (Kraft)	1 oz.	84	.3
Natural, low moisture, part skim, pizza (Kraft)	1 oz.	79	.3
Muenster, natural (Kraft)	1 oz.	100	.3
Muenster, process, slices (Kraft)	1 oz.	102	.6
Neufchâtel:			
Process (Borden)	1 oz.	73	6.5
Loaf (Kraft)	1 oz.	69	.7
Natural (Kraft) *Calorie-Wise*	1 oz.	70	.7
Swankyswigs (Kraft):			
Olive-pimiento	1 oz.	70	1.2
Pimiento	1 oz.	67	1.4
Pineapple	1 oz.	70	2.7
Relish	1 oz.	71	3.3
Roka	1 oz.	80	.6
Nippy Whipped (Kraft)	1 oz.	82	.9
Nuworld, natural (Kraft)	1 oz.	103	.7
Old English, process, loaf or slices (Kraft)	1 oz.	105	.5
Parmesan:			
Natural:			
(USDA)	1 oz.	111	.8
(Frigo)	1 oz.	107	.8
(Kraft)	1 oz.	107	.8

Food and Description	Measure or Quantity	Calories	Carbo-hydrates (grams)
(Stella)	1 oz.	103	.9
Grated:			
(USDA) loosely packed	1 cup (3.7 oz.)	417	3.1
(USDA) loosely packed	1 T. (7 grams)	26	.2
(Borden)	1 oz.	143	8.8
(Buitoni)	1 oz.	118	.8
(Frigo)	1 T. (6 grams)	27	.2
(Kraft)	1 oz.	127	1.0
Shredded (Kraft)	1 oz.	114	.9
Parmesan & Romano, grated:			
(Borden)	1 oz.	143	.9
(Borden)	1 T.	31	.2
Pepato (Frigo)	1 oz.	110	.8
Pimiento American, process:			
(USDA)	1 oz.	105	.5
(Borden)	1 oz.	104	.5
Loaf or slices (Kraft)	1 oz.	103	.4
Pizza:			
(Frigo)	1 oz.	73	.3
(Kraft)	1 oz.	73	.3
Shredded (Kraft)	1 oz.	86	.4
Port du Salut (Foremost Blue Moon)	1 oz.	100	Tr.
Port du Salut, natural (Kraft)	1 oz.	100	.3
Primost, natural (Kraft)	1 oz.	134	13.0
Provolone (Frigo)	1 oz.	99	.5
Provolone or Provoloncini, natural (Kraft)	1 oz.	99	.5
Ricotta cheese (Sierra)	1 oz.	50	1.3
Romano:			
Natural:			
(Borden) Italian pecorino	1 oz.	114	.8
(Frigo)	1 oz.	110	.8
(Stella)	1 oz.	106	.6
Grated:			
(Buitoni)	1 oz.	123	1.1
(Frigo)	1 T. (6 grams)	29	.2
(Kraft)	1 oz.	134	1.0

(USDA): United States Department of Agriculture
DNA: Data Not Available
* Prepared as Package Directs

Food and Description	Measure or Quantity	Calories	Carbo- hydrates (grams)
Shredded (Kraft)	1 oz.	121	.9
Roquefort, natural:			
(USDA)	1 oz.	104	.6
(Borden) Napolean	1 oz.	107	.6
(Kraft)	1 oz.	105	.5
Sap Sago, natural (Kraft)	1 oz.	76	1.7
Sardo Romano, natural			
(Kraft)	1 oz.	109	.8
Scamorze (Frigo)	1 oz.	79	.3
Scamorze, natural (Kraft)	1 oz.	100	.3
Swiss, domestic:			
Natural:			
(USDA)	1 oz.	105	.5
(Foremost Blue Moon)	1 oz.	105	1.0
(Kraft)	1 oz.	104	.5
(Sealtest)	1 oz.	105	.5
Process:			
(USDA)	1 oz.	101	.5
(Borden)	1-oz. slice	96	.9
Loaf (Kraft)	1 oz.	92	.5
Slices (Kraft)	1 oz.	95	.6
With Muenster (Kraft)	1 oz.	98	.6
Swiss, imported, natural:			
(Borden) Finland	1 oz.	104	.5
(Borden) Switzerland	1 oz.	104	.5
Washed curd, natural			
(Kraft)	1 oz.	107	.6
CHEESE CAKE, frozen (Mrs. Smith's)	⅛ of 8″ cake (4 oz.)	306	38.8
CHEESE CAKE MIX:			
*(Jell-O)	⅛ of cake including crust (3.3 oz.)	255	31.4
*(Royal) *No-Bake*	⅛ of 9″ cake including crust (3.2 oz.)	240	28.8
CHEESE DIP (See **DIP**)			
CHEESE FONDUE, home recipe (USDA)	4 oz.	301	11.3

Food and Description	Measure or Quantity	Calories	Carbo-hydrates (grams)
CHEESE FOOD, process:			
American			
(USDA)	1 oz.	92	2.0
(Borden)	1-oz. slice	93	2.3
Grated, used in *Kraft*			
Dinner	1 oz.	129	8.4
Slices (Kraft)	1 oz.	94	2.4
(Foremost Blue Moon)	1 oz.	87	1.5
With bacon (Kraft)	1 oz.	101	.7
Blue, cold pack (Kraft)	1 oz.	89	2.2
Cheddar, cold pack (Kraft)	1 oz.	90	2.4
Links (Kraft) *Handi-Snack:*			
Bacon	1 oz.	93	2.2
Nippy	1 oz.	92	2.2
Smokelle	1 oz.	93	2.2
Swiss	1 oz.	90	1.4
Loaf:			
Munst-ett (Kraft)	1 oz.	100	1.7
Pimiento *Velveeta* (Kraft)	1 oz.	90	2.5
Pizzalone (Kraft)	1 oz.	90	.5
Sharp (Kraft)	1 oz.	97	1.1
Super blend (Kraft)	1 oz.	92	1.6
Swiss (Borden)	1 oz.	92	1.7
Velveeta, California only			
(Kraft)	1 oz.	90	2.5
CHEESE PIE:			
(Tastykake)	4 oz. pie	357	51.2
Frozen, pineapple (Mrs. Smith's)	⅛ of 8″ pie (4 oz.)	273	36.4
CHEESE PUFF, hors d'oeuvres, frozen (Durkee)	1 piece (.5 oz.)	59	2.9
CHEESE SOUFFLE:			
Home recipe (USDA)	¼ of 7″ soufflé (3.9 oz.)	240	6.8
Frozen (Stouffer's)	12-oz. pkg.	730	35.0

(USDA): United States Department of Agriculture
DNA: Data Not Available
* Prepared as Package Directs

Food and Description	Measure or Quantity	Calories	Carbo- hydrates (grams)
CHEESE SPREAD:			
American, process:			
(USDA)	1 oz.	82	2.3
(Borden)	1 oz.	82	2.3
(Kraft) *Swankyswig*	1 oz.	77	1.7
(Nabisco) *Snack Mate*	1 tsp. (5 grams)	15	.4
Bacon (Borden) cheese 'n bacon	1 oz.	80	1.2
Cheddar (Nabisco) *Snack Mate*	1 tsp. (5 grams)	15	.4
Cheese & bacon (Kraft) *Swankyswig*	1 oz.	92	.6
Cheez Whiz, process (Kraft)	1 oz.	76	1.7
Garlic, process (Kraft) *Swankyswig*	1 oz.	86	2.2
Imitation (Kraft) *Calorie-Wise*	1 oz.	48	3.6
Jalapeno (Kraft) *Cheez Whiz*	1 oz.	76	1.9
Limburger (Kraft)	1 oz.	69	.3
Neufchâtel:			
Bacon & horseradish (Kraft) *Party Snacks*	1 oz.	74	.7
Chipped beef (Kraft) *Party Snacks*	1 oz.	67	1.2
Chive (Kraft) *Party Snacks*	1 oz.	69	.8
Clam (Kraft) *Party Snacks*	1 oz.	67	.8
Onion (Kraft) *Party Snacks*	1 oz.	66	1.6
Pimiento (Kraft) *Party Snacks*	1 oz.	67	1.4
Old English (Kraft) *Swankyswig*	1 oz.	96	.6
Onion flavor, French (Nabisco) *Snack Mate*	1 tsp. (5 grams)	15	.4
Parmesan & Romano, grated:			
(Kraft)	1 oz.	130	1.0
Phenix or *Phenix Pimento* (Kraft)	1 oz.	80	2.3
Pimiento:			
(Sealtest)	1 oz.	77	1.7
(Nabisco) *Snack Mate*	1 tsp. (5 grams)	15	.4

Food and Description	Measure or Quantity	Calories	Carbo-hydrates (grams)
Cheez Whiz (Kraft)	1 oz.	76	1.7
Neufchâtel (Kraft)	1 oz.	67	1.4
Process (Kraft) *Swankyswig*	1 oz.	77	1.7
Velveeta, process (Kraft)	1 oz.	84	2.6
Pinconning, natural (Kraft)	1 oz.	113	.7
Pizza (Borden)	1 oz.	85	.8
Pizza, low fat, part skim, shredded (Kraft)	1 oz.	86	.4
Ricotta (Breakstone)	1 tablespoon (.6 oz.)	25	.7
Sharpie, process (Kraft)	1 oz.	90	.5
Smokelle Swankyswig, process (Kraft)	1 oz.	90	.5
Velveeta, process (Kraft)	1 oz.	84	2.6
CHEESE STRAW:			
(USDA)	1 oz.	128	9.8
(Durkee)	1 piece (8 grams)	29	1.2
CHELOIS WINE (Great Western) 12% alcohol	3 fl. oz.	78	2.2
CHENIN BLANC WINE (Louis M. Martini) dry, 12½% alcohol	3 fl. oz.	90	.2
CHERIMOYA, raw (USDA):			
Whole	1 lb. (weighed with skin & seeds)	247	63.1
Flesh only	4 oz.	107	27.2
CHERI SUISSE, Swiss liqueur (Leroux) 60 proof	1 fl. oz.	90	10.2
CHERRY:			
Sour:			
Fresh (USDA):			
Whole	1 lb. (weighed with stems)	213	52.5

(USDA): United States Department of Agriculture
DNA: Data Not Available
* Prepared as Package Directs

Food and Description	Measure or Quantity	Calories	Carbohydrates (grams)
Whole	1 lb. (weighed without stems)	242	59.7
Pitted	½ cup (2.7 oz.)	45	11.0
Canned, syrup pack, pitted (USDA):			
Light syrup	4 oz. (with liq.)	84	21.2
Heavy syrup	½ cup (with liq.)	116	29.5
Extra heavy syrup	4 oz. (with liq.)	127	32.4
Canned, water pack, pitted, solids & liq.:			
(USDA)	½ cup (4.3 oz.)	52	13.1
(Musselman's)	½ cup (4.5 oz.)	61	D.N.A.
(Stokely-Van Camp)	½ cup	49	12.2
Frozen, pitted (USDA):			
Sweetened	½ cup (4.6 oz.)	146	36.1
Unsweetened	4 oz.	62	15.2
Sweet:			
Fresh (USDA):			
Whole	1 lb. (weighed with stems)	286	71.0
Whole, with stems	½ cup (2.3 oz.)	41	10.2
Pitted	½ cup (2.9 oz.)	57	14.3
Canned, water pack, pitted, (USDA):			
Light syrup	4 oz. (with liq.)	74	18.7
Heavy syrup	½ cup (with liq., 4.2 oz.)	96	24.2
Extra heavy syrup	4 oz. (with liq.)	113	29.0
Canned, water or dietetic pack, pitted:			
Solids & liq. (USDA)	½ cup (4.3 oz.)	52	13.1
Solids & liq. (Blue Boy)	4 oz.	52	10.4
Dark, Bing (Yes Madame)	½ cup	63	11.3
Dark, solids & liq. (S and W) Nutradiet	4 oz.	60	14.4
Royal Anne:			
Solids & liq. (Diet Delight)	½ cup (4.4 oz.)	65	15.0
Unsweetened (S and W) Nutradiet	14 whole cherries (3.5 oz.)	47	10.8
(White Rose)	4 oz.	64	15.0
(Yes Madame)	½ cup	61	14.0

Food and Description	Measure or Quantity	Calories	Carbo-hydrates (grams)
Frozen, quick thaw (Birds Eye)	½ cup (5 oz.)	122	30.8
CHERRY ALMOND CAKE (Van de Kamp's)	1 cake	1227	D.N.A.
CHERRY, BLACK, SOFT DRINK:			
Sweetened:			
(Canada Dry)	6 fl. oz.	96	24.0
(Dr. Brown's)	6 fl. oz.	81	20.2
(Hoffman)	6 fl. oz.	87	21.9
(Key Food)	6 fl. oz.	81	20.1
(Kirsch)	6 fl. oz.	88	22.1
(Shasta)	6 fl. oz.	88	22.2
(Waldbaum)	6 fl. oz.	81	20.1
Unsweetened or low calorie:			
(Dr. Brown's) *Slim-Ray*	6 fl. oz.	2	.4
(Hoffman)	6 fl. oz.	2	.4
(No-Cal)	6 fl. oz.	2	0.
(Shasta)	6 fl. oz.	<1	.1
CHERRY CAKE MIX:			
*(Duncan Hines)	½₁₂ of cake (2.6 oz.)	193	34.8
*Chip (Betty Crocker)	½₁₂ of cake	198	37.6
CHERRY, CANDIED:			
(USDA)	1 oz.	96	24.6
(Liberty)	1 oz.	93	22.6
CHERRY DRINK:			
(Hi-C)	6 fl. oz.	92	22.7
*Mix (Wyler's)	6 fl. oz.	64	15.8
Cherry-apple (BC)	6 fl. oz.	102	D.N.A.
CHERRY EXTRACT, imitation (Ehlers)	1 tsp.	8	D.N.A.
CHERRY FRUIT ROLL, frozen (Chun King)	1 oz.	64	10.4

(USDA): United States Department of Agriculture
DNA: Data Not Available
* Prepared as Package Directs

Food and Description	Measure or Quantity	Calories	Carbohydrates (grams)
CHERRY FRUIT SPREAD			
(Vita):			
With brandy wine flavor	1 T.	9	D.N.A.
With papaya	1 T.	9	D.N.A.
CHERRY HEERING, Danish liqueur, 49 proof	1 fl. oz.	80	10.0
CHERRY JELLY (Slenderella)	1 T.	24	6.0
CHERRY KARISE, liqueur (Leroux) 49 proof	1 fl. oz.	71	7.6
CHERRY KIJAFA, Danish wine, 17.5% alcohol	3 fl. oz.	148	15.3
CHERRY LIQUEUR:			
(Bols) 60 proof	1 fl. oz.	96	8.9
(Hiram Walker) 60 proof	1 fl. oz.	82	8.2
(Leroux) 60 proof	1 fl. oz.	80	7.6
CHERRY, MARASCHINO:			
(USDA)	1 oz. (with liq.)	33	8.3
(Liberty)	1 average cherry	8	1.9
CHERRY PIE:			
Home recipe, 2 crusts			
(USDA)	⅙ of 9″ pie (5.6 oz.)	412	60.7
Cherry-apple (Tastykake)	4-oz. pie	373	56.8
Frozen:			
(Unbaked (USDA)	5 oz.	364	55.4
Baked (USDA)	5 oz.	413	63.0
(Banquet)	5 oz.	352	50.2
(Morton)	⅙ of 20-oz. pie	250	35.7
(Mrs. Smith's)	⅙ of 8″ pie (4.3 oz.)	274	35.4
CHERRY PIE FILLING:			
(Comstock)	1 cup (10¾ oz.)	334	84.6
(Lucky Leaf)	8 oz.	242	58.2
*CHERRY-PLUM DANISH DESSERT (Junket)	½ cup	138	33.8

Food and Description	Measure or Quantity	Calories	Carbo-hydrates (grams)
CHERRY PRESERVE, dietetic, morello or cherry-pineapple (Dia-Mel)	1 T.	22	5.4
CHERRY SOFT DRINK, sweetened:			
(Canada Dry)	6 fl. oz.	96	24.0
Fanta	6 fl. oz.	85	21.9
(Mission)	6 fl. oz.	94	23.0
(Nedick's)	6 fl. oz.	81	20.1
(White Rock)	6 fl. oz.	89	D.N.A.
(Yoo-Hoo)	6 fl. oz.	90	18.0
High-Protein (Yoo-Hoo)	6 fl. oz.	114	24.6
(Yukon Club)	6 fl. oz.	86	21.5
CHERRY SYRUP, dietetic:			
(Dia-Mel)	1 T.	22	5.5
(No-Cal) black	1 tsp. (5 grams)	<1	0.
CHERRY TURNOVER, frozen (Pepperidge Farm)	1 turnover (3.3 oz.)	342	30.3
CHERRY WINE (Mogen David) 12% alcohol	3 fl. oz.	126	16.9
CHERVIL, raw (USDA)	1 oz.	16	3.3
CHESTNUT (USDA):			
Fresh, in shell	1 lb. (weighed in shell)	713	154.7
Fresh, shelled	4 oz.	220	47.7
Dried, in shell	1 lb. (weighed in shell)	1402	292.4
Dried, shelled	4 oz.	428	89.1
CHESTNUT FLOUR (See FLOUR, CHESTNUT)			
CHEWING GUM:			
Sweetened:	1 stick (3 grams)	10	2.9

(USDA): United States Department of Agriculture
DNA: Data Not Available
* Prepared as Package Directs

Food and Description	Measure or Quantity	Calories	Carbo-hydrates (grams)
(USDA)	1 piece	18	4.5
Bazooka, bubble, 1¢ size	1 piece	85	21.2
Bazooka, bubble, 5¢ size	1 tablet (2 grams)	6	1.6
Beechies	1 stick (3 grams)	10	2.3
Beech-Nut	1 stick	9	2.3
Beemans	1 stick	9	2.3
Black Jack	1 piece	6	1.1
Chiclets	5¢ pkg.	65	D.N.A.
Chiclets, tiny size	1 stick	10	2.3
Cinnamint	1 stick	9	2.3
Clove	1 piece	4	1.2
Dentyne	1 stick	8	2.3
Doublemint	1 stick	10	2.3
Fruit Punch	1 stick	9	2.4
Juicy Fruit	1 stick	10	2.3
Peppermint (Clark)	1 piece	10	D.N.A.
Sour (Warner-Lambert)	1 stick	10	2.3
Sour lemon (Clark)	1 stick (3 grams)	8	2.2
Spearmint (Wrigley's)	1 stick	10	2.3
Teaberry			
Unsweetened or dietetic:			
All flavors (Clark)	1 stick	7	1.7
All flavors (Estee)	1 stick	8	2.0
Bazooka, bubble, sugarless	1 piece	16	Tr.
Bubble (Estee)	1 piece	3	.6
(Harvey's)	1 stick	4	1.0
Peppermint (Amurol)	1 stick	5	1.8

CHIANTI WINE:

(Antinori):			
Classico, 12½% alcohol	3 fl. oz.	87	6.3
1955, 12½% alcohol	3 fl. oz.	87	6.3
Vintage, 12½% alcohol	3 fl. oz.	87	6.3
Brolio Classico, 13% alcohol	3 fl. oz.	66	.3
(Gancia) Classico, 12½% alcohol	3 fl. oz.	75	D.N.A.
(Italian Swiss Colony):			
Gold Medal, 12.1% alcohol	3 fl. oz.	65	1.4
Private Stock, Tipo, 12% alcohol	3 fl. oz.	59	<.1
(Louis M. Martini) 12½% alcohol	3 fl. oz.	90	.2

Food and Description	Measure or Quantity	Calories	Carbohydrates (grams)
CHICKEN (See also **CHICKEN, CANNED**) (USDA):			
Broiler, cooked, meat only	4 oz.	154	0.
Capon, raw, with bone	1 lb. (weighed ready-to-cook)	937	0.
Fryer:			
Raw:			
Ready-to-cook	1 lb. (weighed ready-to-cook)	382	0.
Breast	1 lb. (weighed with bone)	394	0.
Leg or drumstick	1 lb. (weighed with bone)	313	0.
Thigh	1 lb. (weighed with bone)	435	0.
Fried. A 2½-pound chicken (weighed before cooking with bone) will give you:			
Back	1 back (2.2 oz.)	139	2.7
Breast	½ breast (3⅛ oz.)	154	1.1
Leg or drumstick	1 leg (2 oz.)	87	.4
Neck	1 neck (2.1 oz.)	121	1.9
Rib	1 rib (.7 oz.)	42	.8
Thigh	1 thigh (2¼ oz.)	118	1.2
Wing	1 wing (1¾ oz.)	78	.8
Fried skin	1 oz.	119	2.6
Hen and cock:			
Raw	1 lb. (weighed ready-to-cook)	987	0.
Stewed:			
Meat only	4 oz.	236	0.
Chopped	½ cup (2.5 oz.)	150	0.
Diced	½ cup (2.4 oz.)	139	0.
Ground	½ cup (2 oz.)	116	0.
Roaster:			
Raw	1 lb. (weighed ready-to-cook)	791	0.
Roasted:			
Dark meat without skin	4 oz.	209	0.

(USDA): United States Department of Agriculture
DNA: Data Not Available
* Prepared as Package Directs

Food and Description	Measure or Quantity	Calories	Carbo-hydrates (grams)
Light meat without skin	4 oz.	206	0.
CHICKEN A LA KING:			
Home recipe (USDA)	1 cup (8.6 oz.)	468	12.2
Canned (College Inn)	1 cup	266	8.9
Canned (Richardson & Robbins)	1 cup (7.9 oz.)	272	14.4
Frozen (Banquet) cookin' bag	5 oz.	140	9.0
CHICKEN BARONET			
(Lipton)	1 pkg.	634	90.6
CHICKEN BOUILLON/ BROTH, cube or powder (See also **CHICKEN SOUP**):			
(Croyden House)	1 tsp.	12	2.5
(Herb-Ox)	1 cube (4 grams)	6	.6
(Herb-Ox)	1 packet (5 grams)	12	1.9
*(Knorr Swiss)	1 cube	13	D.N.A.
(Maggi)	1 cube or 1 tsp.	8	1.1
(Steero)	1 cube (4 grams)	6	.4
(Wyler's)	1 cube or 1 tsp.	6	.7
CHICKEN CACCIATORE			
(Hormel)	1-lb. can	386	8.2
CHICKEN, CANNED:			
Boned:			
(USDA)	½ cup (3 oz.)	168	0.
(College Inn)	4 oz.	299	0.
(Lynden Farms) solids & liq.	5-oz. jar	229	0.
(Richardson & Robbins)	4 oz.	239	.9
(Swanson) with broth	5-oz. can	223	0.
Whole (Lynden Farms)	4 oz.	359	0.
CHICKEN, CREAMED, frozen (Stouffer's)	11½-oz. pkg.	613	16.2
CHICKEN DINNER:			
Canned:			
Noodle (Heinz)	8½-oz. can	186	18.9
Noodle (Lynden Farms)	14-oz. jar	413	31.8

Food and Description	Measure or Quantity	Calories	Carbo-hydrates (grams)
Noodle with vegetables (Lynden Farms)	15-oz. can	434	38.2
Frozen:			
Cantonese (Chun King)	11-oz. dinner	302	D.N.A.
Chicken & dumplings:			
Buffet (Banquet)	2-lb. pkg.	1306	110.8
(Tom Thumb)	3-lb. 8-oz. tray	1920	112.6
Fried:			
With mashed potato, carrots, peas, corn & beans (USDA)	12 oz.	588	38.4
(Banquet)	11-oz. dinner	542	48.2
(Morton)	11-oz. dinner	482	37.2
(Swanson)	11½-oz. dinner	600	46.6
(Swanson) 3-course	15-oz. dinner	639	62.6
CHICKEN & DUMPLINGS (See **CHICKEN DINNER**)			
CHICKEN FRICASSEE:			
Home recipe (USDA)	1 cup (8.5 oz.)	386	7.7
Canned (College Inn)	1 cup	234	14.8
Canned (Richardson & Robbins)	1 cup (7.9 oz.)	256	15.1
CHICKEN, FRIED, frozen With whipped potato (Swanson)	7-oz. pkg.	412	27.0
CHICKEN, GIZZARD (USDA):			
Raw	2 oz.	64	.4
Simmered	2 oz.	84	.4
CHICKEN LIVER (See **LIVER**)			
CHICKEN LIVER, CHOPPED (Mrs. Kornberg's)	6-oz. pkg.	260	D.N.A.

(USDA): United States Department of Agriculture
DNA: Data Not Available
* Prepared as Package Directs

Food and Description	Measure or Quantity	Calories	Carbo-hydrates (grams)
CHICKEN LIVER PUFF, hors d'oeuvres, frozen (Durkee)	1 piece (.5 oz.)	64	3.1
CHICKEN & NOODLES:			
Home recipe (USDA)	1 cup (8.5 oz.)	367	25.7
Frozen (Banquet) buffet	2-lb. pkg.	735	61.2
Frozen, escalloped (Stouffer's)	11½-oz. pkg.	589	35.9
CHICKEN PIE:			
Baked, home recipe (USDA)	8 oz. (4¼" dia.)	533	41.5
Frozen:			
Commercial, unheated (USDA)	8-oz. pie	497	50.4
(Banquet)	8-oz. pie	412	37.8
(Morton)	8-oz. pie	445	35.4
(Stouffer's)	10-oz. pie	722	44.2
(Swanson)	8-oz. pie	445	40.0
(Van de Kamp's)	10½-oz. pie	601	D.N.A.
CHICKEN PUFF, hors d'oeuvres, frozen (Durkee)	1 piece (.5 oz.)	49	3.0
CHICKEN RAVIOLI (Lynden Farms)	14½-oz. can	452	74.0
CHICKEN SOUP, canned:			
*Barley (Manischewitz)	8 oz. (by wt.)	83	12.3
Broth:			
*(Campbell)	1 cup	53	.9
*Diet, condensed (Claybourne)	1 cup	9	0.
(College Inn)	1 cup	30	.1
Low calorie (College Inn)	8 oz.	9	.1
(Richardson & Robbins)	1 cup (8.1 oz.)	32	1.6
With noodles (College Inn)	8 oz.	20	2.2
With rice (College Inn)	8 oz.	44	7.7
With rice (Richardson & Robbins)	1 cup (8.1 oz.)	48	5.0
Consommé:			
Condensed (USDA)	8 oz. (by wt.)	41	3.4
*Prepared with equal volume water (USDA)	1 cup (8.5 oz.)	22	1.9

Food and Description	Measure or Quantity	Calories	Carbo-hydrates (grams)
Cream of:			
Condensed (USDA)	8 oz. (by wt.)	179	15.2
*Prepared with equal volume milk (USDA)	1 cup (8.6 oz.)	179	14.5
*Prepared with equal volume water (USDA)	1 cup (8.5 oz.)	94	7.9
*(Campbell)	1 cup	87	7.2
*(Heinz)	1 cup (8.5 oz.)	93	8.3
(Heinz) *Great American*	1 cup (8.5 oz.)	108	9.0
*& Dumplings (Campbell)	1 cup	95	4.8
Egg drop, frozen (Temple)	8 oz.	49	D.N.A.
Gumbo:			
Condensed (USDA)	8 oz. (by wt.)	104	13.8
*Prepared with equal volume water (USDA)	1 cup (8.5 oz.)	55	7.4
*(Campbell)	1 cup	55	8.3
& Noodle:			
Condensed (USDA)	8 oz. (by wt.)	120	15.0
*Prepared with equal volume water (USDA)	1 cup (8.5 oz.)	65	8.2
*(Campbell)	1 cup	62	8.2
*Noodle-O's (Campbell)	1 cup	67	9.0
*(Heinz)	1 cup (8.5 oz.)	75	9.5
*(Manischewitz)	1 cup (8.1 oz.)	46	4.2
(Tillie Lewis) dietetic	1 cup (8 oz.)	53	6.8
With dumplings (Heinz) *Great American*	1 cup (8.5 oz.)	89	8.9
*With stars (Campbell)	1 cup	57	6.9
*With stars (Heinz)	1 cup (8.5 oz.)	66	7.9
& Rice:			
Condensed (USDA)	8 oz. (by wt.)	89	10.7
*Prepared with equal volume water (USDA)	1 cup (8.5 oz.)	48	5.8
*(Campbell)	1 cup	49	5.6
*(Heinz)	1 cup (8.5 oz.)	61	6.7
*(Manischewitz)	8 oz. (by wt.)	47	5.3
With mushrooms (Heinz), *Great American*	1 cup (8.5 oz.)	96	11.6

(USDA): United States Department of Agriculture
DNA: Data Not Available
* Prepared as Package Directs

Food and Description	Measure or Quantity	Calories	Carbo-hydrates (grams)
Vegetable:			
Condensed (USDA)	8 oz. (by wt.)	141	17.5
*Prepared with equal volume water (USDA)	1 cup (8.6 oz.)	76	9.6
*(Campbell)	1 cup	68	8.6
*(Heinz)	1 cup (8.5 oz.)	85	9.3
*(Manischewitz)	1 cup	55	7.8
*With Kasha (Manischewitz)	1 cup	41	5.4
CHICKEN SOUP MIX:			
& Noodle:			
(USDA)	2-oz. pkg.	218	33.1
*(USDA)	1 cup (8.1 oz.)	51	7.4
*(Golden Grain)	1 cup	58	8.8
(Lipton)	1 pkg. (2 oz.)	217	29.3
With diced chicken (Lipton)	1 pkg. (1.9 oz.)	204	26.8
*(Wyler's)	6 fl. oz.	33	4.2
& Rice:			
(USDA)	1 oz.	100	17.6
*(USDA)	1 cup (8 oz.)	46	8.0
*(Lipton)	1 cup	63	7.9
*Rice-A-Roni	1 cup	63	10.9
*(Wyler's)	6 fl. oz.	37	6.4
Vegetable (Lipton)	1 pkg. (2 oz.)	218	30.4
*Vegetable (Wyler's)	6 fl. oz.	28	4.0
CHICKEN SPREAD:			
(Swanson)	5-oz. can	283	2.0
(Underwood)	1 T. (.5 oz.)	31	.5
CHICKEN STEW:			
Canned:			
(B&M)	1 cup (7.9 oz.)	128	15.3
(Bounty)	1 cup	166	16.3
With dumplings (Heinz)	8½-oz. can	202	22.1
Frozen, in white wine cream sauce (Swanson)	6-oz. pkg.	243	3.7
CHICK-PEAS or GARBANZOS			
Dry (USDA)	1 cup (7.1 oz.)	720	122.0

Food and Description	Measure or Quantity	Calories	Carbo-hydrates (grams)
CHICORY GREENS, raw (USDA):			
Untrimmed	½ lb. (weighed untrimmed)	37	7.0
Trimmed	4 oz.	23	4.3
CHICORY, WITLOOF, Belgian or French endive, raw, bleached head (USDA):			
Untrimmed	½ lb. (weighed untrimmed)	30	6.4
Trimmed, cut	½ cup (.9 oz.)	4	.8
CHILI or CHILI CON CARNE:			
Canned, beans only, spiced (Gebhardt)	1 cup	184	D.N.A.
Canned, with beans:			
(USDA)	1 cup (8.8 oz.)	332	30.5
(Armour Star)	15½-oz. can	692	59.3
(Austex)	15½-oz. can (1¾ cups)	584	53.6
(Chef Boy-Ar-Dee)	¼ of 30-oz. can	307	24.1
(College Inn)	8 oz.	465	18.6
(Heinz)	8¾-oz. can	352	28.2
(Hormel)	2-lb. 8-oz. can	1406	106.6
(Hormel)	1-lb. 8-oz. can	775	44.2
(Hormel)	15-oz. can	625	41.6
(Hormel)	8-oz. can	275	17.5
(Nalley's) mild or hot	8 oz.	363	26.8
(Rosarita)	8 oz.	376	27.2
(Rutherford)	6 oz.	284	D.N.A.
(Silver Skillet)	8 oz.	334	19.6
(Swanson)	1 cup	270	21.8
(Van Camp)	1 cup (8 oz.)	304	28.0
(Wilson)	½ of 15½-oz. can	315	26.4
Canned, without beans:			
(USDA)	1 cup (9 oz.)	510	14.8
(Armour Star)	15½-oz. can	835	25.5

(USDA): United States Department of Agriculture
DNA: Data Not Available
* Prepared as Package Directs

Food and Description	Measure or Quantity	Calories	Carbohydrates (grams)
(Austex)	15-oz. can (1¾ cups)	851	24.7
(Bunker Hill)	10¼-oz. can	657	D.N.A.
(Chef Boy-Ar-Dee)	½ of 15¼-oz. can	328	14.0
(Hormel)	15-oz. can	774	15.7
(Morton House)	15-oz. can	1065	D.N.A.
(Nalley's)	8 oz.	352	12.9
(Rutherford)	6 oz.	335	D.N.A.
(Van Camp)	1 cup	460	13.2
(Wilson)	½ of 15½-oz. can	420	12.7
Frozen, with beans:			
(Banquet)	8-oz. bag	310	21.5
Dinner (Swanson)	11¼-oz. dinner	459	58.6
CHILI BEEF SOUP, canned:			
*(Campbell)	1 cup	149	20.8
*(Heinz)	1 cup (8¾ oz.)	161	21.2
(Heinz) *Great American*	1 cup (8¾ oz.)	179	22.0
CHILI CON CARNE MIX:			
*With meat & beans			
(Durkee)	2½ cups (2¼-oz. dry pkg.)	1720	94.0
*Without meat & beans			
(Durkee)	1¼ cups (2¼-oz. dry pkg.)	196	44.6
(Chili Products)	1 oz.	94	15.6
(Mexene)	1 oz.	97	16.1
*CHILI DOG SAUCE MIX			
(McCormick)	.9-oz. serving	18	4.0
CHILI POWDER, with added seasonings (USDA)	1 T. (.5 oz.)	51	8.5
CHILI SAUCE:			
(USDA)	1 T.	16	3.7
(Heinz)	1 T.	17	3.8
(Hunt's)	1 T. (.6 oz.)	21	4.9
CHILI SEASONING MIX:			
Chili-O (French's)	1¾-oz. pkg.	125	24.0
(Lawry's)	1.6-oz. pkg.	137	23.6
(Wyler's)	1⅝-oz. pkg.	D.N.A.	22.0

Food and Description	Measure or Quantity	Calories	Carbo-hydrates (grams)
CHINESE DATE (See **JUJUBE**)			
CHINESE DINNER, frozen (Swanson)	11-oz. dinner	356	40.9
CHIPS (See **CRACKERS** for **CORN CHIPS** and **POTATO CHIPS**)			
CHITTERLINGS, canned (Hormel)	1 lb. 2-oz. can	832	.5
CHIVES, raw (USDA)	½ lb.	64	13.2
CHOCO FIZZ (Dia-Mel)	1 tsp.	7	.7
CHOCOLATE, BAKING:			
Bitter or unsweetened:			
(USDA)	1 oz.	143	8.2
(Baker's)	1 oz. (1 sq.)	136	7.7
Pre-melted, *Choco-Bake*	1-oz. packet	172	10.2
(Hershey's)	1 oz.	169	6.6
Sweetened:			
German's sweet (Baker's)	1 oz. (4½ sq.)	141	16.9
Semisweet (Baker's)	1 oz. (1 sq.)	132	16.2
Chips, semisweet (Baker's)	¼ cup (1½ oz.)	191	28.5
Chips, semisweet (Ghirardelli)	⅓ cup (2 oz.)	299	35.6
Chips, milk (Hershey's)	1 oz.	152	15.9
Chips, semisweet (Hershey's)	1 oz.	145	17.2
Morsels, milk (Nestlé's)	1 oz.	152	18.0
Morsels, semisweet (Nestlé's)	1 oz.	137	18.1
Morsels, semisweet mint (Nestlé's)	1 oz.	136	18.0

(USDA): United States Department of Agriculture
DNA: Data Not Available
* Prepared as Package Directs

Food and Description	Measure or Quantity	Calories	Carbohydrates (grams)
CHOCOLATE CAKE:			
Home recipe (USDA):			
Without icing	3 oz.	311	44.2
With chocolate icing	1/16 of 10″ cake (4.2 oz.)	443	67.0
With uncooked white icing	1/16 of 10″ cake (4.2 oz.)	443	71.0
Almond (Van de Kamp's)	2 layer cake	3377	D.N.A.
Fudge layer, frozen (Pepperidge Farm)	1/8 of cake (3 oz.)	315	43.4
Golden, frozen (Pepperidge Farm)	1/8 of cake (3 oz.)	320	43.6
Milk (Van de Kamp's)	2 layer cake	2825	D.N.A.
Pecan (Van de Kamp's)	2 layer cake	3366	D.N.A.
CHOCOLATE CAKE MIX (See also **FUDGE CAKE MIX**):			
Chocolate loaf (Pillsbury)	1 oz.	120	21.8
Chocolate malt (USDA)	1 oz.	116	22.4
Chocolate malt (Betty Crocker)	1-lb. 2.5-oz. pkg.	2183	418.1
*Chocolate malt (Betty Crocker)	1/12 of cake	200	35.8
*Chocolate malt, uncooked white icing (USDA)	4 oz.	392	75.5
*Chocolate pudding (Betty Crocker)	1/8 of cake	221	44.0
*Deep chocolate (Duncan Hines)	1 cake	2412	410.4
*Deep chocolate (Duncan Hines)	1/12 of cake (2.7 oz.)	201	34.2
*German chocolate (Betty Crocker)	1/2 of cake	200	35.9
German chocolate (Pillsbury)	1 oz.	121	22.0
*German chocolate (Swans Down)	1/12 of cake	187	35.8
*Milk chocolate (Betty Crocker)	1/2 of cake	199	35.0
*Swiss chocolate			

Food and Description	Measure or Quantity	Calories	Carbo-hydrates (grams)
(Duncan Hines)	1/12 of cake (2.7 oz.)	201	34.2
CHOCOLATE CANDY (See CANDY)			
CHOCOLATE DRINK (Borden):			
Dutch	1 qt.	724	106.8
Dutch, canned	9½-oz. can	232	32.1
CHOCOLATE DRINK MIX: Dutch, instant (Borden):			
*With water	6 fl. oz.	87	18.8
*With skim milk	6 fl. oz.	188	27.6
*With whole milk	6 fl. oz.	207	27.4
Hot (USDA)	1 cup (4.9 oz.)	545	102.7
Hot (USDA)	1 oz.	111	21.0
Hot (Hershey's)	1 oz.	116	20.9
Quik (Nestlé's) regular or fudge	2 heaping tsp.	56	14.4
CHOCOLATE, GROUND (Ghirardelli)	¼ cup (1.3 oz.)	163	30.4
CHOCOLATE, HOT, home recipe (USDA)	1 cup (8.8 oz.)	238	26.0
CHOCOLATE ICE CREAM (See also individual brands):			
(Sealtest)	¼ pt. (2.3 oz.)	136	17.3
French (Prestige)	¼ pt. (2.6 oz.)	182	18.0
CHOCOLATE ICE CREAM MIX (Junket)	6 serving pkg. (4 oz.)	380	94.4
CHOCOLATE PIE: Chiffon, home recipe (USDA)	1/6 of 9″ pie (4.9 oz.)	459	61.2

(USDA): United States Department of Agriculture
DNA: Data Not Available
* Prepared as Package Directs

Food and Description	Measure or Quantity	Calories	Carbo- hydrates (grams)
Meringue, home recipe (USDA)	⅛ of 9" pie (4.9 oz.)	353	46.9
Nut (Tastykake)	4½-oz. pie	451	64.3
Frozen, cream:			
(Banquet)	2½-oz. serving	202	28.5
(Morton)	¼ of 14.5-oz. pie	290	40.6
(Mrs. Smith's)	⅛ of 8" pie	214	25.5
CHOCOLATE PIE FILLING:			
*Regular, fudge (Jell-O)	½ cup (5.2 oz.)	175	28.1
*Cream (Jell-O)	⅛ of 8" pie (including crust)	336	42.4
(My-T-Fine)	1 oz.	122	25.5
Almond (My-T-Fine)	1 oz.	123	25.6
Fudge (My-T-Fine)	1 oz.	124	25.5
CHOCOLATE PUDDING,			
Sweetened:			
Home recipe with starch base (USDA)	½ cup (4.6 oz.)	192	33.4
Canned:			
(Betty Crocker)	½ cup	175	29.8
(Hunt's)	5-oz. can	239	30.5
*(Thank You)	½ cup	175	29.2
Dutch (Bounty)	4 oz.	173	31.8
Fudge (Betty Crocker)	½ cup	175	30.0
Fudge (Del Monte)	5-oz. can	199	32.5
Fudge (Hunt's)	5-oz. can	229	28.9
Milk chocolate (Del Monte)	5-oz. can	200	33.1
Chilled (Sealtest)	4 oz.	136	22.8
CHOCOLATE PUDDING or PIE FILLING MIX:			
Sweetened:			
Regular:			
Dry (USDA)	1 oz.	102	26.0
*Prepared with milk (USDA)	½ cup (4.6 oz.)	161	29.6
*(Jell-O)	½ cup (5.2 oz.)	174	29.5
*(My-T-Fine)	½ cup	187	31.3
*(Royal)	½ cup (5.1 oz.)	190	30.7
*(Royal) *Dark 'N' Sweet*	½ cup (5.1 oz.)	194	30.5

Food and Description	Measure or Quantity	Calories	Carbo-hydrates (grams)
*Almond (My-T-Fine)	½ cup	196	31.2
*Fudge (Jell-O)	½ cup (5.2 oz.)	174	29.5
*Fudge (My-T-Fine)	½ cup (5 oz.)	190	31.2
*Tapioca (Royal)	½ cup (5.1 oz.)	185	29.2
Instant:			
Dry (USDA)	1 oz.	101	25.7
*Prepared with milk, without cooking (USDA)	4 oz.	142	27.7
*(Jell-O)	½ cup (5.4 oz.)	190	33.4
*(Royal)	½ cup (5.1 oz.)	195	31.9
*(Royal) *Dark 'N' Sweet*	½ cup (5.1 oz.)	195	31.9
*Fudge (Jell-O)	½ cup (5.4 oz.)	190	33.4
Low calorie or dietetic:			
*With nonfat milk (Dia-Mel)	4 oz.	53	8.2
*With whole milk (Dia-Mel)	4 oz.	90	8.1
*With nonfat milk (D-Zerta)	½ cup (4.5 oz.)	67	11.6
*With whole milk (D-Zerta)	½ cup (4.6 oz.)	102	11.0

CHOCOLATE RENNET CUSTARD MIX (Junket):

Powder:			
Dry	1 oz.	116	25.2
*With sugar	4 oz.	113	14.9
Tablet:			
Dry	1 tablet	1	.2
*With sugar	4 oz.	101	13.4

CHOCOLATE SOFT DRINK:

Cocoa Cooler (Hoffman)	6 fl. oz.	89	22.3
Cream (Mission)	6 fl. oz.	92	22.0
(Yoo-Hoo)	6 fl. oz.	90	18.0
High protein (Yoo-Hoo)	6 fl. oz.	114	24.6

(USDA): United States Department of Agriculture
DNA: Data Not Available
* Prepared as Package Directs

Food and Description	Measure or Quantity	Calories	Carbo-hydrates (grams)
CHOCOLATE SYRUP:			
Sweetened:			
Fudge (USDA)	1 T. (.7 oz.)	63	10.3
Thin type (USDA)	1 T. (.7 oz.)	47	11.9
(Cocoa Marsh)	1 T.	50	D.N.A.
(Hershey's)	1 T. (1 oz.)	69	16.7
Low calorie, *Choco Sip*			
(Dia-Mel)	1 T.	14	3.5
CHOP SUEY:			
Home recipe, with meat			
(USDA)	1 cup (8.8 oz.)	300	12.8
Canned:			
With meat (USDA)	1 cup (8.8 oz.)	155	10.5
Beef (Chun King)	4 oz.	61	D.N.A.
Chicken (Hung's)	4 oz.	60	6.2
Meatless (Hung's)	4 oz.	56	5.6
Vegetable (Hung's)	¾ cup	30	4.6
Frozen, beef (Banquet)	7-oz. bag	121	9.5
CHOP SUEY VEGETABLES,			
canned, drained (Hung's)	4 oz.	20	3.0
CHOW CHOW:			
Sour (USDA)	1 oz.	8	1.2
Sweet (USDA)	1 oz.	33	7.7
(Crosse & Blackwell)	1 T. (.6 oz.)	6	1.0
CHOW MEIN:			
Home recipe, chicken, with-out noodles (USDA)	4 oz.	116	4.5
Canned:			
Without noodles (USDA)	4 oz.	43	8.1
Chicken:			
(Chun King)	1 cup	100	11.2
(Hung's)	8 oz.	104	10.4
& noodles (Chun King)	8 oz.	111	D.N.A.
Subgum (Chun King)	8 oz.	78	D.N.A.
Meatless:			
(Chun King)	1 cup	83	9.4
(Hung's)	8 oz.	96	8.8
& noodles (Chun King)	8 oz.	74	D.N.A.
Frozen:			
Chicken (Chun King)	½ of 15-oz. pkg.	163	11.0

Food and Description	Measure or Quantity	Calories	Carbo-hydrates (grams)
Chicken (Temple)	11-oz. pkg.	178	D.N.A.
Meatless (Chun King)	8 oz.	94	15.4
Shrimp (Chun King)	½ of 15-oz. pkg.	95	13.5
Shrimp (Temple)	1 cup	132	15.0
Vegetable (Temple)	1 cup	68	12.0

CHOW MEIN NOODLES
(See **NOODLES, CHOW MEIN**)

CHUB, raw (USDA):
Whole	1 lb. (weighed whole)	217	0.
Meat only	4 oz.	164	0.

CHUTNEY, *Major Grey's*
(Crosse & Blackwell) | 1 T. (.8 oz.) | 53 | 13.1 |

CIDER (See **APPLE CIDER**)

CINNAMON, GROUND
(Information supplied by
General Mills Laboratory) | 1 oz. | 114 | 25.1 |

CINNAMON STICKS, frozen
(Aunt Jemima) | 3 pieces (1¾ oz.) | 145 | 21.9 |

CITRON, CANDIED:
(USDA)	1 oz.	89	22.7
(Liberty)	1 oz.	93	22.6

CITRUS COOLER (Hi-C) | 6 fl. oz. | 92 | 22.7 |

CITRUS SALAD, canned (See
**GRAPEFRUIT & ORANGE
SECTIONS**)

CITRUS SOFT DRINK,
low calorie (No-Cal) | 6 fl. oz.* | 2 | 0. |

(USDA): United States Department of Agriculture
DNA: Data Not Available
* Prepared as Package Directs

Food and Description	Measure or Quantity	Calories	Carbo-hydrates (grams)
CLACKERS, cereal (General Mills)	1 cup (1 oz.)	111	22.1
CLAM:			
Raw, meat only (USDA)	4 med. clams	65	1.7
Raw, hard or round, meat & liq. (USDA)	1 lb (weighed in shell)	71	6.1
Raw, soft, meat & liq. (USDA)	1 lb. (weighed in shell)	142	5.3
Raw, soft, meat only (USDA)	4 oz.	93	1.5
Canned, all kinds:			
Solids & liq. (USDA)	4 oz.	59	3.2
Meat only (USDA)	½ cup (2.8 oz.)	78	1.5
Chopped & minced, solids & liq. (Doxsee)	4 oz.	59	3.2
Chopped & liq. (Doxsee)	4 oz.	66	D.N.A.
Chopped, meat only (Doxsee)	4 oz.	111	2.1
Steamed, meat & broth (Doxsee)	1 pt. 8 fl. oz.	152	D.N.A.
Steamed, meat only (Doxsee)	1 pt. 8 fl. oz.	66	D.N.A.
Whole (Doxsee)	4 oz.	62	D.N.A.
CLAM CHOWDER:			
Manhattan, canned:			
Condensed (USDA)	8 oz. (by wt.)	150	22.7
*Prepared with equal volume water (USDA)	1 cup (8.6 oz.)	81	12.2
*(Campbell)	1 cup	72	10.5
(Crosse & Blackwell)	6½ oz. (½ can)	61	12.9
*(Doxsee)	1 cup (8.6 oz.)	112	17.7
(Heinz) *Great American*	1 cup (8½ oz.)	111	14.2
New England:			
Canned:			
*(Campbell)	1 cup	157	16.4
(Crosse & Blackwell)	6½ oz. (½ can)	101	10.3
*(Doxsee)	1 cup (8.6 oz.)	214	27.0
(Snow)	1 cup	148	16.9
Frozen:			
Condensed (USDA)	8 oz. (by wt.)	243	19.5

Food and Description	Measure or Quantity	Calories	Carbo-hydrates (grams)
*Prepared with equal volume water (USDA)	1 cup (8.5 oz.)	130	10.6
*Prepared with equal volume milk (USDA)	1 cup (8.6 oz.)	211	16.4
CLAM COCKTAIL (Sau-Sea)	4 oz.	80	19.1
CLAM FRITTERS, home recipe (USDA)	1.4-oz. fritter (2" x 1¾")	124	12.4
CLAM JUICE/LIQUOR, canned:			
(USDA) (Doxsee)	1 cup (8.3 oz.)	45	5.0
	8 oz.	43	D.N.A.
CLAM STEW, frozen (Mrs. Paul's)	8 oz.	244	20.0
CLAM STICKS, frozen (Mrs. Paul's)	4 oz.	229	D.N.A.
CLARET WINE:			
(Gold Seal) 12% alcohol	3 fl. oz.	82	.4
(Italian Swiss Colony-Gold Medal) 12.3% alcohol	3 fl oz.	63	.7
(Louis M. Martini) 12.5% alcohol	3 fl. oz.	90	.2
(Taylor) 12.5% alcohol	3 fl. oz.	72	D.N.A.
CLARISTINE LIQUEUR (Leroux) 86 proof	1 fl. oz.	114	10.8
CLORETS:			
Chewing gum	1 piece	6	1.3
Mint	1 piece	6	1.6
CLUB SODA SOFT DRINK, any brand:			
Regular	6 fl. oz.	0	0.
Dietetic	6 fl. oz.	0	0.

(USDA): United States Department of Agriculture
DNA: Data Not Available
* Prepared as Package Directs

Food and Description	Measure or Quantity	Calories	Carbohydrates (grams)
COCOA, dry:			
Low fat (USDA)	1 T. (5 grams)	10	3.1
Medium low fat (USDA)	1 T. (5 grams)	12	2.9
Medium high fat (USDA)	1 T. (5 grams)	14	2.8
High fat (USDA)	1 T.	16	2.6
Unsweetened (Droste)	1 T. (7 grams)	21	2.9
(Hershey's)	1 cup (3 oz.)	337	40.1
(Hershey's)	1 T. (5 grams)	20	2.4
COCOA, HOME RECIPE			
(USDA)	1 cup (8.8 oz.)	242	27.2
COCOA KRISPIES, cereal			
(Kellogg's)	1 cup (1 oz.)	111	25.2
COCOA MIX:			
With nonfat dry milk (USDA)	1 oz.	102	20.1
Without nonfat dry milk (USDA)	1 oz.	98	25.3
(Nestlé's) *EverReady*	3 heaping tsp. (.8 oz.)	105	19.6
Instant (Hershey's)	1 oz.	105	25.3
Instant, milk chocolate (Carnation)	1-oz. pkg.	120	20.5
Instant (Swiss Miss)	1 oz.	106	20.4
COCOA PEBBLES, cereal			
(Post)	⅞ cup (1 oz.)	111	25.0
COCOA PUFFS, cereal			
(General Mills)	1 cup (1 oz.)	109	25.2
COCONUT:			
Fresh (USDA):			
Whole	1 lb. (weighed in shell)	816	22.2
Meat only	4 oz.	392	10.7
Meat only	2″ x 2″ x ½″ piece (1.6 oz.)	156	4.2
Grated or shredded, loosely packed	½ cup (1.4 oz.)	225	6.1
Dried, canned or packaged:			
Unsweetened, shredded (USDA)	½ cup (1.6 oz.)	305	10.6

Food and Description	*Measure or Quantity*	*Calories*	*Carbo-hydrates (grams)*
Sweetened, shredded (USDA)	½ cup (1.6 oz.)	252	24.5
Angel Flake (Baker's)	¼ cup (.7 oz.)	89	7.4
Cookie (Baker's)	¼ cup (1 oz.)	140	11.6
COCONUT CAKE, frozen (Pepperidge Farm)	⅙ of cake (3 oz.)	323	46.0
COCONUT CAKE MIX:			
Toasted (Betty Crocker)	1-lb. 3.5-oz. pkg.	2360	436.8
*(Duncan Hines)	1/12 of cake (2.7 oz.)	200	35.0
COCONUT PIE:			
Cream:			
(Tastykake)	4-oz. pie	467	48.4
Frozen:			
(Banquet)	2½ oz.	209	24.2
(Morton)	¼ of 14.4-oz. pie	278	37.1
(Mrs. Smith's)	⅙ of 8″ pie (2.3 oz.)	212	24.5
Custard:			
Home recipe (USDA)	⅙ of 9″ pie (5.4 oz.)	357	37.8
Frozen:			
Baked (USDA)	5 oz.	354	41.9
Unbaked (USDA)	5 oz.	291	38.5
(Banquet)	5 oz.	294	39.8
(Morton)	⅙ of 20-oz. pie	203	27.7
(Mrs. Smith's)	⅙ of 8″ pie (4 oz.)	272	31.7
COCONUT PIE FILLING MIX (Also see **COCONUT PUDDING MIX**):			
Custard & pie, dry (USDA)	1 oz.	133	20.0
*Custard, prepared with egg yolk & milk (USDA)	5 oz. (including crust)	288	41.3

(USDA): United States Department of Agriculture
DNA: Data Not Available
* Prepared as Package Directs

Food and Description	Measure or Quantity	Calories	Carbo-hydrates (grams)
COCONUT PUDDING MIX:			
*Cream, regular (Jell-O)	½ cup (5.2 oz.)	175	25.8
*Cream, instant (Jell-O)	½ cup (5.3 oz.)	188	29.0
*Toasted, instant (Royal)	½ cup (5.1 oz.)	186	28.4
COCONUT SOFT DRINK (Yoo-Hoo):			
Regular	6 fl. oz.	90	18.0
High protein	6 fl. oz.	114	24.6
COCO WHEATS, cereal	2 T. (.6 oz.)	82	16.8
COD:			
Raw, whole (USDA)	1 lb. (weighed whole)	110	0.
Raw, meat only (USDA)	4 oz.	88	0.
Broiled (USDA)	4 oz.	193	0.
Canned (USDA)	4 oz.	96	0.
Dehydrated, lightly salted (USDA)	4 oz.	425	0.
Dried, salted (USDA)	5½" x 1½" x ½" (2.8 oz.)	104	0.
Frozen, fillets (Taste O'Sea)	4 oz.	80	0.
Frozen, Alaska (Van de Kamp's)	1 pkg.	473	0.
COFFEE:			
Max Pax	¾ cup	2	.5
*Regular (Maxwell House)	¾ cup	2	.4
*Regular (Yuban)	¾ cup	2	.4
Instant:			
Dry (USDA)	1 rounded tsp. (2 grams)	3	.9
*(USDA)	1 cup (8.4 oz.)	3	.9
*(Chase & Sanborn)	5 fl. oz.	1	Tr.
Kava (Borden)	1 tsp. (1 gram)	3	.5
*(Maxwell House)	¾ cup	4	.9
Nescafé	1 slightly rounded tsp. (2 grams)	4	.7
*(Yuban)	¾ cup	4	.9
Decaffeinated:			
Decaf	1 tsp. (2 grams)	4	.6
Sanka, regular	¾ cup	2	.4
Siesta	5 fl. oz.	1	Tr.

Food and Description	Measure or Quantity	Calories	Carbo-hydrates (grams)
Freeze-dried:			
*Maxim	¾ cup	4	.9
Taster's Choice	1 slightly rounded tsp. (2 grams)	4	.7
COFFEE CAKE:			
(Drake's) junior	1 pkg. (1.1 oz.)	149	22.0
(Drake's) large	11-oz. cake	1426	211.6
(Drake's) small	2¼-oz. cake	290	43.1
Almond brittle (Van de Kamp's)	9½-oz. cake	1449	D.N.A.
Almond crispy (Van de Kamp's)	1 piece (3 oz.)	449	D.N.A.
Apple (Van de Kamp's)	9-oz. cake	977	D.N.A.
Bear claw (Van de Kamp's)	1 piece (2.2 oz.)	127	D.N.A.
Butterfly (Mrs. Smith's)	1 piece (2¾ oz.)	250	28.4
Butter horn (Van de Kamp's)	1 piece (2.2 oz.)	287	D.N.A.
Cinnamon, 1-lb. loaf (Van de Kamp's)	1 slice (.8 oz.)	85	D.N.A.
Danish cluster (Van de Kamp's)	1 piece (1 oz.)	150	D.N.A.
Danish pastry (USDA)	1″ x 4¼″ dia. (2.3 oz.)	274	29.6
Dutch ring (Van de Kamp's)	10-oz. cake	1107	D.N.A.
French pecan (Van de Kamp's)	12-oz. cake	1458	D.N.A.
Rosette (Van de Kamp's)	1 piece (2.5 oz.)	349	D.N.A.
Swedish twist (Van de Kamp's)	12-oz. cake	1356	D.N.A.
Walnut swirl (Van de Kamp's)	1 piece (1.5 oz.)	266	D.N.A.
COFFEE CAKE MIX:			
Dry (USDA)	1 oz.	122	21.9
*Prepared with egg & milk (USDA)	2 oz.	183	29.7
*(Aunt Jemima)	⅛ of cake (1.8 oz.)	182	29.5
COFFEE FLAVORING, low calorie (Coffee Time)	1 fl. oz.	<1	.1

(USDA): United States Department of Agriculture
DNA: Data Not Available
* Prepared as Package Directs

Food and Description	Measure or Quantity	Calories	Carbo-hydrates (grams)
COFFEE-MATE, cream substitute	1 tsp.	11	1.0
COFFEE-RICH, cream substitute	1 tsp.	8	.7
COFFEE SOFT DRINK, low calorie (No-Cal)	6 fl. oz.	3	<.1
COFFEE SOUTHERN, liqueur	1 fl. oz.	85	7.0
COGNAC (See **DISTILLED LIQUOR**)			
COLA SOFT DRINK:			
Sweetened:			
(Canada Dry) Jamaica	6 fl. oz.	75	19.2
(Clicquot Club)	6 fl. oz.	83	20.0
Coca-Cola	6 fl. oz.	73	18.5
(Cott)	6 fl. oz.	83	20.0
(Dr. Brown's)	6 fl. oz.	81	20.1
(Hoffman)	6 fl. oz.	81	20.1
(Key Food)	6 fl. oz.	77	19.4
(Kirsch)	6 fl. oz.	80	20.1
(Mission)	6 fl. oz.	83	20.0
Mr. Cola	6 fl. oz.	79	20.3
Pepsi-Cola	6 fl. oz.	78	19.7
(Royal Crown)	6 fl. oz.	81	20.4
(Shasta)	6 fl. oz.	76	19.4
(Waldbaum)	6 fl. oz.	81	20.1
(White Rock)	6 fl. oz.	80	D.N.A.
Cherry (Shasta)	6 fl. oz.	76	19.4
Low calorie:			
(Canada Dry)	6 fl. oz.	<1	<.1
Diet Pepsi-Cola	6 fl. oz.	35	8.8
Diet-Rite	6 fl. oz.	36	9.0
(Dr. Brown's)	6 fl. oz.	1	.2
(Hoffman)	6 fl. oz.	1	.2
(No-Cal)	6 fl. oz.	<1	<.1
(Shasta)	6 fl. oz.	<1	<.1
Cherry (Shasta)	6 fl. oz.	<1	<.1
Tab	6 fl. oz.	<1	<.1

Food and Description	Measure or Quantity	Calories	Carbo-hydrates (grams)
COLA SYRUP, dietetic (No-Cal)	1 tsp. (5 grams)	<1	Tr.
COLD DUCK WINE, (Italian Swiss Colony—Private Stock) 12% alcohol	3 fl. oz.	75	4.3
COLESLAW, not drained (USDA):			
Prepared, with commercial French dressing	4 oz.	108	8.6
Prepared with homemade French dressing	4 oz.	146	5.8
Prepared with mayonnaise	4 oz.	163	5.4
Prepared with mayonnaise-type salad dressing	4 oz.	112	8.1
Prepared with mayonnaise-type salad dressing	1 cup (4.2 oz.)	118	8.5
COLLARDS:			
Raw (USDA):			
Leaves including stems	1 lb.	181	32.7
Leaves only	½ lb.	70	11.6
Boiled, drained (USDA):			
Leaves, cooked in large amount water	½ cup (3.4 oz.)	29	4.6
Leaves & stems, cooked in small amount water	4 oz.	33	5.6
Leaves & stems, cooked in small amount water	½ cup (3.4 oz.)	31	4.8
Frozen:			
Not thawed (USDA)	10-oz. pkg.	91	16.4
Boiled, chopped, drained (USDA)	½ cup (3 oz.)	26	4.8
Chopped (Birds Eye)	⅓ pkg. (3.3 oz.)	29	4.5
COLLINS MIX (Bar-Tender's)	1 serving (⅝ oz.)	70	17.4
COLLINS MIXER, SOFT DRINK (See **TOM COLLINS SOFT DRINK**)			

(USDA): United States Department of Agriculture
DNA: Data Not Available
* Prepared as Package Directs

Food and Description	Measure or Quantity	Calories	Carbohydrates (grams)
CONCENTRATE, cereal			
(Kellogg's)	⅓ cup (1 oz.)	108	15.3
CONCORD WINE:			
(Gold Seal) 13–14% alcohol	3 fl. oz.	125	9.8
(Mogen David) 12% alcohol	3 fl. oz.	120	16.0
(Mogen David) dry, 12% alcohol	3 fl. oz.	24	1.8
CONSOMME MADRILENE, canned, clear or red			
(Crosse & Blackwell)	6½ oz. (½ can)	33	2.4
COOK-IN-A-BOWL, cereal (Ralston Purina):			
Apple-cinnamon	1 packet (1.1 oz.)	125	D.N.A.
Whole wheat	1 packet (1 oz.)	112	D.N.A.
COOKIE. The following are listed by type or brand name:			
Almond toast, Mandel (Stella D'oro)	1 piece (.5 oz.)	49	9.6
Angelica Goodies (Stella D'oro)	1 piece (.8 oz.)	100	14.6
Angel puffs, dietetic (Stella D'oro)	1 piece	17	1.4
Anginetti (Stella D'oro)	1 piece (5 grams)	28	2.4
Animal cracker:			
(USDA)	1 oz.	122	22.7
(Nabisco) *Barnum's*	1 piece (3 grams)	12	2.0
(Sunshine) regular	1 piece (2 grams)	10	1.7
(Sunshine) iced	1 piece (5 grams)	26	3.7
Anisette sponge (Stella D'oro)	1 piece (.5 oz.)	39	10.0
Anisette toast (Stella D'oro)	1 piece (.4 oz.)	39	7.8
Applesauce (Sunshine)	1 piece (.6 oz.)	86	11.9
Apple strudel (Nabisco)	1 piece (.4 oz.)	48	6.8
Assortments:			
(USDA)	1 oz.	136	20.1
(Nabisco) *Famous*	1 piece (.5 oz.)	71	9.1
(Nabisco), *Pride* sandwich	1 piece (.4 oz.)	54	7.3
(Stella D'oro) *Lady Stella Assortment*	1 piece (8 grams)	37	5.0

Food and Description	Measure or Quantity	Calories	Carbohydrates (grams)
(Sunshine) *Lady Joan Party Assortment*	1 piece (9 grams)	42	5.8
Bordeaux (Pepperidge Farm)	1 piece (8 grams)	36	5.1
Breakfast Treats (Stella D'oro)	1 piece (.8 oz.)	99	15.0
Brown edge wafers (Nabisco)	1 piece (6 grams)	28	4.1
Brownie:			
(Tastykake)	1 pkg. (2¼ oz.)	242	34.0
Chocolate nut (Pepperidge Farm)	1 piece (.4 oz.)	54	6.3
Nut fudge (Nab) *Bake Shop*	1 pkg. (2 oz.)	265	33.6
Peanut butter (Tastykake)	1 pkg. (1¾ oz.)	239	32.0
Pecan fudge (Keebler)	1 pkg. (1.8 oz.)	230	27.9
Pecan fudge, bulk (Keebler)	.9-oz. square	115	13.9
Frozen, with nuts & chocolate icing (USDA)	1 oz.	119	17.2
Brown sugar (Nabisco) *Family Favorites*	1 piece (5 grams)	25	3.0
Brussels (Pepperidge Farm)	1 piece (8 grams)	42	4.6
Butter:			
Thin, rich (USDA)	1 oz.	130	20.1
(Burry's)	1 piece	23	D.N.A.
(Nabisco)	1 piece (5 grams)	23	3.6
(Sunshine)	1 piece (5 grams)	23	3.5
Buttercup (Keebler)	1 piece (5 grams)	24	3.6
Butterscotch Fudgies (Tastykake)	1 pkg. (1¾ oz.)	251	35.0
Capri (Pepperidge Farm)	1 piece (.6 oz.)	82	9.7
Caramel peanut logs (Nabisco) *Hey Days*	1 piece (.8 oz.)	122	13.4
Chocolate & chocolate-covered:			
(USDA)	1 oz.	126	20.3
(Van de Kamp's)	1 piece (.7 oz.)	79	D.N.A.
Kings (Sunshine)	1 piece (1.1 oz.)	135	19.6
Melody (Nabisco)	1 piece (7 grams)	31	5.1
Nuggets (Sunshine)	1 piece (4 grams)	23	3.3

(USDA): United States Department of Agriculture
DNA: Data Not Available
* Prepared as Package Directs

Food and Description	Measure or Quantity	Calories	Carbohydrates (grams)
Peanut bars (Nabisco)			
Ideal	1 piece (.6 oz.)	94	10.3
Pinwheel cakes (Nabisco)	1 piece (1.1 oz.)	139	20.9
Puffs (Sunshine)	1 piece (.5 oz.)	63	10.6
Snaps (Nabisco)	1 piece (4 grams)	18	2.7
Wafers (Nabisco) *Famous*	1 piece (6 grams)	28	4.7
Wafers (Sunshine)	1 piece (3 grams)	13	2.6
Wafers (Sunshine) Ice Box	1 piece (7 grams)	30	4.8
Chocolate chip:			
(USDA)	1 oz.	134	19.8
(Keebler)	1 piece (.6 oz.)	80	11.0
(Nab)	1.2-oz. pkg. (6 pieces)	176	23.6
(Nabisco)	1 piece (7 grams)	33	4.5
(Nabisco) *Chips Ahoy*	1 piece (.4 oz.)	51	7.5
(Nabisco) *Family Favorites*	1 piece (7 grams)	33	4.5
Snaps (Nabisco)	1 piece (4 grams)	21	3.4
(Pepperidge Farm)	1 piece (.4 oz.)	52	6.2
(Sunshine) *Chip-A-Roos*	1 piece (.4 oz.)	63	7.7
Coconut (Sunshine)	1 piece (.5 oz.)	76	9.9
(Tastykake) *Choc-O-Chip*	1¾-oz. pkg. (4 pieces)	283	34.8
(Van de Kamp's)	1 piece (.5 oz.)	66	D.N.A.
Cinnamon sugar (Pepperidge Farm)	1 piece (.4 oz.)	52	7.0
Cinnamon toast (Sunshine)	1 piece (3 grams)	13	2.3
Clover Leaves (Sunshine)	1 piece (5 grams)	25	3.7
Coco Creme (Wise)	1 piece (9 grams)	39	6.5
Coconut:			
Bars (USDA)	1 oz.	140	18.1
Bars (Nabisco)	1 piece (9 grams)	45	6.3
Bars (Sunshine)	1 piece (.4 oz.)	47	6.2
Chocolate chip (Nabisco)	1 piece (.5 oz.)	77	9.0
Chocolate drop (Keebler)	1 piece (.5 oz.)	75	8.5
Coconut Kiss (Tastykake)	1¾-oz. pkg. (4 pieces)	318	33.2
Family Favorites (Nabisco)	1 piece (3 grams)	16	2.2
Como Delight (Stella D'oro)	1 piece (1.1 oz.)	153	18.3
Cowboys and Indians (Nabisco)	1 piece (2 grams)	10	1.8
Creme Wafer Stick (Dutch Twin)	1 piece (7 grams)	36	5.9

Food and Description	Measure or Quantity	Calories	Carbohydrates (grams)
Creme Wafer Stick (Nabisco)	1 piece (9 grams)	50	5.9
Crests Cakes (Nabisco)	1 piece (.5 oz.)	54	10.4
Cup Custard, vanilla (Sunshine)	1 piece (.5 oz.)	71	9.3
Danish Swirls (Nabisco)	1 piece (.4 oz.)	49	7.0
Danish Wedding (Keebler)	1 piece (6 grams)	33	5.0
Date and nut (Sunshine)	1 piece (¾ oz.)	82	14.7
Devil's food cake:			
(Nab)	1¼-oz. pkg. (2 pieces)	135	26.8
(Nabisco)	1 piece (.5 oz.)	49	9.8
(Sunshine)	1 piece (.5 oz.)	55	10.9
Dresden (Pepperidge Farm)	1 piece (.6 oz.)	83	10.0
Dutch Apple (Keebler)	1 piece (6 grams)	34	4.7
Dutch Crunch (Keebler)	1 piece (10 grams)	44	6.7
Dutch Girl (Van de Kamp's)	1 piece (.3 oz.)	53	D.N.A.
Egg Jumbo (Stella D'oro)	1 piece (.4 oz.)	40	7.6
Fig bar:			
(USDA)	1 oz.	101	21.4
(Keebler)	1 piece (.7 oz.)	71	14.4
(Nab) *Fig Newton*	2-oz. pkg. (2 pieces)	208	40.4
Nabisco) *Fig Newton*	1 piece (.6 oz.)	57	11.2
(Sunshine)	1 piece (.4 oz.)	45	9.2
Fortune (Chun King)	1 piece	31	4.6
Frosted cake (Sunshine)	1 piece (.6 oz.)	68	14.8
Fruit:			
California fruit bar (Stella D'oro)	1 piece	72	11.6
Golden fruit (Sunshine)	1 piece (⅔ oz.)	73	16.2
Iced fruit (Nabisco)	1 piece (.6 oz.)	71	13.5
Fudge:			
Chip (Pepperidge Farm)	1 piece (.4 oz.)	51	6.7
Eton Fudge Stick (Keebler)	1 piece (.4 oz.)	55	6.3
Fudge Stripes (Keebler)	1 piece (.4 oz.)	57	7.5
Fudgetown, chocolate or vanilla base (Burry's)	1 piece	67	D.N.A.
Penguin Fudge (Keebler)	1 piece (.8 oz.)	111	14.0
Gaucho (Burry's)	1 piece	72	D.N.A.

(USDA): United States Department of Agriculture
DNA: Data Not Available
* Prepared as Package Directs

Food and Description	Measure or Quantity	Calories	Carbo-hydrates (grams)
Gingersnap:			
(USDA)	1 oz.	119	22.6
Crumbs (USDA)	1 cup (4.1 oz.)	483	91.8
(Sunshine)	1 piece (6 grams)	24	4.4
Old fashioned (Nabisco)	1 piece (7 grams)	29	5.4
Zu Zu (Nabisco)	1 piece (4 grams)	16	3.1
Golden bars (Stella D'oro)	1 piece (1 oz.)	123	16.0
Golden fruit (Sunshine)	1 piece (.7 oz.)	61	14.4
Graham Cracker (See **CRACKER,** Graham)			
Hermit bar, frosted (Tastykake)	1 pkg. (2 oz.)	321	60.8
Hydrox (Sunshine)	1 piece (.4 oz.)	48	7.1
Jumble (Drake's)	1 piece	78	11.8
Kreemlined wafers (Sunshine)	1 piece (8 grams)	45	6.2
Ladyfingers (USDA)	1 oz.	102	18.3
Lemon:			
Creme sandwich (Keebler)	1 piece	85	12.0
Jumble rings (Nabisco)	1 piece (.5 oz.)	68	11.0
Nut crunch (Pepperidge Farm)	1 piece (.4 oz.)	57	6.4
Punch (Burry's)	1 piece	62	D.N.A.
Snaps (Nabisco)	1 piece (4 grams)	17	3.1
Lickety Splits, chocolate or vanilla base (Burry's)	1 piece	57	D.N.A.
Lido (Pepperidge Farm)	1 piece (.6 oz.)	91	10.0
Lisbon (Pepperidge Farm)	1 piece (5 grams)	28	3.3
Macaroon:			
(USDA)	1 oz.	135	18.7
(Sunshine)	1 piece (.6 oz.)	85	12.1
Almond (Tastykake)	2-oz. pkg. (2 pieces)	336	35.1
Butter-flavored (Sunshine)	1 piece (8 grams)	39	4.9
Coconut (Nabisco) Bake Shop	1 piece (.7 oz.)	87	12.1
Coconut (Sunshine)	1 piece (.7 oz.)	81	12.8
Coconut (Van de Kamp's)	1 piece (.7 oz.)	89	D.N.A.
Sandwich (Nabisco)	1 piece (.5 oz.)	71	9.5
Marble sponge (Stella D'oro)	1 piece	50	D.N.A.
Margherite, chocolate (Stella D'oro)	1 piece (.6 oz.)	73	10.6
Margherite, vanilla (Stella D'oro)	1 piece (.6 oz.)	73	10.5

Food and Description	Measure or Quantity	Calories	Carbo-hydrates (grams)
Marquisette (Pepperidge Farm)	1 piece (8 grams)	45	5.0
Marshmallow:			
(USDA)	1 oz.	116	20.5
Mallomar (Nabisco)	1 piece (.5 oz.)	60	8.7
Mallo Puff (Sunshine)	1 piece (.6 oz.)	63	12.2
Puffs (Nabisco)	1 piece (.7 oz.)	94	12.8
Sandwich (Nabisco)	1 piece (8 grams)	32	5.7
Twirls (Nabisco)	1 piece (1.1 oz.)	133	21.9
Milano (Pepperidge Farm)	1 piece (.4 oz.)	62	7.2
Milano, mint (Pepperidge Farm)	1 piece (.5 oz.)	76	8.4
Milco, dandies (Sunshine)	1 piece (.6 oz.)	91	12.3
Milco, sugar wafers (Sunshine)	1 piece (.5 oz.)	80	10.1
Minarets (Nabisco)	1 piece (10 grams)	46	5.6
Minarets cakes (Nab)	1-oz. pkg. (3 pieces)	144	17.9
Mint sandwich (Nabisco) *Mystic*	1 piece (.6 oz.)	88	10.6
Molasses (USDA)	1 oz.	120	21.5
Mr. Chips (Burry's), coconut, mint, oatmeal or regular	1 piece	42	D.N.A.
Naples (Pepperidge Farm)	1 piece (6 grams)	33	3.7
Nassau (Pepperidge Farm)	1 piece (.6 oz.)	83	9.2
Nut Sundae (Sunshine)	1 piece (.6 oz.)	74	12.0
Oatmeal:			
(Drake's)	1 piece	83	12.5
(Nabisco)	1 piece (.6 oz.)	82	12.3
(Nabisco) *Family Favorites*	1 piece (5 grams)	24	3.8
(Sunshine)	1 piece (.4 oz.)	58	8.9
(Van de Kamp's)	1 piece (.6 oz.)	59	D.N.A.
Iced (Sunshine)	1 piece (.5 oz.)	69	11.6
Irish (Pepperidge Farm)	1 piece (.4 oz.)	50	7.1
Old fashioned (Keebler)	1 piece (.6 oz.)	79	11.7
Peanut butter (Sunshine)	1 piece (.6 oz.)	79	10.5
Raisin (USDA)	1 oz.	128	20.8
Raisin (Nabisco) *Bake Shop*	1 piece (.6 oz.)	77	11.5

(USDA): United States Department of Agriculture
DNA: Data Not Available
* Prepared as Package Directs

Food and Description	Measure or Quantity	Calories	Carbo-hydrates (grams)
Raisin bar (Tastykake)	1 pkg. (2¼ oz.)	298	47.6
Raisin, iced (Nabisco)	1 piece (.4 oz.)	57	8.2
Raisin, old fashioned (Pepperidge Farm)	1 piece (.4 oz.)	55	7.5
Old Country Treats (Stella D'oro)	1 piece (.5 oz.)	64	7.1
Orleans (Pepperidge Farm)	1 piece (6 grams)	30	3.5
Peanut & peanut butter:			
(USDA)	1 oz.	134	19.0
(Sunshine)	1 piece (6 grams)	33	3.8
Bars, cocoa-covered (Nabisco) Crowns	1 piece (.6 oz.)	92	10.0
Crunch (Sunshine)	1 piece (.5 oz.)	68	8.1
Creme patties (Nab)	½-oz. pkg. (3 pieces)	74	8.4
Creme patties (Nabisco)	1 piece (7 grams)	34	3.9
Creme patties, cocoa-covered (Nabisco) Fancy	1 piece (.4 oz.)	60	6.4
Creme sticks, cocoa-covered (Nabisco)	1 piece (9 grams)	48	5.8
Patties (Sunshine)	1 piece (7 grams)	33	4.2
Pecan Krunch (Sunshine)	1 piece (.5 oz.)	78	8.4
Pecan Sandies (Keebler)	1 piece (.6 oz.)	85	9.2
Pfefferneuse (Stella D'oro)	1 piece	40	D.N.A.
Pirouettes (Pepperidge Farm):			
Chocolate	1 piece (7 grams)	38	4.5
Original or lemon	1 piece (7 grams)	38	4.6
Pitter Patter (Keebler)	1 piece (.6 oz.)	84	10.9
Pizzelle Carolines (Stella D'oro)	1 piece (.4 oz.)	49	6.7
Raisin:			
(USDA)	1 oz.	107	22.9
Bar, iced (Keebler)	1 piece (.6 oz.)	81	11.0
Fruit biscuit (Nabisco)	1 piece (.5 oz.)	58	12.3
Rich 'n' Chips (Keebler)	1 piece (.5 oz.)	73	8.9
Sandwich, creme:			
(USDA)	1 oz.	140	19.6
Cameo (Nabisco)	1 piece (.5 oz.)	68	10.5
Chocolate fudge:			
(Keebler)	1 piece (.7 oz.)	99	13.0
(Nabisco) Cookie Break	1 piece (.4 oz.)	52	7.0
(Sunshine)	1 piece (.5 oz.)	74	9.3
Empire (Keebler)	1 piece (.6 oz.)	80	11.3
Lemon (Keebler)	1 piece	85	12.0

Food and Description	Measure or Quantity	Calories	Carbohydrates (grams)
Orbit (Sunshine)	1 piece (.4 oz.)	51	7.0
Oreo (Nab)	1⅝-oz. pkg. (6 pieces)	228	32.7
Oreo (Nabisco)	1 piece (.4 oz.)	51	7.3
Oreo & Swiss (Nab)	1⅝-oz. pkg. (6 pieces)	230	31.4
Oreo & Swiss creme (Nabisco)	1 piece (.4 oz.)	51	7.0
Social Tea (Nabisco)	1 piece (.4 oz.)	51	7.2
Swiss (Nab)	1¾-oz. pkg. (6 pieces)	252	31.9
Vanilla (Nabisco)	1 piece (.4 oz.)	52	7.0
Vanilla, French (Keebler)	1 piece (.6 oz.)	82	11.1
Vienna Finger (Sunshine)	1 piece (.5 oz.)	71	10.5
Scooter Pies (Burry's) any flavor	1 piece	162	D.N.A.
Scooter Puffs (Burry's) any flavor	1 piece	62	D.N.A.
Sesame, Regina (Stella D'oro)	1 piece (.4 oz.)	51	6.9
Shortbread or shortcake:			
(USDA)	1¾″ sq. (8 grams)	40	5.2
(Nabisco) *Dandy*	1 piece (.4 oz.)	46	7.7
Cherry nut (Van de Kamp's)	1 piece (.4 oz.)	59	D.N.A.
Lorna Doone (Nab)	1½-oz. pkg. (6 pieces)	207	28.5
Lorna Doone (Nabisco)	1 piece (7 grams)	38	4.4
Pecan (Nabisco)	1 piece (.5 oz.)	80	9.0
Scotties (Sunshine)	1 piece (8 grams)	39	5.0
Striped (Nabisco)	1 piece (10 grams)	50	6.8
Vanilla (Tastykake)	2¼-oz. pkg. (6 pieces)	352	43.8
Sierra Eclairs (Burry's), any flavor	1 piece	62	D.N.A.
Smack Wafers (Sunshine)	1 piece (2 grams)	10	1.2
Social Tea Biscuit (Nabisco)	1 piece (5 grams)	21	3.5
Spiced wafers (Nabisco)	1 piece (10 grams)	41	7.4
Sprinkles (Sunshine)	1 piece (.6 oz.)	57	11.4
Sugar cookie:			
(Van de Kamp's)	1 piece (.6 oz.)	79	D.N.A.

(USDA): United States Department of Agriculture
DNA: Data Not Available
* Prepared as Package Directs

Food and Description	Measure or Quantity	Calories	Carbo-hydrates (grams)
Brown, old fashioned (Pepperidge Farm)	1 piece (.4 oz.)	48	6.9
Old fashioned (Keebler)	1 piece (.6 oz.)	78	12.4
Old fashioned (Pepperidge Farm)	1 piece (.4 oz.)	51	7.0
Rings (Nabisco)	1 piece (.5 oz.)	69	10.7
Sugar wafer:			
(USDA)	1 oz.	137	20.8
(Nab)	⅞-oz. pkg. (3 pieces)	128	17.5
(Nabisco) *Biscos*	1 piece (4 grams)	19	2.5
(Sunshine)	1 piece (9 grams)	43	6.6
Assorted (Dutch Twin)	1 piece	34	4.7
Chocolate (Keebler)	1 piece (6 grams)	31	3.5
Krisp Kreem (Keebler)	1 piece (6 grams)	31	3.7
Regent (Sunshine)	1 piece (5 grams)	23	3.4
Strawberry (Keebler)	1 piece (6 grams)	31	3.7
Vanilla (Keebler)	1 piece (6 grams)	31	3.7
Swedish Kreme (Keebler)	1 piece (.7 oz.)	98	12.2
Tahiti (Pepperidge Farm)	1 piece (.5 oz.)	84	8.6
Toy (Sunshine)	1 piece (3 grams)	13	2.1
Vanilla creme (Wise)	1 piece (7 grams)	33	5.0
Vanilla snap (Nabisco)	1 piece (3 grams)	13	2.3
Vanilla wafer:			
(USDA)	1 oz.	131	21.1
(Keebler)	1 piece (4 grams)	19	2.6
Nilla (Nabisco)	1 piece (4 grams)	18	2.9
(Sunshine)	1 piece (3 grams)	15	2.2
Venice (Pepperidge Farm)	1 piece (.4 oz.)	57	6.3
Waffle creme (Dutch Twin)	1 piece	44	6.1
Waffle creme (Nabisco)			
Biscos	1 piece (8 grams)	42	6.0
Yum Yums (Sunshine)	1 piece (.5 oz.)	83	10.4
COOKIE DIETETIC:			
Almond chocolate wafer (Estee)	1 wafer	27	2.6
Angel puffs (Stella D'oro)	1 piece (3 grams)	17	1.5
Apple pastry (Stella D'oro)	1 piece (.8 oz.)	94	13.6
Assorted (Estee)	1 piece	31	4.8
Assorted filled wafers (Estee)	1 piece	25	3.2
Beljuin Treats (Estee)	1 piece	32	3.2
Chocolate chip (Dia-Mel)	1 piece (9 grams)	40	3.7
Chocolate chip (Estee)	1 piece	32	3.6

Food and Description	Measure or Quantity	Calories	Carbo-hydrates (grams)
Chocolate continental (Stella D'oro)	1 piece	21	D.N.A.
Chocolate Holland-filled wafer (Estee)	1 piece	22	2.0
Chocolate mint wafer (Dia-Mel)	1 piece (9 grams)	43	3.2
Chocolate & vanilla wafer (Estee)	1 piece	27	3.2
Coconut bar continental (Stella D'oro)	1 piece	34	D.N.A.
Coconut tea (Dia-Mel)	1 piece (7 grams)	32	2.8
Expresso Wafers (Estee)	1 piece	22	1.9
Fig pastry (Stella D'oro)	1 piece (.9 oz.)	100	15.5
Fruit flavored wafer (Estee)	1 piece	22	2.0
Fudge nut (Estee)	1 piece	12	1.6
Have-A-Heart (Stella D'oro)	1 piece (.7 oz.)	97	11.3
Kichel (Stella D'oro)	1 piece (1 gram)	8	.7
Metrecal (Drackett) any flavor	1 piece (6 grams)	25	3.0
Monties (Estee)	1 piece	38	2.5
Oatmeal raisin (Estee)	1 piece	36	4.4
Oatmeal raisin (Dia-Mel)	1 piece (7 grams)	29	2.7
Peach-apricot pastry (Stella D'oro)	1 piece (.8 oz.)	104	15.2
Prune pastry (Stella D'oro)	1 piece (.8 oz.)	92	14.3
Ripple Supreme (Dia-Mel)	1 piece (12 grams)	54	4.4
Royal Nuggets (Stella D'oro)	1 piece (<1 gram)	2	.1
Sandwich, duplex (Estee)	1 piece	42	4.8
Sandwich, lemon (Estee)	1 piece	69	7.8
Sandwich (Dia-Mel)	1 piece (9 grams)	44	3.2
Vanilla continental (Stella D'oro)	1 piece	24	D.N.A.
Vanilla filled wafer (Estee)	1 piece	25	3.2
Vanilla Holland-filled wafer (Estee)	1 piece	22	2.0

COOKIE DOUGH,
refrigerated:

Unbaked, plain (USDA)	1 oz.	127	16.7

(USDA): United States Department of Agriculture
DNA: Data Not Available
* Prepared as Package Directs

Food and Description	Measure or Quantity	Calories	Carbo-hydrates (grams)
(Pillsbury):			
Brownie	1 oz.	110	17.3
Butterscotch nut	1 oz.	128	15.2
Chocolate chip	1 oz.	116	17.0
Fudge nut	1 oz.	119	15.9
Oatmeal raisin	1 oz.	116	16.8
Peanut butter	1 oz.	129	16.0
Sugar	1 oz.	125	16.1
COOKIE, HOME RECIPE:			
Brownie with nuts (USDA)	1 oz.	137	14.4
Chocolate chip (USDA)	1 oz.	146	17.0
Sugar, soft, thick (USDA)	1 oz.	126	19.3
COOKIE MIX:			
Plain, dry (USDA)	1 oz.	140	18.9
*Plain, prepared with egg & water (USDA)	1 oz.	140	18.4
*Plain, prepared with milk (USDA)	1 oz.	139	18.9
Brownie:			
Dry, with egg (USDA)	1 oz.	119	22.3
*Dry, with egg, prepared with water & nuts (USDA)	1 oz.	114	17.0
Dry, without egg (USDA)	1 oz.	125	21.5
*Dry, without egg, prepared with egg, water & nuts (USDA)	1 oz.	121	17.9
*Chewy fudge, regular size (Duncan Hines)	1/16 of cake (1.2 oz.)	147	20.5
*Butterscotch (Betty Crocker)	1½" sq.	59	9.6
*Butterscotch, chocolate chip (Betty Crocker)	1 lb. pkg.	2096	332.8
*Fudge (Betty Crocker)	1½" sq.	58	9.6
*Fudge, supreme (Betty Crocker)	1½" sq.	59	9.9
Fudge (Pillsbury)	1 oz.	125	21.7
*German chocolate (Betty Crocker)	1½" sq.	70	12.0
*Walnut (Betty Crocker)	1½" sq.	63	9.5
Walnut (Pillsbury)	1 oz.	125	21.7

Food and Description	Measure or Quantity	Calories	Carbo-hydrates (grams)
*Date bar (Betty Crocker)	2″ x 1″ bar	58	8.8
*Macaroon, coconut (Betty Crocker)	1¾″ macaroon	73	10.2
*Toll House with morsels (Nestlé's)	1 piece (.4 oz.)	52	7.2
*Toll House without morsels (Nestlé's)	1 piece (8 grams)	42	5.7
*Vienna Dream bar (Betty Crocker)	2″ x 1⅛″	87	10.3

COOKING FATS (See **FATS**)

COOL 'N CREAMY (Birds Eye) ½ cup (4.4 oz.)   172   27.7

CORDIAL (See individual kinds of liqueur by flavor or brand name)

CORDON D'ALSACE,
Alsatian wine, 12% alcohol (Willm)   3 fl. oz.   66   3.6

CORDON DE BORDEAUX,
French Bordeaux, red or white (Chanson) 11½% alcohol   3 fl. oz.   60   6.3

CORDON DE BOURGOGNE,
French white Burgundy, (Chanson) 11½% alcohol   3 fl. oz.   81   6.3

CORDON DU RHONE,
French red Rhone wine, (Chanson) 12% alcohol   3 fl. oz.   84   6.3

CORN:
Fresh, white or yellow (USDA):
Raw, untrimmed, on cob   1 lb. (weighed in husk)   157   36.1

(USDA): United States Department of Agriculture
DNA: Data Not Available
* Prepared as Package Directs

Food and Description	Measure or Quantity	Calories	Carbo-hydrates (grams)
Raw, trimmed, on cob	1 lb. (husk removed)	240	55.1
Boiled, kernels, cut from cob, drained	1 cup (5.9 oz.)	138	31.2
Boiled, whole	4.9-oz. ear (5" x 1¾")	70	16.2
Canned, regular pack:			
Golden or yellow, whole kernel:			
Solids & liq., vacuum pack (USDA)	½ cup (3.7 oz.)	88	21.7
Solids & liq., wet pack (USDA)	½ cup (4.5 oz.)	84	20.1
Drained solids, wet pack (USDA)	½ cup (3 oz.)	72	17.0
Drained solids (Butter Kernel)	½ cup (4.1 oz.)	75	18.0
Drained solids (Cannon)	4 oz.	95	22.5
(Fall River)	½ cup	75	18.0
(Green Giant) Niblets, vacuum pack	⅓ of 12-oz. can	100	21.8
With red & green sweet pepper (Del Monte)	½ cup (3.7 oz.)	78	19.3
White, whole kernel:			
Solids & liq., wet pack (USDA)	½ cup (4.5 oz.)	84	20.1
Drained solids, wet pack (USDA)	½ cup (2.8 oz.)	67	15.8
Drained liq., wet pack (USDA)	4 oz.	29	7.8
(Fall River)	½ cup	70	16.4
Canned, white or yellow, whole kernel, dietetic pack:			
Solids & liq., wet pack (USDA)	4 oz.	65	15.4
Drained solids (USDA)	4 oz.	86	20.4
Drained liq. (USDA)	4 oz. (by wt.)	19	4.9
Solids & liq. (Blue Boy)	4 oz.	78	16.0
Solids & liq. (Diet Delight)	½ cup (4.4 oz.)	70	16.9
(S and W) Nutradiet	4 oz.	59	12.2
(Tillie Lewis)	½ cup (4.5 oz.)	82	16.8
Canned, cream style, white or yellow, regular pack:			

Food and Description	Measure or Quantity	Calories	Carbo-hydrates (grams)
Solids & liq. (USDA)	½ cup (4.4 oz.)	102	25.0
(Butter Kernel)	½ cup (4.1 oz.)	92	22.5
Golden (Del Monte)	½ cup (4.4 oz.)	102	26.1
Golden (Green Giant)			
Niblets	½ of 8.5-oz. can	106	23.7
White (Fall River)	½ cup	91	21.9
White or golden			
(Stokely-Van Camp)	½ cup (4.1 oz.)	94	23.0
Canned, cream style, dietetic pack:			
Solids & liq. (USDA)	4 oz.	93	21.0
Solids & liq. (Blue Boy)	4 oz.	105	20.6
(S and W) *Nutradiet*	4 oz.	95	20.1
Frozen:			
On the cob:			
Not thawed (USDA)	4 oz.	111	25.6
Boiled, drained (USDA)	4 oz.	107	24.5
(Birds Eye)	1 ear (3.5 oz.)	98	21.7
Kernel, cut off cob:			
Not thawed (USDA)	4 oz.	93	22.3
Boiled, drained solids			
(USDA)	½ cup (3.2 oz.)	72	17.1
(Birds Eye)	½ cup (3.3 oz.)	77	17.8
Sweet, white (Birds			
Eye)	½ cup (3.3 oz.)	77	17.9
(Blue Goose)	4 oz.	102	20.6
In butter sauce:			
Niblets (Green Giant)			
boil-in-the-bag	⅓ of 10-oz. pkg.	87	14.6
White Shoe Peg (Green			
Giant) boil-in-the-bag	⅓ of 12-oz. pkg.	109	19.4
Mexicorn (Green Giant)			
boil-in-the-bag	⅓ of 10-oz. pkg.	89	15.1
Cream style:			
(Birds Eye)	½ cup (3.3 oz.)	79	19.2
(Green Giant) *Niblets*	⅓ of 10-oz. pkg.	65	15.4
With peas & tomatoes			
(Birds Eye)	½ cup (3.3 oz.)	67	15.0
With sweet pepper &			

(USDA): United States Department of Agriculture
DNA: Data Not Available
* Prepared as Package Directs

Food and Description	Measure or Quantity	Calories	Carbohydrates (grams)
swiss cheese casserole (Green Giant)	⅓ of 10-oz. pkg.	87	15.8
CORNBREAD:			
Corn pone, home recipe, prepared with white, whole-ground cornmeal (USDA)	4 oz.	231	41.1
Corn sticks, frozen (Aunt Jemima)	3 pieces (1¾ oz.)	134	19.2
Johnnycake, home recipe, prepared with yellow, degermed cornmeal (USDA)	4 oz.	303	51.6
Southern-style, home recipe, prepared with degermed cornmeal (USDA)	4 oz.	254	39.3
Southern-style, home recipe, prepared with whole-ground cornmeal (USDA)	4 oz.	235	33.0
Spoonbread, home recipe, prepared with white whole-ground cornmeal (USDA)	4 oz.	221	19.2
CORNBREAD MIX:			
Dry (USDA)	1 oz.	122	20.1
*Prepared with egg & milk (USDA)	2⅜" muffin (1.4 oz.)	93	13.2
(*Aunt Jemima)	⅙ of cornbread (2.4 oz.)	226	34.5
(Pillsbury) *Ballard*	1 oz.	103	19.2
CORN BURSTS, cereal	1 cup (1 oz.)	110	25.6
CORN CHEX, cereal	1¼ cups (1 oz.)	107	24.2
CORN CHIPS (See **CRACKERS**)			
CORNED BEEF:			
Uncooked, boneless, medium fat (USDA)	1 lb.	1329	0.

Food and Description	Measure or Quantity	Calories	Carbohydrates (grams)
Cooked, boneless, medium fat (USDA)	4 oz.	422	0.
Canned:			
Lean (USDA)	4 oz.	210	0.
Medium fat (USDA)	4 oz.	245	0.
Fat (USDA)	4 oz.	298	0.
(Vienna)	4 oz.	272	.4
CORNED BEEF HASH, canned:			
With potato (USDA)	4 oz.	205	12.1
(Armour Star)	15½-oz. can	831	36.0
(Austex)	15-oz. can	769	45.5
(Bounty)	4 oz.	209	12.1
(Hormel)	15-oz. can	574	30.6
(Morton House)	15-oz. can	890	D.N.A.
(Nalley's)	4 oz.	209	9.1
(Silver Skillet)	4 oz.	217	10.9
(Wilson)	15½-oz. can	792	31.6
CORNED BEEF HASH DINNER, frozen (Swanson)	12½-oz. dinner	511	55.0
CORNED BEEF SPREAD (Underwood)	1 T. (.5 oz.)	27	.5
CORN FLAKES, cereal:			
(USDA)	1 cup (1 oz.)	112	24.7
Crushed (USDA)	1 cup (2.5 oz.)	270	59.7
Frosted (USDA)	1 cup (1.4 oz.)	154	36.5
Country (General Mills)	1¼ cups (1 oz.)	111	24.3
(Kellogg's)	1⅛ cups (1 oz.)	108	24.3
(Ralston Purina)	1 cup (1 oz.)	108	24.4
(Van Brode)	1 oz.	106	24.2
Dietetic (Van Brode)	1 oz.	109	24.9
CORN FRITTER:			
Home recipe (USDA)	4 oz.	428	45.0
Frozen (Mrs. Paul's)	12-oz. pkg.	846	123.3
CORN GRITS (See **HOMINY**)			

(USDA): United States Department of Agriculture
DNA: Data Not Available
* Prepared as Package Directs

Food and Description	Measure or Quantity	Calories	Carbo- hydrates (grams)
CORNMEAL, WHITE or YELLOW:			
Dry:			
Bolted (USDA)	1 cup (4.3 oz.)	442	90.9
Degermed:			
(USDA)	1 cup (4.9 oz.)	502	108.2
(USDA)	1 oz.	103	22.2
Self-rising degermed (USDA)	1 cup (5 oz.)	491	105.9
Self-rising whole-ground (USDA)	1 cup (5 oz.)	489	101.4
Whole-ground, unbolted (USDA)	1 cup (4.3 oz.)	433	90.0
Cooked:			
(USDA)	1 cup (8.5 oz.)	120	25.7
Degermed (Albers)	1 cup	119	25.5
Bolted (Aunt Jemima/ Quaker)	⅔ cup	82	17.0
Degermed (Aunt Jemima/ Quaker)	⅔ cup	82	17.6
CORN PUDDING, home recipe (USDA)	1 cup (8.6 oz.)	255	31.9
CORN SALAD, raw (USDA):			
Untrimmed	1 lb. (weighed untrimmed)	91	15.7
Trimmed	4 oz.	24	4.1
CORN SOUFFLE, frozen (Stouffer's)	12-oz. pkg.	492	57.0
CORNSTARCH:			
(USDA)	1 cup (4.5 oz.)	463	112.1
(USDA)	1 T. (8 grams)	29	7.0
(Argo)	1 T. (8 grams)	28	7.0
(Kingsford)	1 T. (8 grams)	28	7.0
(Duryeas)	1 T. (8 grams)	28	7.0
CORN STICK (See **CORNBREAD**)			
CORN SYRUP, light & dark blend (USDA)	1 T. (.7 oz.)	61	15.8

Food and Description	Measure or Quantity	Calories	Carbo-hydrates (grams)
CORN TOTAL, cereal	1 oz.	111	24.3
COTTAGE PUDDING, home recipe (USDA):			
Without sauce	2 oz.	195	30.8
With chocolate sauce	2 oz.	180	32.1
With strawberry sauce	2 oz.	166	27.4
COUGH DROP:			
(Beech-Nut)	1 drop (2 grams)	10	2.4
(F & F)	1 drop	11	D.N.A.
(H-B)	1 drop	8	1.9
(Luden's):			
Honey lemon	1 drop	8	D.N.A.
Honey licorice	1 drop	8	D.N.A.
Menthol	1 drop	9	2.1
Wild cherry	1 drop	9	D.N.A.
(Pine Bros.)	1 drop	10	2.5
(Smith Brothers)	1 drop	7	2.1
COUNTRY-STYLE SAUSAGE, smoked links (USDA)	1 oz.	98	0.
COWPEA (USDA):			
Immature seeds:			
Raw, whole	1 lb. (weighed in pods)	317	54.4
Raw, shelled	½ cup (2.5 oz.)	91	15.7
Boiled, drained solids	½ cup (2.9 oz.)	88	14.8
Canned, solids and liq.	4 oz.	79	14.1
Frozen (See **BLACK-EYED PEAS,** frozen)			
Young pods with seeds:			
Raw, whole	1 lb. (weighed untrimmed)	182	39.2
Boiled, drained solids	4 oz.	39	7.9
Mature seeds, dry:			
Raw	1 lb.	1556	279.9
Raw	½ cup (3 oz.)	288	51.8
Boiled	½ cup (4.4 oz.)	94	17.1

(USDA): United States Department of Agriculture
DNA: Data Not Available
* Prepared as Package Directs

Food and Description	Measure or Quantity	Calories	Carbo-hydrates (grams)
CRAB, all species:			
Fresh:			
Steamed, whole (USDA)	1 lb. (weighed in shell)	202	1.1
Steamed, meat only (USDA)	4 oz.	105	.6
(Epicure)	½ cup	50	.6
Canned:			
Drained solids (USDA)	4 oz.	115	1.2
(Del Monte)	7½-oz. can	202	3.6
(Harris Atlantic)	4 oz.	115	1.3
Alaska King, drained solids (Icy Point)	7½-oz. can	215	2.3
Alaska King, drained solids (Pillar Rock)	7½-oz. can	215	2.3
Frozen, Alaska King, thawed & drained (Wakefield's)	4 oz.	96	.6
CRAB APPLE, fresh (USDA):			
Whole	1 lb. (weighed whole)	284	74.3
Flesh only	4 oz.	77	20.2
CRAB COCKTAIL, King crab (Sau-Sea)	4-oz. jar	80	18.4
CRAB, DEVILED:			
Home recipe (USDA)	1 cup (8.5 oz.)	451	31.9
Frozen (Mrs. Paul's)	4 oz.	230	D.N.A.
CRAB IMPERIAL, home recipe (USDA)	1 cup (7.8 oz.)	323	8.6
CRAB NEWBURG, Alaska King, frozen (Stouffer's)	12-oz. pkg.	562	13.6
CRAB SOUP (Crosse & Blackwell)	6½ oz. (½ can)	59	8.3
CRACKER, PUFFS & CHIPS:			
Appeteasers (Nabisco):			
Crescent roll shaped	1 piece (<1 gram)	3	.5
Ham tasting, shaped	1 piece (<1 gram)	2	.4

Food and Description	Measure or Quantity	Calories	Carbohydrates (grams)
Onion shaped	1 piece (<1 gram)	2	.3
Arrowroot biscuit (Nabisco)	1 piece (5 grams)	22	3.5
Arrowroot biscuit (Sunshine)	1 piece (4 grams)	15	2.9
Bacon flavored thins (Nabisco)	1 piece (2 grams)	11	1.2
Bacon toast (Keebler)	1 piece (3 grams)	15	2.0
Barbecue snack wafer (Sunshine)	1 piece (3 grams)	17	2.0
Barbecue Vittles (General Mills)	32 pieces (½ oz.)	67	9.1
Bows (General Mills)	22 pieces (½ oz.)	81	7.5
Bugles (General Mills)	15 pieces (½ oz.)	81	7.5
Butter (USDA)	1 oz.	130	19.1
Butter thins (Nabisco)	1 piece (3 grams)	15	2.4
Buttons (General Mills)	48 pieces (½ oz.)	73	7.8
Cheese flavored (See also individual brand names in this grouping): (USDA)	1 oz.	136	17.1
Cheese 'n Bacon flavored sandwich (Nab)	1.4-oz. pkg. (6 pieces)	179	18.9
Cheese-N-Cheese (Wise)	1 piece (6 grams)	32	3.8
Cheese Nips (Nab)	⅞-oz. pkg. (24 pieces)	114	16.5
Cheese Nips (Nabisco)	1 piece (1 gram)	5	.7
Cheese on Rye sandwich (Nab)	1.4-oz. pkg. (6 pieces)	209	19.3
Chee Tos, cheese-flavored puffs	1 oz.	156	15.2
Cheez Doodles (Old London)	1⅛-oz. bag	170	18.5
Cheez-Its (Sunshine)	1 piece (1 gram)	6	.6
Che-zo (Keebler)	1 piece (<1 gram)	5	.6
Combo Cheez sandwich (Austin's)	1 piece	26	D.N.A.
Cheese Pixies (Wise)	1-oz. bag	163	13.4
Cheez Waffles (Austin's)	1 piece	26	D.N.A.

(USDA): United States Department of Agriculture
DNA: Data Not Available
* Prepared as Package Directs

Food and Description	Measure or Quantity	Calories	Carbo-hydrates (grams)
Cheez Waffles (Old London)	1 piece (2 grams)	11	1.3
Ritz cheese (Nabisco)	1 piece (3 grams)	17	1.9
Sesame cheese snack (Sunshine)	1 cracker (3 grams)	16	2.2
Shapies, dip delights (Nabisco)	1 piece (2 grams)	9	.8
Shapies, shells (Nabisco)	1 piece (2 grams)	10	.9
Skinny Dips (Keebler)	1 piece (1 gram)	5	.7
Thins (Pepperidge Farm)	2 pieces (5 grams)	23	3.5
Thins, dietetic (Estee)	1 thin	6	.9
Tid-Bit (Nab)	1⅛-oz. pkg. (32 pieces)	150	19.7
Tid Bit (Nabisco)	1 piece (<1 gram)	4	.6
Toast (Keebler)	1 piece (3 grams)	16	1.9
Twists (Nalley's)	1 oz.	137	14.2
Twists (Wonder)	1 oz.	154	14.7
Cheese & peanut butter sandwich:			
(USDA)	1 oz.	139	15.9
(Austin's)	1 piece	43	4.5
(Nab) *O-So-Gud*	1 oz. (4 pieces)	141	16.3
(Nab) *Squares*	1½-oz. pkg. (6 pieces)	208	22.1
(Nab) *Variety Pack*	1½-oz. pkg. (6 pieces)	209	22.7
(Wise)	1 piece (7 grams)	34	3.5
Chicken in a Biskit (Nabisco)	1 piece (2 grams)	10	1.2
Chippers (Nabisco)	1 piece (3 grams)	14	1.8
Chipsters (Nabisco)	1 piece (<1 gram)	2	.3
Cinnamon Crisp (Keebler)	1 section (4 grams)	17	2.7
Club, with or without salt (Keebler)	1 section (3 grams)	15	2.0
Corn Chips:			
(Fritos)	1 oz.	164	15.2
(Old London)	1¾-oz. bag	263	27.3
(Wise)	1¾-oz. bag	276	27.6
Barbecue flavored (Wise)	1¾-oz. bag	274	27.5
Crown Pilot (Nabisco)	1 piece (.6 oz.)	73	12.4
Dipsy Doodles (Old London)	1¾-oz. bag	276	26.4
Doo Dads (Nabisco)	1 piece (<1 gram)	2	.3
Duet (Nabisco)	1 piece (4 grams)	17	2.3

Food and Description	Measure or Quantity	Calories	Carbo-hydrates (grams)
Euphrates (Burry's), original, onion or rye	1 cracker	22	D.N.A.
Flings, cheese-flavored curls (Nabisco)	1 piece (2 grams)	11	.6
Flings, Swiss- & ham-flavored curls (Nabisco)	1 piece (2 grams)	10	.8
French Fried Potato Crisps (General Mills)	16 pieces (½ oz.)	78	7.5
Goldfish (Pepperidge Farm):			
Cheddar cheese	10 pieces (6 grams)	28	3.3
Lightly salted	10 pieces	28	3.6
Onion	10 pieces (6 grams)	28	3.6
Pretzel	10 pieces (7 grams)	29	5.0
Graham:			
(USDA)	1 oz.	109	20.8
(USDA)	2½″ square (7 grams)	27	5.1
(Nabisco)	1 piece (7 grams)	30	5.4
(Sunshine)	1 piece (4 grams)	17	3.0
Chocolate or cocoa-covered:			
(USDA)	1 oz.	135	19.2
(Burry's) Crunchy	1 piece	46	D.N.A.
(Keebler) *Deluxe*	1 piece (9 grams)	42	5.6
(Nabisco)	1 piece (.4 oz.)	55	7.0
(Nabisco) *Fancy*	1 piece (.5 oz.)	68	9.0
(Nabisco) *Pantry*	1 piece (.4 oz.)	62	8.5
(Sunshine) *Sweet Tooth*	1 piece (.4 oz.)	45	6.4
Sugar-honey coated:			
(USDA)	1 oz.	117	21.7
(Keebler)	1 section (4 grams)	17	2.8
(Nabisco) *Honey Maid*	1 piece (7 grams)	30	5.3
(Sunshine)	1 piece (7 grams)	30	5.2
Hi-Ho (Sunshine)	1 piece (4 grams	18	2.1
Krispy, salted tops (Sunshine)	1 piece (3 grams)	12	2.1
Krispy, unsalted tops (Sunshine)	1 piece (3 grams)	12	2.0

(USDA): United States Department of Agriculture
DNA: Data Not Available
* Prepared as Package Directs

Food and Description	Measure or Quantity	Calories	Carbohydrates (grams)
Matzo (See **MATZO**)			
Melba toast (See **MELBA**)			
Milk lunch (Burry's)	1 piece	36	D.N.A.
Milk lunch (Nabisco)			
Royal Lunch	1 piece (.4 oz.)	55	7.9
New Daisys (General Mills)	28 pieces (½ oz.)	68	8.8
Onion flavored:			
French (Nabisco)	1 piece (2 grams)	12	1.6
Rings (Old London)	½-oz. bag	68	10.4
Rings (Wise)	½-oz. bag	65	11.1
Skinny Dips (Keebler)	1 piece (1 gram)	5	.7
Tam (Manischewitz)	1 piece	14	D.N.A.
Toast (Keebler)	1 piece (3 grams)	18	2.1
Onion Waffies (Old London)	1 oz.	138	13.4
OTC (Original Trenton Cracker) regular or wine	1 piece	23	4.4
Oyster:			
(USDA)	1 cup (1 oz.)	124	20.0
(Keebler)	1 piece (<1 gram)	2	.2
Oysterettes (Nabisco)	1 piece (<1 gram)	3	.6
Soup & oyster (Nabisco)			
Dandy	1 piece (<1 gram)	3	.5
(Sunshine)	1 piece (<1 gram)	4	.7
Party Toast (Keebler)	1 piece (3 grams)	15	1.9
Peanut butter sandwich:			
& jelly flavored (Nabisco)	1.3-oz. pkg. (6 pieces)	180	23.9
Malted milk (Nab)	1⅜-oz. pkg. (6 pieces)	189	22.1
Toaster crackers (Wise)	1 piece (6 grams)	30	3.7
Toasty (Austin's)	1 piece	37	D.N.A.
Peanut butter & cheese (See Cheese & Peanut Butter Sandwich)			
Pizza Spins (General Mills)	½ oz. (32 pieces)	72	8.0
Pizza Wheels (Wise)	¾-oz. bag	90	16.1
Ritz (Nabisco)	1 piece (3 grams)	16	2.1
Ry Brot (Burry's)	1 piece	67	D.N.A.
Rye thins (Pepperidge Farm)	2 pieces	21	3.9
Rye toast (Keebler)	1 piece (4 grams)	17	2.2
Saltine:			
(USDA)	4 crackers (.4 oz.)	48	7.9

Food and Description	Measure or Quantity	Calories	Carbo- hydrates (grams)
Regular (Flavor Kist)	1 piece	12	2.2
Premium (Nab)	¾-oz. pkg. (8 pieces)	91	15.3
Premium (Nabisco)	1 piece (3 grams)	12	2.0
Premium (Nabisco), unsalted tops	1 piece (3 grams)	12	2.0
Rye (Flavor Kist)	1 piece	13	2.2
Sesame (Flavor Kist)	1 piece	13	2.2
Zesta (Keebler)	1 section (3 grams)	12	2.0
Sea Toast (Keebler)	1 piece (.5 oz.)	62	11.1
Sesa Wheat (Austin's)	1 piece	34	3.7
Sesame bread wafer (Keebler)	1 piece (3 grams)	16	2.0
Sesame bread wafer (Nabisco) Meal Mates	1 piece (5 grams)	21	3.2
Sip 'N Chips snacks (Nabisco)	1 piece (2 grams)	9	1.0
Sociables (Nabisco)	1 piece (2 grams)	10	1.3
Soda (USDA)	1 oz.	124	20.0
Soda (USDA)	2 crackers, 2½" sq. (.4 oz.)	48	7.8
Souperfish (Burry's)	1 piece	9	D.N.A.
Swedish rye wafers (Keebler)	1 piece (5 grams)	5	3.8
Tam Tam (Manischewitz)	1 piece	13	1.7
Toasted wafers (Sunshine)	1 wafer (2 grams)	10	1.2
Tomato onion (Sunshine)	1 piece (3 grams)	15	2.5
Tortilla chips (Frito-Lay) Doritos	1 oz.	140	18.7
Tortilla chips (Old London)	1½-oz. bag	207	27.8
Town House (Keebler)	1 piece (3 grams)	18	2.0
Triangle Thins (Nabisco)	1 piece (2 grams)	8	1.1
Triscuit wafers (Nabisco)	1 piece (4 grams)	21	3.0
Uneeda Biscuit, unsalted tops (Nabisco)	1 piece (5 grams)	22	3.7
Wafer-ets (Hol-Grain):			
Rice, salted or unsalted	1 piece (3 grams)	12	2.5
Wheat, salted or unsalted	1 piece (2 grams)	7	1.4
Waldorf low salt (Keebler)	1 piece (3 grams)	14	2.4
Waverly wafers (Nabisco)	1 piece (4 grams)	18	2.6

(USDA): United States Department of Agriculture
DNA: Data Not Available
* Prepared as Package Directs

Food and Description	Measure or Quantity	Calories	Carbo-hydrates (grams)
Wheat *Skinny Dips* (Keebler)	1 piece (1 gram)	5	.7
Wheat thins (Nabisco)	1 piece (2 grams)	9	1.2
Wheat toast (Keebler)	1 piece (3 grams)	16	2.0
Whistles (General Mills)	17 pieces (½ oz.)	71	8.0
White thins (Pepperidge Farm)	2 pieces (5 grams)	23	4.0
Whole wheat (USDA)	1 oz.	114	19.3
Whole wheat, natural (Froumine)	1 piece (.4 oz.)	46	7.5
CRACKER CRUMBS:			
Graham (USDA)	1 cup (3 oz.)	330	63.0
Graham (Keebler)	3 oz.	368	64.1
Graham (Nabisco)	9″ pie shell (1½ cups, 4.6 oz.)	563	100.3
CRACKER JACK (See **POPCORN**)			
CRACKER MEAL:			
(USDA)	3 oz.	373	60.0
(USDA)	1 T. (.4 oz.)	44	7.1
(Keebler):			
Fine, medium or coarse	3 oz.	316	68.5
Zesty	3 oz.	363	61.5
(Nabisco) salted	1 cup (3 oz.)	309	65.7
(Nabisco) unsalted	1 cup (3 oz.)	319	67.9
CRACKER PIE CRUST MIX (See **PIECRUST MIX**)			
CRANBERRY:			
Fresh:			
Untrimmed (USDA)	1 lb. (weighed with stems)	200	47.0
Stems removed (USDA)	1 cup (4 oz.)	52	12.2
(Ocean Spray)	1 oz.	15	2.7
Dehydrated (USDA)	1 oz.	104	23.9
CRANBERRY APPLE JUICE DRINK			
(Ocean Spray) *Cranapple*	½ cup (4.5 oz.)	94	23.0

Food and Description	Measure or Quantity	Calories	Carbo-hydrates (grams)
CRANBERRY JUICE COCKTAIL:			
(USDA)	½ cup (4.4 oz.)	81	20.6
(Ocean Spray)	½ cup (4.4 oz.)	83	19.7
CRANBERRY-ORANGE RELISH:			
Uncooked (USDA)	4 oz.	202	51.5
(Ocean Spray)	4 oz.	209	51.8
CRANBERRY-PAPAYA FRUIT SPREAD (Vita)	1 T.	9	D.N.A.
CRANBERRY PIE (Tastykake)	4-oz. pie	376	57.7
CRANBERRY SAUCE:			
Home recipe, sweetened, unstrained (USDA)	4 oz.	202	51.6
Canned:			
Sweetened, strained (USDA)	½ cup (4.8 oz.)	199	51.0
Sweetened, strained (USDA)	4 oz.	166	42.5
Jellied (Ocean Spray)	4 oz.	184	42.9
Whole berry (Ocean Spray)	4 oz.	191	44.3
CRANBREAKER MIX (Bar-Tender's)	1 serving (⅝ oz.)	70	17.4
CRANPRUNE JUICE DRINK (Ocean Spray)	½ cup (4.4 oz.)	82	20.1
CRAPPIE, white, raw, meat only (USDA)	4 oz.	90	0.
CRAYFISH, freshwater (USDA):			
Raw, in shell	1 lb. (weighed in shell)	39	.7
Raw, meat only	4 oz.	82	1.4

(USDA): United States Department of Agriculture
DNA: Data Not Available
* Prepared as Package Directs

Food and Description	Measure or Quantity	Calories	Carbo-hydrates (grams)
CREAM:			
Half and half:			
(USDA)	1 cup (8.5 oz.)	324	11.1
(USDA)	1 T. (.5 oz.)	20	.7
10.5% fat (Sealtest)	½ cup (4.2 oz.)	148	5.1
12.0% fat (Sealtest)	½ cup (4.2 oz.)	161	5.0
Light, table, or coffee:			
(USDA)	1 cup (8.5 oz.)	506	10.3
(USDA)	1 T. (.5 oz.)	32	.6
18% fat (Sealtest)	1 T. (.5 oz.)	28	.6
25% fat (Sealtest)	1 T. (.5 oz.)	37	.5
Light whipping:			
(USDA)	1 cup (8.4 oz.)	717	8.6
(USDA)	1 T. (.5 oz.)	45	.5
30% fat (Sealtest)	1 T. (.5 oz.)	44	.5
Whipped topping, pressurized:			
(USDA)	1 cup (2.1 oz.)	155	.6
(USDA)	1 T. (3 grams)	10	Tr.
Heavy whipping:			
Unwhipped (USDA)	1 cup (8.4 oz.)	838	7.4
(USDA)	1 T. (.5 oz.)	53	.5
36% fat (Sealtest)	1 T. (.5 oz.)	52	.5
Sour:			
(USDA)	1 cup (8.1 oz.)	485	9.9
(USDA)	1 T. (.4 oz.)	25	.5
(Borden)	1 T. (.5 oz.)	28	.5
(Breakstone)	1 T. (.5 oz.)	29	.6
(Sealtest)	1 T. (.5 oz.)	28	.5
Imitation:			
(Borden) *Zest,* 13.5% vegetable fat	1 pt.	776	28.0
(Borden) *Zest,* 13.5% vegetable fat	2 T.	97	3.5
Sour cream, dried (Information supplied by General Mills Laboratory)	1 oz.	188	8.1
Sour dressing, cultured (Breakstone)	1 T.	27	.7
CREAMIES (Tastykake):			
Banana cake	1 pkg. (1⅞ oz.)	238	34.5
Chocolate	1 pkg. (1⅞ oz.)	290	29.3
Koffee Kake	1 pkg. (1⅞ oz.)	303	47.2
Vanilla	1 pkg. (1⅞ oz.)	292	32.3

Food and Description	Measure or Quantity	Calories	Carbo-hydrates (grams)
CREAM OF RICE, cereal	4 oz.	82	17.9
CREAMSICLE (Popsicle Industries)	3 fl. oz.	96	20.0
CREAM or CREME SOFT DRINK:			
Sweetened:			
(Canada Dry) vanilla	6 fl. oz.	97	24.1
(Dr. Brown's)	6 fl. oz.	84	20.9
(Fanta)	6 fl. oz.	94	24.2
(Hoffman)	6 fl. oz.	85	21.3
(Key Food)	6 fl. oz.	84	20.9
(Kirsch)	6 fl. oz.	77	19.6
(Shasta)	6 fl. oz.	84	21.3
(Waldbaum)	6 fl. oz.	84	20.9
(Yukon Club)	6 fl. oz.	85	21.3
Low calorie:			
(Dr. Brown's)	6 fl. oz.	1	.2
(Hoffman)	6 fl. oz.	1	.2
(No-Cal)	6 fl. oz.	2	<.1
(Shasta)	6 fl. oz.	<1	<.1
CREAM SUBSTITUTE (See individual brand names)			
CREAM OF WHEAT, cereal:			
Instant or quick, dry	1 oz. (¾ cup cooked)	99	21.2
Mix'n Eat, regular, dry	3½ T. (1 oz.)	99	20.8
Regular, dry	1 oz. (¾ cup cooked)	102	21.7
CREME D'AMANDE LIQUEUR (Garnier) 60 proof	1 fl. oz.	111	15.6
CREME D'APRICOT LIQUEUR (Old Mr. Boston) 42 proof	1 fl. oz.	66	6.0

(USDA): United States Department of Agriculture
DNA: Data Not Available
* Prepared as Package Directs

Food and Description	Measure or Quantity	Calories	Carbo-hydrates (grams)
CREME DE BANANE LIQUEUR:			
(Garnier) 60 proof	1 fl. oz.	80	8.0
(Old Mr. Boston) 42 proof	1 fl. oz.	66	6.0
CREME DE BLACKBERRY LIQUEUR (Old Mr. Boston) 42 proof	1 fl. oz.	66	6.0
CREME DE CACAO LIQUEUR, brown or white:			
(Bols) 54 proof	1 fl. oz.	101	11.8
(Garnier) 54 proof	1 fl. oz.	97	13.1
(Hiram Walker) 54 proof	1 fl. oz.	104	15.0
(Leroux) brown, 54 proof	1 fl. oz.	101	14.3
(Leroux) white, 54 proof	1 fl. oz.	98	13.3
(Old Mr. Boston) 42 proof	1 fl. oz.	84	7.0
(Old Mr. Boston) 54 proof	1 fl. oz.	95	7.0
CREME DE CAFE LIQUEUR (Leroux) 60 proof	1 fl. oz.	104	13.6
CREME DE CASSIS LIQUEUR:			
(Garnier) 36 proof	1 fl. oz.	83	13.5
(Leroux) 35 proof	1 fl. oz.	88	14.9
CREME DE CHERRY LIQUEUR black cherry (Old Mr. Boston) 42 proof	1 fl. oz.	66	6.0
CREME DE COFFEE LIQUEUR (Old Mr. Boston) 42 proof	1 fl. oz.	66	6.0
CREME DE MENTHE LIQUEUR, green or white:			
(Bols) 60 proof	1 fl. oz.	112	13.0
(Garnier) 60 proof	1 fl. oz.	110	15.3
(Hiram Walker) 60 proof	1 fl. oz.	94	11.2
(Leroux) green, 60 proof	1 fl. oz.	110	15.2
(Leroux) white, 60 proof	1 fl. oz.	101	12.8

Food and Description	Measure or Quantity	Calories	Carbo-hydrates (grams)
(Old Mr. Boston) 42 proof	1 fl. oz.	66	6.0
(Old Mr. Boston) 60 proof	1 fl. oz.	94	8.5
CREME DE NOYAUX LIQUEUR:			
(Bols) 60 proof	1 fl. oz.	115	13.7
(Leroux) 60 proof	1 fl. oz.	108	14.6
CREME DE PEACH LIQUEUR (Old Mr. Boston) 42 proof	1 fl. oz.	66	6.0
CREME SOFT DRINK (See **CREAM SOFT DRINK**)			
CREMORA, non-dairy (Borden)	1 tsp.	11	1.1
CRESS, GARDEN (USDA):			
Raw, whole	1 lb. (weighed untrimmed)	103	17.7
Boiled in small amount of water, short time, drained	1 cup (6.3 oz.)	41	6.8
Boiled in large amount of water, long time, drained	1 cup (6.3 oz.)	40	6.5
CRISP RICE (Van Brode):			
Regular	1 oz.	106	24.7
Dietetic	1 oz.	109	25.5
CRISPY CRITTERS, cereal	1 cup (1 oz.)	113	23.0
CROAKER (USDA): Atlantic:			
Raw, whole	1 lb. (weighed whole)	148	0.
Raw, meat only	4 oz.	109	0.
Baked	4 oz.	151	0.

(USDA): United States Department of Agriculture
DNA: Data Not Available
* Prepared as Package Directs

Food and Description	Measure or Quantity	Calories	Carbo- hydrates (grams)
White, raw, meat only	4 oz.	95	0.
Yellowfin, raw, meat only	4 oz.	101	0.

CRULLER (See **DOUGHNUT**)

CUCUMBER, fresh (USDA):

Eaten with skin	½ lb. (weighed whole)	32	7.4
Eaten without skin	½ lb. (weighed with skin)	23	5.3
Unpared, 10-oz. cucumber	7½″ x 2″ pared cucumber (7.3 oz.)	29	6.6
Pared	6 slices (2″ x ⅛″)	7	1.6
Pared & diced	½ cup (2.5 oz.)	10	2.3

CUPCAKE:

Home recipe (USDA):

Without icing	1.4-oz. cupcake (2¾″)	146	22.4
With chocolate icing	1.8-oz. cupcake (2¾″)	184	29.7
With boiled white icing	1.8-oz. cupcake (2¾″)	176	30.9
With uncooked white icing	1.8-oz. cupcake (2¾″)	184	31.6

Commercial:

Chocolate (Tastykake)	1 cupcake (1 oz.)	192	33.0
Chocolate, chocolate creme filled (Tastykake)	1 cupcake (1¼ oz.)	128	23.2
Chocolate, creme filled (Drake's)	1 cupcake (1½ oz.)	187	25.6
Coconut (Tastykake)	1 cupcake (¾ oz.)	92	16.7
Creme filled, chocolate butter cream (Tastykake)	1 cupcake (1⅛ oz.)	161	23.1
Lemon creme filled (Tastykake)	1 cupcake (⅞ oz.)	124	17.1
Orange (Hostess) 2 to pkg.	1 cupcake (1.5 oz.)	150	26.7

Food and Description	Measure or Quantity	Calories	Carbo-hydrates (grams)
Orange creme filled (Tastykake)	1 cupcake (⅞ oz.)	133	17.1
Vanilla creme filled (Tastykake)	1 cupcake (⅞ oz.)	123	16.4
Vanilla *Triplets* (Tastykake)	1 cupcake (.8 oz.)	101	16.1
CUPCAKE MIX:			
(USDA)	4 oz.	497	86.0
*Prepared with eggs, milk, without icing (USDA)	.8-oz. cupcake	88	14.0
*Prepared with eggs, milk, with chocolate icing (USDA)	1.2-oz. cupcake (2½" dia.)	129	21.3
*(Flako)	.8-oz. cupcake (1/16 of pkg.)	101	15.9
CURACAO LIQUEUR:			
Curaçao-Blue (Bols) 64 proof	1 fl. oz.	105	10.3
Curaçao-Orange (Bols) 64 proof	1 fl. oz.	100	8.8
(Garnier) 60 proof	1 fl. oz.	100	12.7
(Hiram Walker) 60 proof	1 fl. oz.	96	11.8
(Leroux) 60 proof	1 fl. oz.	84	9.5
CURRANT, fresh (USDA):			
Black European:			
Whole	1 lb. (weighed with stems)	240	58.2
Stems removed	4 oz.	61	14.9
Red & white:			
Whole	1 lb. (weighed with stems)	220	53.2
Stems removed	1 cup (3.9 oz.)	55	13.3
*CURRANT-RASPBERRY DANISH DESSERT (Junket)	½ cup	138	33.8

(USDA): United States Department of Agriculture
DNA: Data Not Available
* Prepared as Package Directs

Food and Description	Measure or Quantity	Calories	Carbohydrates (grams)
CURRY POWDER (Crosse & Blackwell)	1 T.	21	3.9
CUSK (USDA)			
Raw, drawn	1 lb. (weighed drawn, head & tail on)	197	0.
Raw, meat only	4 oz.	85	0.
Steamed	4 oz.	120	0.
CUSTARD:			
Home recipe, baked (USDA)	½ cup (4.7 oz.)	152	14.7
Chilled (Sealtest)	4 oz.	149	24.3
CUSTARD APPLE, bullock's-heart, raw (USDA):			
Whole	1 lb. (weighed with skin & seeds)	266	66.3
Flesh only	4 oz.	115	28.6
CUSTARD PIE:			
Home recipe (USDA)	⅙ of 9″ pie (5.4 oz.)	331	35.6
Frozen (Banquet)	5 oz.	274	41.2
CUSTARD PUDDING MIX:			
Dry, with vegetable gum base (USDA)	1 oz.	109	28.0
*Prepared with whole milk (USDA)	4 oz.	149	25.6
*Jell-O	½ cup (5 oz.)	165	22.9
Real egg (Lynden Farms)	4-oz. pkg.	441	69.2
*Regular (Royal)	½ cup (5.1 oz.)	152	22.5

Food and Description	Measure or Quantity	Calories	Carbo- hydrates (grams)

D

DAIQUIRI COCKTAIL:
(Calvert) 60 proof	3 fl. oz.	190	9.5
(Hiram Walker) 52.5 proof	3 fl. oz.	177	12.0
(National Distillers) *Duet,* 12% alcohol	8-fl.-oz. can	280	24.0

DAIQUIRI MIX (Bar-Tender's)
	1 serving (⅝ oz.)	70	17.2

DAMSON PLUM (See **PLUM**)

DANDELION GREENS, raw (USDA):
Trimmed	1 lb.	204	41.7
Boiled, drained	½ cup (3.2 oz.)	30	5.8

DANISH PASTRY (See **COFFEE CAKE**)

DANISH-STYLE VEGETABLES, frozen (Birds Eye)
	⅓ pkg. (3⅓ oz.)	92	7.6

DATE, dry:
Domestic:
With pits (USDA)	1 lb. (weighed with pits)	1081	287.7
Without pits (USDA)	4 oz.	311	82.7
Without pits, chopped (USDA)	1 cup (6.1 oz.)	477	126.8
California (Cal-Date)	2 oz.	161	42.8
California (Cal-Date)	1 date (8 oz.)	62	16.4
California (Garden of the Setting Sun)	5 dates	152	40.5
Chopped (Dromedary)	1 cup (5 oz.)	493	114.2
Pitted (Dromedary)	1 cup (5 oz.)	470	112.3

(USDA): United States Department of Agriculture
DNA: Data Not Available
* Prepared as Package Directs

Food and Description	Measure or Quantity	Calories	Carbo-hydrates (grams)
Imported (Bordo):			
Iraq	4 oz.	370	99.5
Iraq	4 average dates	76	19.3
Dehydrated (Vacu-Dry)	1 oz.	98	26.1
DELAWARE WINE:			
(Gold Seal) 12% alcohol	3 fl oz.	87	2.6
(Great Western) 12% alcohol	3 fl. oz.	82	3.0
DEVIL DOGS (Drake's)	1 cake (1½ oz.)	170	24.5
DEVIL'S FOOD CAKE:			
Home recipe (USDA):			
Without icing	3″ x 2″ x 1½″ (1.9 oz.)	201	28.6
With chocolate icing	¹⁄₁₆ of 10″ layer cake (4.2 oz.)	443	67.0
With uncooked white icing	¹⁄₁₆ of 10″ layer cake (4.2 oz.)	443	71.0
Commercial, frozen:			
With chocolate icing (USDA)	2 oz.	215	31.5
With whipped cream filling & chocolate icing (USDA)	2 oz.	210	24.8
(Pepperidge Farm)	⅛ of cake (3.1 oz.)	326	47.0
DEVIL'S FOOD CAKE MIX:			
Dry (USDA)	1 oz.	115	21.8
*With chocolate icing (USDA)	¹⁄₁₆ of 9″ cake	234	40.2
*(Betty Crocker)	¹⁄₁₂ of cake	199	35.8
*Butter recipe (Betty Crocker)	¹⁄₁₂ of cake	269	37.0
*(Duncan Hines)	¹⁄₁₂ of cake (2.7 oz.)	205	35.0
Red Devil (Pillsbury)	1 oz.	119	21.5
*(Swans Down)	¹⁄₁₂ of cake (2.4 oz.)	184	35.3

DEWBERRY, fresh (See BLACKBERRY, fresh)

Food and Description	Measure or Quantity	Calories	Carbo-hydrates (grams)
DIAMOND WINE (Great Western) 12% alcohol	3 fl. oz.	76	1.7
DING DONG (Hostess):			
Dark chocolate	1 cake (1.4 oz.)	167	21.6
Milk chocolate, 2 to pkg.	1 cake (1.4 oz.)	166	21.6
Milk chocolate, 12 to pkg.	1 cake (1.3 oz.)	162	20.9
DINNER, frozen (See individual listings such as **BEEF DINNER, CHICKEN DINNER, CHINESE DINNER, ENCHILADA DINNER,** etc.)			
DIP:			
Bacon-horseradish, neufchâtel cheese (Kraft) *Ready Dip*	1 oz.	71	.8
Bacon-horseradish (Kraft) *Teez*	1 oz.	57	1.6
Blue cheese, neufchâtel cheese (Kraft) *Ready Dip*	1 oz.	69	1.6
Blue cheese (Kraft) *Teez*	1 oz.	51	1.3
Clam, neufchâtel cheese (Kraft) *Ready Dip*	1 oz.	67	1.8
Clam, sour cream (Kraft) *Teez*	1 oz.	45	1.5
Dill pickle & neufchâtel cheese (Kraft) *Ready Dip*	1 oz.	67	2.4
Garlic (Kraft) *Teez*	1 oz.	47	1.5
Green Goddess (Kraft) *Teez*	1 oz.	46	1.5
Onion:			
(Borden)	1 oz.	48	1.8
Neufchâtel cheese (Kraft) *Ready Dip*	1 oz.	68	2.0
French onion (Kraft) *Teez*	1 oz.	43	1.5
French onion (Sealtest) *Dip 'n Dressing*	1 oz.	46	2.2
Tasty Tartar (Borden)	1 oz.	48	1.8
Western Bar B-Q (Borden)	1 oz.	48	1.8

(USDA): United States Department of Agriculture
DNA: Data Not Available
* Prepared as Package Directs

Food and Description	Measure or Quantity	Calories	Carbo-hydrates (grams)
DIP MIX:			
Bacon onion (Fritos)	1 pkg. (.6 oz.)	47	7.2
Bleu cheese (Fritos)	1 pkg. (.6 oz.)	48	8.1
Chili con queso (Fritos)	1 pkg. (.6 oz.)	72	7.5
Green onion (Lawry's)	1 pkg. (.6 oz.)	50	10.6
Guacamole	1 pkg. (.6 oz.)	60	5.5
Toasted onion (Lawry's)	1 pkg. (.6 oz.)	48	9.8
DISTILLED LIQUOR. The values below apply to un-flavored bourbon whiskey, brandy, Canadian whisky, gin, Irish whiskey, rum, rye whiskey, Scotch whisky, te-quila, and vodka. The caloric content of distilled liquors depends on the percentage of alcohol. The proof is twice the alcohol percent and the following values apply to all brands. (USDA):			
80 proof	1 fl. oz.	65	Tr.
86 proof	1 fl. oz.	70	Tr.
90 proof	1 fl. oz.	74	Tr.
94 proof	1 fl. oz.	77	Tr.
100 proof	1 fl. oz.	83	Tr.
DOCK, including **SHEEP SORREL:** Raw, whole (USDA)	1 lb. (weighed untrimmed)	89	17.8
Boiled, drained (USDA)	4 oz.	22	4.4
DOGFISH, spiny, raw, meat only (USDA)	4 oz.	177	0.
DOLLY VARDEN, raw, meat & skin (USDA)	4 oz.	163	0.
DOUGHNUT: Cake type:			
(USDA)	4 oz.	443	58.2
(USDA)	1 piece (1.1 oz.)	125	16.4

Food and Description	Measure or Quantity	Calories	Carbo-hydrates (grams)
(Van de Kamp's)	1 piece (1½ oz.)	174	D.N.A.
Chocolate:			
(Hostess) 10 to pkg.	1 piece (1.2 oz.)	139	18.2
Coated gem (Hostess)	1 piece (.6 oz.)	110	D.N.A.
Long John (Van de Kamp's)	1 piece (2.1 oz.)	179	D.N.A.
Cruller (Van de Kamp's)	1 piece (1½ oz.)	161	D.N.A.
Cruller, old-fashioned (Hostess)	1 piece	100	D.N.A.
Powdered, frozen (Morton)	1 piece (.6 oz.)	82	9.2
Sugared (Hostess):			
Regular	1 piece (1.8 oz.)	233	D.N.A.
Gem, mini	1 piece (½ oz.)	95	D.N.A.
Gem, chocolate inside	1 piece (½ oz.)	100	D.N.A.
Sugar & spice, frozen (Morton)	1 piece (.6 oz.)	82	8.6
Yeast-leavened (USDA)	4 oz.	469	42.8
DRAMBUIE LIQUEUR, 80 proof (Hiram Walker)	1 fl. oz.	110	11.0
DR. BROWN'S CEL-RAY TONIC, soft drink	6 fl. oz.	66	16.5
DREAMSICLE (Popsicle Industries)	3 fl. oz.	87	D.N.A.
DR. PEPPER, soft drink:			
Regular	6 fl. oz.	71	17.4
Sugar free	6 fl. oz.	2	.4
DRUM, raw (USDA):			
Freshwater:			
Whole	1 lb. (weighed whole)	143	0.
Meat only	4 oz.	137	0.
Red:			
Whole	1 lb. (weighed whole)	149	0.
Meat only	4 oz.	91	0.

(USDA): United States Department of Agriculture
DNA: Data Not Available
* Prepared as Package Directs

Food and Description	Measure or Quantity	Calories	Carbohydrates (grams)
DUCK, raw (USDA):			
Domesticated:			
Ready-to-cook	1 lb. (weighed with bones)	1213	0.
Meat only	4 oz.	187	0.
Wild:			
Dressed	1 lb. (weighed dressed)	613	0.
Meat only	4 oz.	156	0.
DUTCH CAKE MIX, Double			
Dutch (Pillsbury)	1 oz.	117	21.5

Food and Description	Measure or Quantity	Calories	Carbohydrates (grams)

E

ECLAIR, home recipe, with custard filling & chocolate icing (USDA) | 4 oz. | 271 | 26.3

EEL (USDA):
Raw, meat only | 4 oz. | 264 | 0.
Smoked, meat only | 4 oz. | 374 | 0.

EGG, CHICKEN (USDA)
Raw:

White only	1 large egg (1.2 oz.)	17	.3
White only	1 cup (9 oz.)	130	2.0
Yolk only	1 large egg (.6 oz.)	59	.1
Yolk only	1 cup (8.5 oz.)	835	1.4
Whole, small	1 egg (1.3 oz.)	60	.3
Whole, medium	1 egg (1.5 oz.)	71	.4
Whole, large	1 egg (1.8 oz.)	81	.4
Whole	1 cup (8.8 oz.)	409	2.3
Whole, extra large	1 egg (2 oz.)	94	.5
Whole, jumbo	1 egg (2.3 oz.)	105	.6

Cooked:

Boiled	1 large egg (1.8 oz.)	81	.4
Fried in butter	1 large egg	99	.1
Omelet, mixed with milk & cooked in fat	1 large egg	107	1.5
Poached	1 large egg	78	.4
Scrambled, mixed with milk & cooked in fat	1 large egg	111	1.5
Scrambled, mixed with milk & cooked in fat	1 cup (7.8 oz.)	381	5.3

Dried:

Whole	1 cup (3.8 oz.)	639	4.4
White, powder	1 oz.	105	1.6
Yolk	1 cup (3.4 oz.)	637	2.4

(USDA): United States Department of Agriculture
DNA: Data Not Available
* Prepared as Package Directs

Food and Description	Measure or Quantity	Calories	Carbo-hydrates (grams)
EGG, DUCK, raw (USDA)	1 egg (2.8 oz.)	153	.6
EGG, GOOSE, raw (USDA)	1 egg (5.8 oz.)	303	2.1
EGG, TURKEY, raw (USDA)	1 egg (3.1 oz.)	150	1.5
EGG FOO YOUNG, frozen (Chun King)	6 oz. (½ pkg.)	120	10.9
EGG NOG:			
Dairy:			
(Borden) 4.69% fat	½ cup (4.2 oz.)	132	16.3
(Borden) 6.0% fat	½ cup (4.2 oz.)	151	16.3
(Borden) 8.0% fat	½ cup (4.2 oz.)	171	16.3
(Sealtest) 6% fat	½ cup (4.6 oz.)	174	18.0
(Sealtest) 8% fat	½ cup (4.6 oz.)	192	17.3
With alcohol (Old Mr. Boston) 30 proof	1 fl. oz.	83	4.5
EGGPLANT:			
Raw, whole (USDA)	1 lb. (weighed untrimmed)	92	20.6
Boiled, drained, diced (USDA)	1 cup (7.1 oz.)	38	8.2
Frozen, parmegiana (Buitoni)	4 oz.	189	16.2
Frozen, sticks (Mrs. Paul's)	7-oz. pkg.	516	57.3
EGG ROLL, frozen:			
Lobster & meat (Chun King)	½-oz. roll	26	3.7
Shrimp (Chun King)	½-oz. roll	24	3.8
Shrimp & meat (Chun King)	½-oz. roll	29	3.7
Shrimp (Hung's)	1 piece	131	15.7
EGGSTRA (Tillie Lewis)	½ of 7-oz. dry pkg. (1 large egg)	42	2.2
ELDERBERRY, fresh (USDA):			
Whole	1 lb. (weighed with stems)	307	69.9
Stems removed	4 oz.	82	18.6
ENCHILADA, frozen:			
Beef:			
With cheese (Banquet)	8 pieces (2 lbs.)	1297	136.0
With sauce (Banquet) cookin' bag	6 oz.	259	29.0
With chili gravy (Patio)	2¾-oz. piece (2 in pkg.)	371	23.7

Food and Description	Measure or Quantity	Calories	Carbo-hydrates (grams)
With chili gravy (Patio)	4-oz. piece (8 in pkg.)	185	5.5
Cheese:			
(Patio)	4-oz. piece (2 in pkg.)	130	18.9
(Van de Kamp's)	1 pkg.	387	D.N.A.
Chicken (Van de Kamp's)	1 pkg.	365	D.N.A.
ENCHILADA DINNER, frozen:			
Beef:			
(Banquet)	12½-oz. dinner	467	61.0
(Patio)	12-oz. dinner	757	87.5
(Rosarita)	12-oz. dinner	511	D.N.A.
(Swanson)	15-oz. dinner	561	59.5
Cheese:			
(Banquet)	12½-oz. dinner	482	58.2
(Patio)	12-oz. dinner	591	88.1
(Rosarita)	12-oz. dinner	436	D.N.A.
ENDIVE, BELGIAN or FRENCH (See **CHICORY, WITLOOF**)			
ENDIVE, CURLY, raw (USDA):			
Untrimmed	1 lb. (weighed untrimmed)	80	16.4
Trimmed	½ lb.	45	9.3
Cut up or shredded	1 cup (2.5 oz.)	14	2.9
ESCAROLE, raw (USDA):			
Untrimmed	1 lb. (weighed untrimmed)	80	16.4
Trimmed	½ lb.	46	9.2
Cut up or shredded	1 cup (2.5 oz.)	14	2.9
EULACHON or SMELT, raw, meat only (USDA)	4 oz.	134	0.
EXTRACT (See individual listings)			

(USDA): United States Department of Agriculture
DNA: Data Not Available
* Prepared as Package Directs

Food and Description	Measure or Quantity	Calories	Carbo-hydrates (grams)

F

FARINA (see also *CREAM OF WHEAT*):
  Regular:
    Dry:

(USDA)	1 cup (6 oz.)	627	130.1
Cream, enriched (H-O)	1 cup (6.2 oz.)	635	135.9
Cream, enriched (H-O)	1 T.	40	8.5
(Pearls of Wheat)	1 cup	608	128.6
Cooked:			
*(USDA)	1 cup (8.4 oz.)	100	20.7
*(USDA)	4 oz.	48	9.9
*(Quaker)	1 cup (1 oz. dry)	100	22.2
Quick-cooking (USDA):			
Dry	1 oz.	103	21.2
Cooked	1 cup (8.6 oz.)	105	21.8
Instant-cooking (USDA):			
Dry	1 oz.	103	21.2
Cooked	4 oz.	62	12.9

FAT, COOKING, vegetable:

(USDA)	1 cup (7.1 oz.)	1768	0.
(USDA)	1 T. (.4 oz.)	106	0.
Snowdrift	1 T.	110	0.
Light Spry	¼ lb.	1002	0.
Light Spry	1 T. (.4 oz.)	94	0.

FENNEL LEAVES, raw
  (USDA):

Untrimmed	1 lb. (weighed untrimmed)	118	21.5
Trimmed	4 oz.	32	5.8

FESTIVAL MAIN MEAL MEAT, Canned (Wilson Sinclair):

Beef roast	3 oz.	100	0.
Corned beef brisket	3 oz.	135	0.
Ham	3 oz.	129	.8
Picnic	3 oz.	137	.8
Pork loin, smoked	3 oz.	114	.8

Food and Description	Measure or Quantity	Calories	Carbo-hydrates (grams)
Pork roast	3 oz.	133	0.
Turkey & dressing	3 oz.	159	8.5
Turkey roast	3 oz.	87	0.
FIG:			
Fresh			
(USDA)	1 lb.	363	92.1
Small (USDA)	1.3-oz. fig (1½" dia.)	30	7.7
Candied (USDA)	1 oz.	85	20.9
Canned, regular pack (USDA):			
Light syrup, solids & liq.	4 oz.	74	19.1
Heavy syrup, solids & liq.	3 figs & 2 T. syrup (4 oz.)	96	24.9
Heavy syrup, solids & liq.	½ cup (4.4 oz.)	106	27.5
Extra heavy syrup, solids & liq.	4 oz.	117	30.3
Canned, unsweetened or dietetic pack:			
Water pack, solids & liq. (USDA)	4 oz.	54	14.1
Kadota, solids & liq. (Diet Delight)	½ cup (4.4 oz.)	76	18.2
Whole, unsweetened (S and W) *Nutradiet*	6 figs (3.5 oz.)	52	12.7
Dehydrated, white, slices (Vacu-Dry)	1 oz.	98	24.4
Dried:			
(USDA)	4 oz.	311	7.8
Chopped (USDA)	1 cup (6 oz.)	469	118.2
(USDA)	.7-oz. fig (2" x 1")	58	14.5
FIG JUICE, *Real Fig*	½ cup (4.5 oz.)	61	15.8
FILBERT or HAZELNUT (USDA):			
Whole	1 lb. (weighed in shell)	1323	34.9
Shelled	1 oz.	180	4.7

(USDA): United States Department of Agriculture
DNA: Data Not Available
* Prepared as Package Directs

Food and Description	Measure or Quantity	Calories	Carbo-hydrates (grams)
FINNAN HADDIE, meat only (USDA)	4 oz.	117	0.
FISH (See individual listings)			
FISH, BREADED, frozen:			
Raw (Sea Pass)	4 oz.	129	D.N.A.
Precooked (Sea Pass)	4 oz.	150	D.N.A.
FISH CAKE:			
Home recipe, fried (USDA)	2 oz.	98	5.3
Frozen:			
Fried, reheated (USDA)	2 oz.	153	9.8
(Commodore)	2 oz.	102	9.8
(Mrs. Paul's)	2 oz.	156	10.0
FISH CRISPS, frozen (Commodore)	1 oz.	64	D.N.A.
FISH DINNER, frozen:			
(Morton)	8¾-oz. dinner	375	42.4
With French fries (Swanson)	9¾-oz. dinner	429	41.4
FISH FILLETS (Mrs. Paul's)	2 oz.	102	3.8
FISH FLAKES, canned (USDA)	4 oz.	126	0.
FISH LOAF, home recipe (USDA)	4 oz.	141	8.3
FISH STICK, frozen:			
Cooked, commercial, 3¾″ x 1″ x ½″ sticks (USDA)	10 sticks (8-oz. pkg.)	400	14.8
Cooked (Booth)	1 oz.	50	1.8
(Commodore)	1 oz.	50	1.9
(Mrs. Paul's)	1 oz.	51	1.9
Precooked, breaded (Sea Pass)	1 oz.	41	D.N.A.
FLICK, instant (Ghirardelli)	1 T.	47	10.8
FLIP, soft drink (Dad's)	6 fl. oz.	75	18.4

Food and Description	Measure or Quantity	Calories	Carbohydrates (grams)
FLORIDA PUNCH, fruit drink (Hi-C)	6 fl. oz.	98	24.1
FLOUNDER:			
Raw:			
Whole (USDA)	1 lb. (weighed whole)	118	0.
Meat only (USDA)	4 oz.	90	0.
Meat only (Booth)	4 oz.	90	0.
Baked (USDA)	4 oz.	229	0.
Frozen, dinner, low calorie (Taste O'Sea)	1 dinner	200	D.N.A.
Frozen, dinner (Weight Watchers)	16-oz. dinner	296	28.8
Frozen, & broccoli (Weight Watchers)	8-oz. luncheon	139	14.0
FLOUR:			
Buckwheat, dark, sifted (USDA)	1 cup (3.5 oz.)	326	70.6
Buckwheat, light, sifted (USDA)	1 cup (3.5 oz.)	340	77.9
Carob or St. John's-bread (USDA)	1 oz.	51	22.9
Chestnut (USDA)	1 oz.	103	21.6
Corn (USDA)	1 cup (3.9 oz.)	405	84.5
Cottonseed (USDA)	1 oz.	101	9.4
Fish, from whole fish (USDA)	1 oz.	95	0.
Lima bean (USDA)	1 oz.	97	17.9
Potato (USDA)	1 oz.	100	22.7
Rye:			
Light:			
Unsifted, spooned (USDA)	1 cup (3.6 oz.)	361	78.7
Sifted, spooned (USDA)	1 cup (3.1 oz.)	314	68.6
Medium (USDA)	1 oz.	99	21.2
Dark:			
(USDA)	1 oz.	93	19.3

(USDA): United States Department of Agriculture
DNA: Data Not Available
* Prepared as Package Directs

Food and Description	Measure or Quantity	Calories	Carbo-hydrates (grams)
Unstirred (USDA)	1 cup (4.5 oz.)	419	87.2
Stirred (USDA)	1 cup (4.5 oz.)	415	86.5
Soybean, defatted, stirred (USDA)	1 cup (3.6 oz.)	329	38.5
Soybean, high fat (USDA)	1 oz.	108	9.4
Sunflower seed, partially defatted (USDA)	1 oz.	96	10.7
Wheat:			
All-purpose:			
(USDA)	1 oz.	103	21.6
Unsifted, dipped (USDA)	1 cup (5 oz.)	521	108.8
Unsifted, spooned (USDA)	1 cup (4.4 oz.)	459	95.9
Sifted, spooned (USDA)	1 cup (4.1 oz.)	422	88.3
Bread:			
(USDA)	1 oz.	103	21.2
Unsifted, dipped (USDA)	1 cup (4.8 oz.)	496	101.6
Unsifted, spooned (USDA)	1 cup (4.3 oz.)	449	91.9
Sifted, spooned (USDA)	1 cup (4.1 oz.)	427	87.4
Cake:			
(USDA)	1 oz.	103	22.5
Unsifted, dipped (USDA)	1 cup (4.2 oz.)	433	94.5
Unsifted, spooned (USDA)	1 cup (3.9 oz.)	404	88.1
Sifted, spooned (USDA)	1 cup (3.5 oz.)	360	78.6
Gluten:			
(USDA)	1 oz.	107	13.4
Unsifted, dipped (USDA)	1 cup (5 oz.)	537	67.0
Unsifted, spooned (USDA)	1 cup (4.8 oz.)	510	63.7
Sifted, spooned (USDA)	1 cup (4.8 oz.)	514	64.2
Self-rising:			
(USDA)	1 oz.	100	21.0
Unsifted, dipped (USDA)	1 cup (4.6 oz.)	458	96.5
Unsifted, spooned (USDA)	1 cup (4.5 oz.)	447	94.2
Sifted, spooned (USDA)	1 cup (3.7 oz.)	373	78.7
Whole (USDA)	1 oz.	94	20.1

Food and Description	Measure or Quantity	Calories	Carbohydrates (grams)
Whole, stirred, spooned (USDA)	1 cup (4.8 oz.)	456	97.3
Gold Medal, regular (Betty Crocker)	1 oz.	101	21.2
Gold Medal, self-rising (Betty Crocker)	1 oz.	96	20.7
Red Band, enriched (Betty Crocker)	1 oz.	103	22.0
Red Band, self-rising (Betty Crocker)	1 oz.	98	21.5
Softasilk (Betty Crocker)	1 oz.	102	22.2
Wondra, enriched (Betty Crocker)	1 oz.	101	21.0
FOLLE BLANCHE WINE (Louis M. Martini) 12.5% alcohol	3 fl. oz.	90	.2
FOURNIER NATURE (Gold Seal) 12% alcohol	3 fl. oz.	82	.4
FRANKFURTER:			
Raw:			
All kinds (USDA)	1 frankfurter (10 per lb.)	140	.8
All meat (USDA)	1 frankfurter (10 per lb.)	134	1.1
With cereal (USDA)	1 frankfurter (10 per lb.)	112	<.1
(American Kosher)	1 frankfurter	125	D.N.A.
All meat (Armour Star)	1 frankfurter (10 per lb.)	155	0.
All beef (Eckrich)	1 frankfurter (1.6 oz.)	152	D.N.A.
All meat (Eckrich)	1 frankfurter (1.6 oz.)	152	D.N.A.
Pure beef (Oscar Mayer)	1 frankfurter (1.6 oz.)	143	1.4
(Vienna)	1 frankfurter	121	1.0
All beef (Wilson)	1 frankfurter (1.6 oz.)	136	.8

(USDA): United States Department of Agriculture
DNA: Data Not Available
* Prepared as Package Directs

Food and Description	Measure or Quantity	Calories	Carbohydrates (grams)
Skinless (Wilson)	1 frankfurter (1.6 oz.)	140	.8
Cooked, all kinds (USDA)	1 frankfurter (10 per lb., raw)	136	.7
Canned (USDA)	2 oz.	125	.1
Canned (Hormel)	12-oz. can	966	2.4
FRANKS & BEANS (See **BEANS & FRANKS**)			
FRANKS-N-BLANKETS, frozen (Durkee)	1 piece (.4 oz.)	45	1.0
FRENCH TOAST, frozen (Aunt Jemima)	1 slice (1.5 oz.)	88	13.9
FRESCA, soft drink	6 fl. oz.	<1	<.1
FROG LEGS, raw (USDA):			
Bone in	1 lb. (weighed with bone)	215	0.
Meat only	4 oz.	83	0.
FROOT LOOPS, cereal (Kellogg's)	1 cup (1 oz.)	116	24.8
FROSTED SHAKE, any flavor (Borden)	9¼-oz. can	320	43.0
FROSTING (See **CAKE ICING**)			
FROSTY O's, cereal	1 cup (1 oz.)	112	24.0
FROZEN CUSTARD (See **ICE CREAM**)			
FRUIT BOWL SOFT DRINK:			
(Hires)	6 fl. oz.	90	22.5
(Nedick's)	6 fl. oz.	90	22.5
FRUIT CAKE (USDA):			
Dark, home recipe	1.1-oz. piece (2″ x 2″ x ½″)	114	17.9

Food and Description	Measure or Quantity	Calories	Carbohydrates (grams)
Light, home recipe	1.1-oz. piece (2" x 2" x ½")	117	17.2
FRUIT COCKTAIL:			
Canned, regular pack, solids & liq.:			
Light syrup (USDA)	4 oz.	68	17.8
Heavy syrup (USDA)	½ cup (4.5 oz.)	97	25.2
Heavy syrup (Del Monte)	½ cup (4.3 oz.)	87	23.5
Extra heavy syrup (USDA)	4 oz.	104	26.9
With 2 tablespoons liq. (Dole)	½ cup	72	D.N.A.
(Hunt's)	½ cup (4.5 oz.)	89	23.9
Canned, unsweetened or dietetic pack, solids & liq.:			
Water pack (USDA)	4 oz.	42	11.0
Solids & liq. (Diet Delight)	½ cup (4.4 oz.)	67	16.0
With 2 tablespoons liq. (Dole)	½ cup	36	D.N.A.
(Libby's)	4 oz.	36	11.0
Unsweetened (S and W) *Nutradiet*	4 oz.	40	12.3
Dehydrated, *Fruit Galaxy* (Vacu-Dry)	1 oz.	96	25.2
FRUITFORT, cereal	1 oz.	111	D.N.A.
FRUIT ICE MIX (See individual sherbet flavors)			
FRUIT, MIXED, frozen, quick thaw (Birds Eye)	½ cup (5 oz.)	111	28.4
FRUIT PUNCH:			
Canned (Del Monte)	6 fl. oz.	83	22.6
*Mix (Wyler's)	6 fl. oz.	64	15.8
FRUIT SALAD:			
Bottled, chilled (Kraft)	4 oz.	57	13.3

(USDA): United States Department of Agriculture
DNA: Data Not Available
* Prepared as Package Directs

Food and Description	Measure or Quantity	Calories	Carbo-hydrates (grams)
Canned, regular pack, solids & liq.:			
Light syrup (USDA)	4 oz.	67	17.6
Heavy syrup (USDA)	½ cup (4.3 oz.)	85	22.0
Extra heavy syrup (USDA)	4 oz.	102	26.5
Tropical (Del Monte)	½ cup (4.4 oz.)	110	29.2
Canned, unsweetened or dietetic pack:			
Water pack, solids & liq. (USDA)	4 oz.	40	10.3
Solids & liq. (Diet Delight)	½ cup (4.4 oz.)	67	16.1
(White Rose)	4 oz.	42	10.1
FRUIT-SICLE (Popsicle Industries)	2½ fl. oz.	59	D.N.A.
FUDGE CAKE MIX:			
*Butter recipe (Duncan Hines)	¹⁄₁₂ of cake (3.3 oz.)	283	35.2
*Cherry (Betty Crocker)	¹⁄₁₂ of cake	199	35.8
Chocolate (Pillsbury)	1 oz.	120	22.1
*Dark chocolate (Betty Crocker)	¹⁄₁₂ of cake	198	35.2
Macaroon (Pillsbury)	1 oz.	124	21.2
*Marble (Duncan Hines)	¹⁄₁₂ of cake (2.7 oz.)	202	35.0
*Sour cream, chocolate flavor (Betty Crocker)	¹⁄₁₂ of cake	195	35.4
Sour cream flavor (Pillsbury)	1 oz.	118	21.2
Toffee, batter cake (Pillsbury)	1 oz.	119	21.7
FUDGE PUDDING (Thank You)	½ cup (4.5 oz.)	202	34.3
FUDGSICLE, chocolate (Popsicle Industries)	2½ fl. oz.	110	22.4

Food and Description	Measure or Quantity	Calories	Carbo- hydrates (grams)

G

GARBANZO, dry (See
  CHICK-PEA, dry)

GARBANZO SOUP, canned
  (Hormel) | 15-oz. can | 459 | 30.6

GARLIC, raw (USDA):
  Whole | 2 oz. (weighed with skin) | 68 | 15.4
  Peeled | 1 oz. | 39 | 8.7

GARLIC SPREAD (Lawry's) | 1 T. (.5 oz.) | 79 | 1.2

GATORADE, soft drink | 6 fl. oz. (6.3 oz.) | 53 | 16.0

GAZPACHO SOUP, canned
  (Crosse & Blackwell) | ½ can (6½ oz.) | 61 | 6.8

GEFILTE FISH, canned:
  (Horowitz-Margareten) | 1 piece | 75 | D.N.A.
  (Manischewitz) 4-portion can | 1 piece (3.7 oz.) | 100 | 3.9
  (Manischewitz) 2-lb. jar | 1 piece (2.4 oz.) | 64 | 2.5
  Fish balls (Manischewitz) | 1 piece (1.5 oz.) | 40 | 1.6
  Fishlet (Manischewitz) | 1 piece (7 grams) | 70 | .3
  Whitefish & pike
    (Manischewitz):
    4-portion can | 1 piece (3.8 oz.) | 87 | 3.3
    2-lb. jar | 1 piece (1.7 oz.) | 40 | 1.5

GELATIN, unflavored, dry:
  (USDA) | 1 envelope (7 grams) | 23 | 0.
  (Knox) | 1 envelope (7 grams) | 28 | 0.

(USDA): United States Department of Agriculture
DNA: Data Not Available
* Prepared as Package Directs

Food and Description	Measure or Quantity	Calories	Carbo-hydrates (grams)
GELATIN DESSERT POWDER:			
Regular:			
(USDA)	3-oz. pkg.	315	74.8
*Prepared (USDA)	4 oz.	67	16.0
*Prepared (USDA)	½ cup (4.2 oz.)	71	16.9
*Prepared with fruit added (USDA)	4 oz.	76	18.6
*Prepared with fruit added (USDA)	½ cup (4.2 oz.)	81	19.8
*All fruit flavors (Jell-O)	½ cup (4.9 oz.)	81	18.2
*All flavors (Jells Best)	½ cup	80	18.7
*All flavors (Royal)	½ cup (4.2 oz.)	82	18.4
Dietetic or low calorie:			
*All flavors except orange (D-Zerta)	½ cup (4.3 oz.)	8	Tr.
*Orange (D-Zerta)	½ cup (4.3 oz.)	9	Tr.
*All flavors (Dia-Mel)	4 oz.	11	0.
GELATIN DRINK, any flavor (Knox)	1 envelope (.7 oz.)	79	14.0
GERMAN DINNER, frozen (Swanson)	11-oz. dinner	405	42.2
GEVREY-CHAMBERTIN, French red Burgundy (Cruse) 12% alcohol	3 fl. oz.	72	D.N.A.
GEWURZTRAMINER WINE:			
(Louis M. Martini) 12.5% alcohol	3 fl. oz.	90	.2
(Willm) Alsatian, 11–14% alcohol	3 fl. oz.	66	3.6
(Willm) *Clos Gaensbronnel,* 11–14% alcohol	3 fl. oz.	66	3.6
GIN, Unflavored (See **DISTILLED LIQUOR**)			
GIN, FLAVORED:			
Lemon (Old Mr. Boston) 70 proof	1 fl. oz.	76	1.4

Food and Description	Measure or Quantity	Calories	Carbohydrates (grams)
Mint (Leroux) 70 proof	1 fl. oz.	70	2.8
Mint (Old Mr. Boston) 70 proof	1 fl. oz.	100	8.0
Orange (Leroux) 70 proof	1 fl. oz.	70	2.8
Orange (Old Mr. Boston) 70 proof	1 fl. oz.	76	1.4
GIN, SLOE:			
(Bols) 66 proof	1 fl. oz.	85	4.7
(Garnier) 60 proof	1 fl. oz.	83	8.5
(Hiram Walker) 60 proof	1 fl. oz.	68	4.8
(Leroux) 60 proof	1 fl. oz.	74	6.0
(Old Mr. Boston) 42 proof	1 fl. oz.	50	2.0
(Old Mr. Boston) 70 proof	1 fl. oz.	76	1.4
GINGER ALE, soft drink:			
Sweetened:			
(Canada Dry)	6 fl. oz.	64	16.5
(Clicquot Club)	6 fl. oz.	62	15.0
(Cott)	6 fl. oz.	62	15.0
(Dr. Brown's)	6 fl. oz.	60	15.0
(Fanta)	6 fl. oz.	62	15.9
(Hoffman)	6 fl. oz.	58	14.6
(Key Food)	6 fl. oz.	60	15.0
(Kirsch)	6 fl. oz.	59	14.8
(Mission)	6 fl. oz.	62	15.0
(Schweppes)	6 fl. oz.	66	16.3
(Shasta)	6 fl. oz.	65	16.5
(Vernors)	6 fl. oz.	70	16.8
(Waldbaum)	6 fl. oz.	60	15.0
(White Rock)	6 fl. oz.	62	D.N.A.
(Yukon Club) golden	6 fl. oz.	64	16.1
Low calorie:			
(Dr. Brown's)	6 fl. oz.	1	.2
(Hoffman)	6 fl. oz.	1	.2
(No-Cal)	6 fl. oz.	2	<.1
(Shasta)	6 fl. oz.	<1	<.1
(Vernors)	6 fl. oz.	1	<.1

(USDA): United States Department of Agriculture
DNA: Data Not Available
* Prepared as Package Directs

Food and Description	Measure or Quantity	Calories	Carbo-hydrates (grams)
GINGER BEER, soft drink:			
(Canada Dry)	6 fl. oz.	71	18.4
(Schweppes)	6 fl. oz.	72	17.6
GINGERBREAD, home recipe (USDA)	1.9-oz. piece (2″ x 2″ x 2″)	174	28.6
GINGERBREAD MIX:			
Dry (USDA)	4 oz.	482	88.7
* Prepared (USDA)	⅑ of 8″ sq. (2.2 oz.)	174	32.2
(Betty Crocker)	14.5-oz. pkg.	1696	323.4
*(Betty Crocker)	⅑ of cake	171	36.1
*(Dromedary)	1.2-oz. piece (2″ x 2″)	100	18.8
(Pillsbury)	1 oz.	110	22.1
GINGER, CANDIED, (USDA)	1 oz.	96	24.7
GINGER ROOT, fresh (USDA):			
With skin	1 oz.	13	2.5
Without skin	1 oz.	14	2.7
GIN SOUR COCKTAIL (Calvert) 60 proof	3 fl. oz.	195	10.4
GOLD-O-MINT LIQUEUR (Leroux) 25 proof	1 fl. oz.	110	15.2
GOOD HUMOR:			
Bar, ice cream:			
Chocolate chip	1 piece (3 fl. oz.)	239	D.N.A.
Chocolate chip candy, *Super Humor*	1 piece	383	D.N.A.
Chocolate eclair	1 piece (3 fl. oz.)	217	D.N.A.
Chocolate fudge cake, *Super Humor*	1 piece	345	D.N.A.
Chocolate malt	1 piece	205	13.6
Toasted almond	1 piece (3 fl. oz.)	234	D.N.A.
Vanilla	1 piece	202	13.2
Cone:			
Ice cream, chocolate burst	1 piece	165	D.N.A.
Ice milk, chocolate	1 piece	88	D.N.A.

Food and Description	Measure or Quantity	Calories	Carbo-hydrates (grams)
Ice milk, vanilla	1 piece	85	D.N.A.
Cup:			
Ice:			
Bon Joy Swirl	1 piece	138	D.N.A.
Italian	1 piece	232	D.N.A.
Venetian	1 piece	115	D.N.A.
Ice cream:			
Chocolate	3 oz.	113	D.N.A.
Chocolate	5 oz.	189	D.N.A.
Vanilla	3 oz.	110	11.6
Vanilla	5 oz.	183	D.N.A.
Frostee Humor bar	1 piece	150	D.N.A.
Frostee shake	1 piece	287	D.N.A.
Humorette	1 piece	103	D.N.A.
Ice Stix:			
Chocolate	1 piece	119	D.N.A.
Chocolate, double	1 piece	151	D.N.A.
Fruit	1 piece	89	D.N.A.
Fruit, double	1 piece	138	D.N.A.
Lollie Jets	1 piece	109	D.N.A.
Wahoos	1 piece	52	D.N.A.
X-5 Jetstars	1 piece	57	D.N.A.
Pint, deluxe French	1 oz.	50	D.N.A.
Sandwich, without crackers:			
Ice cream, grocery pack:			
Chocolate	1 piece	53	D.N.A.
Vanilla	1 piece	51	D.N.A.
Ice milk	1 piece	88	D.N.A.
Sundae:			
Bittersweet	1 piece	282	D.N.A.
Chocolate nut fudge			
supreme	1 piece	448	D.N.A.
Strawberry	1 piece	221	D.N.A.
Whammy:			
Fruit ice	1 piece (1¾ fl. oz.)	40	D.N.A.
Ice cream	1 piece (1¾ fl. oz.)	140	D.N.A.
Ice milk	1 piece (1¾ fl. oz.)	128	D.N.A.

(USDA): United States Department of Agriculture
DNA: Data Not Available
* Prepared as Package Directs

Food and Description	Measure or Quantity	Calories	Carbohydrates (grams)
GOOSE, domesticated (USDA):			
Raw	1 lb. (weighed ready-to-cook)	1172	0.
Roasted, meat & skin	4 oz.	500	0.
Roasted, meat only	4 oz.	264	0.
GOOSEBERRY (USDA):			
Fresh	1 lb.	177	44.0
Fresh	1 cup (5.3 oz.)	58	14.6
Canned, water pack, solids & liq.	4 oz.	29	7.5
GOOSE, GIZZARD, raw (USDA)	4 oz.	158	0.
GOULASH DINNER (Chef Boy-Ar-Dee)	7⅛-oz. pkg.	262	32.4
GRAACHER HIMMELREICH, German Moselle (Julius Kayser) 10% alcohol	3 fl. oz.	60	2.5
GRAHAM CRACKER (See CRACKER)			
GRANADILLA (See PASSION FRUIT)			
GRAPE:			
Fresh:			
American type (slip skin), Concord, Delaware, Niagara, Catawba & Scuppernong:			
(USDA)	½ lb. (weighed with stem, skin & seeds)	98	22.4
(USDA)	½ cup (2.7 oz.)	52	11.9
(USDA)	3½" x 3" bunch (3.5 oz.)	43	9.9
European type (adherent skin), Malaga, Muscat, Thompson seedless,			

Food and Description	Measure or Quantity	Calories	Carbo-hydrates (grams)
Emperor & Flame Tokay: (USDA)	½ lb. (weighed with stem & seeds)	135	34.9
Whole (USDA)	20 grapes (¾″ dia.)	54	13.8
Whole (USDA)	½ cup (3. oz.)	58	15.1
Halves (USDA)	½ cup (3. oz.)	58	14.9
Canned, solids & liq. (USDA):			
Thompson seedless, heavy syrup	4 oz.	87	22.7
Thompson seedless, water pack	4 oz.	58	15.4
GRAPEADE, chilled (Sealtest)	6 fl. oz.	96	24.2
GRAPE DRINK (Hi-C)	6 fl. oz.	88	21.8
***GRAPE DRINK MIX:**			
(Salada)	6 fl. oz.	80	19.4
(Wyler's)	6 fl. oz.	64	15.8
GRAPE JAM, dietetic			
(Dia-Mel)	1 T.	22	5.4
GRAPE JELLY, dietetic or low calorie:			
(Dia-Mel)	1 T.	22	5.4
Concord (Diet Delight)	1 T. (.6 oz.)	21	5.3
(Kraft)	1 oz.	34	8.4
(Slenderella)	1 T. (.6 oz.)	22	5.6
(Tillie Lewis)	1 T. (.5 oz.)	10	2.4
GRAPE JUICE:			
Canned:			
(USDA)	½ cup (4.4 oz.)	83	20.9
(Heinz)	5½-fl.-oz. can	130	31.3
(Seneca)	½ cup (4.4 oz.)	115	29.0
Sweetened (Seneca)	½ cup	104	26.0

(USDA): United States Department of Agriculture
DNA: Data Not Available
* Prepared as Package Directs

Food and Description	Measure or Quantity	Calories	Carbohydrates (grams)
Unsweetened (S and W) Nutradiet	4 oz. (by wt.)	68	17.5
Frozen, concentrate, sweetened:			
(USDA)	6-fl.-oz. can	395	100.0
*Diluted (USDA)	½ cup (4.4 oz.)	66	16.6
*(Minute Maid)	½ cup (4.2 oz.)	66	16.7
*(Seneca)	½ cup (4.4 oz.)	66	17.2
*(Snow Crop)	½ cup (4.2 oz.)	66	16.7
GRAPE JUICE DRINK, canned:			
Approx. 30% grape juice (USDA)	1 cup (8.8 oz.)	135	34.5
Grape-apple (BC)	6 fl. oz.	108	D.N.A.
GRAPE-NUTS, cereal	¼ cup (1 oz.)	104	23.0
GRAPE-NUTS FLAKES, cereal	⅔ cup (1 oz.)	101	22.0
GRAPE PIE (Tastykake)	4-oz. pie	369	51.8
GRAPE SOFT DRINK: Sweetened:			
(Canada Dry)	6 fl. oz.	95	23.9
(Clicquot Club)	6 fl. oz.	105	25.1
(Cott)	6 fl. oz.	105	25.1
(Dr. Brown's)	6 fl. oz.	87	21.9
(Dr. Pepper)	6 fl. oz.	102	25.8
(Fanta)	6 fl. oz.	92	23.9
Grapette	6 fl. oz.	91	23.4
(Hoffman)	6 fl. oz.	93	23.2
(Key Food)	6 fl. oz.	87	21.9
(Mission)	6 fl. oz.	105	25.1
(Nedick's)	6 fl. oz.	93	23.2
(Shasta)	6 fl. oz.	88	22.2
(Waldbaum)	6 fl. oz.	87	21.9
(White Rock)	6 fl. oz.	89	D.N.A.
(Yoo-Hoo)	6 fl. oz.	90	18.0
High-protein (Yoo-Hoo)	6 fl oz.	114	24.6
(Yukon Club)	6 fl. oz.	93	23.2
Low calorie:			
(Hoffman)	6 fl. oz.	2	.4

Food and Description	Measure or Quantity	Calories	Carbo-hydrates (grams)
(No-Cal)	6 fl. oz.	2	0.
(Shasta)	6 fl. oz.	<1	.1
GRAPE SYRUP, dietetic			
(No-Cal)	1 tsp. (5 grams)	<1	0.
GRAPEFRUIT:			
Fresh:			
White:			
Seeded type (USDA)	1 lb. (weighed with seeds & skin)	84	22.0
Seedless type (USDA)	1 lb. (weighed with skin)	87	22.4
Seeded type (USDA)	½ med. grapefruit (3¾″ dia., 8.5 oz.)	44	11.7
(Sunkist)	½ grapefruit (8.5 oz.)	44	11.0
Sections, seedless (USDA)	1 cup (7 oz.)	78	20.2
Pink and red:			
Seeded type (USDA)	1 lb. (weighed with seeds & skin)	87	22.6
Seedless type (USDA)	1 lb. (weighed with skin)	93	24.1
Seeded type (USDA)	½ med. grapefruit, (3¾″ dia., 8.5 oz.)	46	12.0
Bottled, chilled sections (Kraft)	4 oz.	53	12.5
Canned, syrup pack, solids & liq. (USDA)	½ cup (4.5 oz.)	90	22.8
Canned, unsweetened or dietetic pack: solids & liq.			
Water pack (USDA)	½ cup (4.2 oz.)	36	9.1
Solids & liq. (Diet Delight)	½ cup (4.3 oz.)	41	9.4
(Tillie Lewis)	½ cup (4.4 oz.)	45	10.4
GRAPEFRUIT DRINK			
(Sealtest)	6 fl. oz.	80	20.0

(USDA): United States Department of Agriculture
DNA: Data Not Available
* Prepared as Package Directs

Food and Description	Measure or Quantity	Calories	Carbohydrates (grams)
GRAPEFRUIT JUICE:			
Fresh, pink, red or white, all varieties (USDA)	½ cup (4.3 oz.)	48	11.3
Bottled, chilled, unsweetened (Kraft)	½ cup (4.3 oz.)	48	11.1
Canned:			
Sweetened:			
(USDA)	½ cup (4.4 oz.)	66	16.0
(Del Monte)	½ cup (4.3 oz.)	48	12.7
(Heinz)	5½-fl.-oz. can	73	16.1
(Stokely-Van Camp)	½ cup (4.4 oz.)	67	16.2
(Treesweet)	½ cup	62	D.N.A.
Unsweetened:			
(USDA)	½ cup (4.4 oz.)	51	12.2
(Del Monte)	½ cup (4.3 oz.)	49	11.6
(Diet Delight)	½ cup (4 oz.)	39	9.5
(Heinz)	5½-fl.-oz. can	56	11.8
Pink (Texsun)	½ cup	52	16.1
Frozen, concentrate:			
Sweetened:			
(USDA)	6-fl.-oz. can	348	84.8
*Diluted with 3 parts water (USDA)	½ cup (4.4 oz.)	58	14.1
*(Minute Maid)	½ cup (4.2 oz.)	57	14.9
*(Snow Crop)	½ cup (4.2 oz.)	57	14.9
*(Treesweet)	½ cup	62	D.N.A.
Unsweetened:			
(USDA)	6-fl.-oz. can	300	71.6
*Diluted with 3 parts water (USDA)	½ cup (4.4 oz.)	51	12.2
*(Birds Eye)	½ cup (4.2 oz.)	48	12.9
*(Florida Diet)	½ cup (4.3 oz.)	50	10.7
*(Minute Maid)	½ cup (4.2 oz.)	50	12.2
*(7L)	½ cup	50	12.0
*(Snow Crop)	½ cup (4.2 oz.)	50	12.2
Dehydrated, crystals:			
(USDA)	4-oz. can	429	102.4
*Reconstituted (USDA)	½ cup (4.4 oz.)	50	11.9

GRAPEFRUIT-ORANGE JUICE (See **ORANGE-GRAPEFRUIT JUICE**)

Food and Description	Measure or Quantity	Calories	Carbohydrates (grams)
GRAPEFRUIT PEEL, CANDIED:			
(USDA)	1 oz.	90	22.9
(Liberty)	1 oz.	93	22.6
GRAPEFRUIT SOFT DRINK:			
Sweetened, golden (Clicquot Club)	6 fl. oz.	83	20.0
Sweetened (Fanta)	6 fl. oz.	84	21.5
Low calorie, pink:			
(Hoffman)	6 fl. oz.	2	.4
(No-Cal)	6 fl. oz.	2	0.
(Shasta)	6 fl. oz.	<1	.1
GRAVES WINE (See also individual regional, vineyard or brand names)			
(Barton & Guestier) 12.5% alcohol	3 fl. oz.	65	.6
(Cruse) 11.5% alcohol	3 fl. oz.	69	D.N.A.
GRAVY, canned:			
Beef (Franco-American)	¼ cup	44	3.6
Chicken (Franco-American)	¼ cup	51	3.2
Chicken giblet (Franco-American)	¼ cup	28	2.8
Giblet (Lynden)	7¾-oz. can	264	16.0
Mushroom (B in B)	1 T.	11	D.N.A.
Mushroom (Franco-American)	¼ cup	27	2.8
GRAVY MASTER	1 fl. oz. (1.3 oz.)	49	8.5
GRAVY with MEAT or TURKEY, canned or frozen:			
Beef chunks (Bunker Hill)	15-oz. can	788	16.0
Chopped beef (Bunker Hill)	10½-oz. can	516	10.0
Sliced beef (Bunker Hill)	15-oz. can	716	16.0

(USDA): United States Department of Agriculture
DNA: Data Not Available
* Prepared as Package Directs

Food and Description	Measure or Quantity	Calories	Carbohydrates (grams)
Sliced beef, buffet, frozen (Banquet)	2 lb.	956	21.2
Sliced beef, cookin' bag, frozen (Banquet)	5 oz.	158	4.2
Sliced beef liver (Bunker Hill)	15-oz. can	398	30.0
Sliced turkey, buffet, frozen (Banquet)	2 lb.	677	27.0
GRAVY MIX:			
Beef:			
(Swiss)	1¼-oz. pkg.	107	22.6
(Swiss)	⅞-oz. pkg.	75	15.8
*(Wyler's)	2-oz. serving	25	3.9
Brown:			
*(Durkee)	1 cup (.9-oz. pkg.)	96	11.2
(French's)	¾-oz. pkg.	72	11.7
*(Kraft)	1 oz.	10	1.4
(Lawry's)	1¼-oz. pkg.	136	16.3
(McCormick)	⅞-oz. pkg.	100	10.0
*(McCormick)	2-oz. serving	25	2.5
Chicken:			
*(Durkee)	1 cup (1.2-oz. pkg.)	96	14.4
(French's)	1¼-oz. pkg.	130	14.7
(Lawry's)	1-oz. pkg.	110	13.6
(McCormick)	⅞-oz. pkg.	95	D.N.A.
*(McCormick)	2-oz. serving	20	3.0
(Swiss)	1¼-oz. pkg.	107	22.7
(Swiss)	⅞-oz. pkg.	75	15.9
*(Wyler's)	2-oz. serving	25	3.7
*Herb (McCormick)	2-oz. serving	22	2.5
Mushroom:			
*(Durkee)	1 cup (1-oz. pkg.)	73	12.1
(French's)	¾-oz. pkg.	62	7.0
(Lawry's)	1.3-oz. pkg.	145	15.6
*(McCormick)	2-oz. serving	17	2.5
*(Wyler's)	2-oz. serving	15	1.8
Onion:			
*(Durkee)	1 cup (1-oz. pkg.)	96	16.5
(French's)	1-oz. pkg.	72	12.3
*(Kraft)	1 oz.	11	1.9
*(McCormick)	2-oz. serving	29	3.5
(Wyler's)	2-oz. serving	17	2.7

Food and Description	Measure or Quantity	Calories	Carbo- hydrates (grams)
GREEN PEA (See **PEA**)			
GRENADINE SYRUP:			
(Garnier) non-alcoholic	1 fl. oz.	103	26.0
(Giroux) non-alcoholic	1 fl. oz.	100	25.0
(Leroux) 25 proof	1 fl. oz.	81	15.2
GRITS (See **HOMINY GRITS**)			
GROUND-CHERRY, Poha or Cape Gooseberry:			
Whole (USDA)	1 lb. (weighed with husks & stems)	221	46.7
Flesh only (USDA)	4 oz.	60	12.7
GROUPER, raw (USDA):			
Whole	1 lb. (weighed whole)	170	0.
Meat only	4 oz.	99	0.
GUAVA, COMMON, fresh:			
Whole (USDA)	1 lb. (weighed untrimmed)	273	66.0
Whole (USDA)	1 guava (2.8 oz.)	48	11.7
Flesh only (USDA)	4 oz.	70	17.0
GUAVA, STRAWBERRY, fresh:			
Whole (USDA)	1 lb. (weighed untrimmed)	289	70.2
Flesh only (USDA)	4 oz.	74	17.9
GUINEA HEN, raw (USDA):			
Ready-to-cook	1 lb. (weighed ready-to-cook)	594	0.
Meat & skin	4 oz.	179	0.

(USDA): United States Department of Agriculture
DNA: Data Not Available
* Prepared as Package Directs

Food and Description	Measure or Quantity	Calories	Carbo-hydrates (grams)

H

HADDOCK:
Raw:

Whole (USDA)	1 lb. (weighed whole)	172	0.
Meat only (USDA)	4 oz.	90	0.
Fried, breaded (USDA)	4" x 3" x ½" fillet (3.5 oz.)	165	5.8
Frozen (Taste O'Sea)	4 oz.	80	0.
*Smoked, canned or not (USDA)	4 oz.	117	0.

HADDOCK MEALS, frozen:

(Banquet)	8.8-oz. dinner	424	44.8
(Swanson)	12¼-oz. dinner	397	36.5
(Taste O'Sea)	12-oz. dinner	245	D.N.A.
(Weight Watchers)	16-oz. dinner	269	19.3
& spinach (Weight Watchers)	8-oz. luncheon	150	7.4

HAKE, raw (USDA):

Whole	1 lb. (weighed whole)	144	0.
Meat only	4 oz.	84	0.

HALF & HALF (milk & cream)
(See **CREAM**)

HALF & HALF SOFT DRINK:
Sweetened:

(Canada Dry)	6 fl. oz.	82	21.4
(Dr. Brown's)	6 fl. oz.	77	19.4
(Hoffman)	6 fl. oz.	77	19.4
(Kirsch)	6 fl. oz.	81	20.3
(Yukon Club)	6 fl. oz.	89	22.1
Low calorie (Hoffman)	6 fl. oz.	3	.8

HALF & HALF WINE:

(Gallo) 20% alcohol	3 fl. oz.	100	5.7
(Lejon) 18.5% alcohol	3 fl. oz.	116	6.7

Food and Description	Measure or Quantity	Calories	Carbo-hydrates (grams)
HALIBUT:			
Atlantic & Pacific:			
Raw:			
Whole (USDA)	1 lb. (weighed whole)	268	0.
Meat only (USDA)	4 oz.	113	0.
Broiled (USDA)	4 oz.	194	0.
Broiled (USDA)	4" x 3" x ½" steak (4.4 oz.)	214	0.
Smoked (USDA)	4 oz.	254	0.
California, raw meat only (USDA)	4 oz.	110	0.
Greenland (See **TURBOT**)			
Frozen, Northern (Van de Kamp's)	1 pkg.	477	D.N.A.
HAM (See also **PORK**):			
Cooked:			
Luncheon meat (USDA)	1 oz.	66	0.
Minced (Oscar Mayer)	1 slice (.9 oz.)	56	.3
Canned:			
(USDA)	1 oz.	55	.3
(Armour Golden Star)	1 oz.	36	0.
(Armour Star)	1 oz.	53	0.
(Hormel)	1 oz. (8-lb. can)	57	.2
(Hormel)	1 oz. (6-lb. can)	44	.2
(Hormel)	1 oz. (4-lb. can)	48	.2
(Hormel)	1 oz. (1-lb. 8-oz. can)	48	.2
(Oscar Mayer) *Jubilee,* boneless	1 lb.	826	4.5
(Wilson)	1 oz.	48	.3
(Wilson) *Tender Made*	1 oz.	44	.3
Chopped or minced, canned:			
(USDA)	1 oz.	65	1.2
(Armour Star)	1 oz.	84	.4
(Hormel)	1 oz. (8-lb. can)	69	.3
(Hormel)	1 oz. (12-oz. can)	71	.4
Deviled, canned:			
(USDA)	1 oz.	100	0.

(USDA): United States Department of Agriculture
DNA: Data Not Available
* Prepared as Package Directs

Food and Description	Measure or Quantity	Calories	Carbo-hydrates (grams)
(USDA)	1 T. (.5 oz.)	46	0.
(Armour Star)	1 oz.	79	0.
(Hormel)	1 oz. (3-oz. can)	73	.2
(Underwood)	1 T. (.5 oz.)	46	Tr.
Frozen, sliced with barbecue sauce (Banquet) cookin' bag	4½ oz.	184	19.0
Smoked, canned (Oscar Mayer)	3 oz.	170	D.N.A.
Spiced or unspiced, canned:			
(USDA)	1 oz.	83	.4
(Hormel)	1 oz. (3-lb. can)	52	.1
(Hormel)	1 oz. (5-lb. can)	78	.4
HAM DINNER, frozen:			
(Banquet)	10-oz. dinner	352	53.2
(Morton)	10-oz. dinner	429	49.1
(Swanson)	10¼-oz. dinner	366	42.1
HAMBURGER (See **BEEF,** Ground)			
HAWAIIAN PUNCH, orange	6 fl. oz.	83	21.6
HAWS, SCARLET, raw (USDA):			
Whole	1 lb. (weighed with core)	316	75.5
Flesh & skin	4 oz.	99	23.6
HAZELNUT (See **FILBERT**)			
HEADCHEESE:			
(USDA)	1 oz.	76	.3
(Sugardale)	1-oz. slice	77	Tr.
HEART (USDA)			
Beef:			
Lean, raw	1 lb.	490	3.2
Lean, braised	4 oz.	213	.8
Lean with visible fat, raw	1 lb.	1148	.5
Lean with visible fat, braised	4 oz.	422	.1
Calf, raw	1 lb.	562	8.2

Food and Description	Measure or Quantity	Calories	Carbo-hydrates (grams)
Calf, braised	4 oz.	236	2.0
Chicken, raw	1 lb.	608	.5
Chicken, simmered	1 heart (5 grams)	9	<.1
Hog, raw	1 lb.	513	1.8
Hog, braised	4 oz.	221	.3
Lamb, raw	1 lb.	735	4.5
Lamb, braised	4 oz.	295	1.1
Turkey, raw	1 lb.	776	.9
Turkey, simmered	4 oz.	245	.2
HERRING (USDA):			
Raw:			
Atlantic, whole	1 lb. (weighed whole)	407	0.
Atlantic, meat only	4 oz.	200	0.
Pacific, meat only	4 oz.	111	0.
Canned:			
Plain, solids & liq.	4 oz.	236	0.
In cream sauce (Vita)	8-oz. jar	397	18.1
In tomato sauce, solids & liq.	4 oz.	200	4.2
In wine sauce, drained (Vita)	8-oz. jar	401	16.6
Pickled, Bismarck type	4 oz.	253	0.
Salted or brined	4 oz.	247	0.
Smoked:			
Bloaters	4 oz.	222	0.
Hard	4 oz.	340	0.
Kippered	4 oz.	239	0.
HICKORY NUT (USDA):			
Whole	1 lb. (weighed in shell)	1068	20.3
Shelled	4 oz.	763	14.5
HI-SPOT, soft drink (Canada Dry)	6 fl. oz.	73	18.8
HO-HO (Hostess):			
2 to pkg.	1 cake (.9 oz.)	103	14.7
10 to carton	1 cake (.9 oz.)	106	15.1

(USDA): United States Department of Agriculture
DNA: Data Not Available
* Prepared as Package Directs

Food and Description	Measure or Quantity	Calories	Carbo-hydrates (grams)
HOMINY GRITS:			
Dry:			
Degermed (USDA)	1 oz.	103	22.1
Degermed (USDA)	½ cup (2.8 oz.)	282	60.9
Instant (Quaker)	8-oz. packet	80	17.6
Cooked:			
Degermed (USDA)	⅔ cup (5.6 oz.)	84	18.0
Enriched (Albers)	⅔ cup	82	17.7
(Aunt Jemima/Quaker)	⅔ cup	100	22.0
HONEY, strained:			
(USDA)	½ cup (5.7 oz.)	496	134.1
(USDA)	1 T. (.7 oz.)	61	16.5
HONEY CAKE (Holland Honey Cake)	½″ slice	63	D.N.A.
HONEYCOMB, cereal (Post)	1 cup	108	25.0
HONEYDEW, fresh (USDA):			
Whole	1 lb. (weighed whole)	94	22.0
Wedge	2″ x 7″ wedge (5.3 oz.)	31	7.2
Flesh only	4 oz.	37	8.7
Flesh only, diced	1 cup (5.9 oz.)	55	12.9
HORSERADISH:			
Raw (USDA):			
Whole	1 lb. (weighed unpared)	288	65.2
Pared	1 oz.	25	5.6
Dehydrated (Heinz)	1 T.	25	5.0
Prepared:			
(USDA)	1 oz.	11	2.7
(Gold's)	1 tsp.	3	D.N.A.
(Kraft)	1 oz.	3	.4
Cream style (Kraft)	1 oz.	9	.7
Oil style (Kraft)	1 oz.	20	.5
*HOT DOG BEAN SOUP			
(Campbell)	1 cup	154	21.0

Food and Description	Measure or Quantity	Calories	Carbohydrates (grams)

HYACINTH BEAN (USDA):
  Young pod, raw:

Whole	1 lb. (weighed untrimmed)	140	29.1
Trimmed	4 oz.	40	8.3
Dry seeds	4 oz.	383	69.2

Food and Description	Measure or Quantity	Calories	Carbohydrates (grams)

I

ICE CREAM and FROZEN CUSTARD (See also listing by flavor or brand name, e.g., **CHOCOLATE ICE CREAM** or *DREAMSICLE* or *GOOD HUMOR*)
Sweetened:

10% fat (USDA)	1 cup (4.7 oz.)	257	27.7
12% fat (USDA)	1 cup (5 oz.)	294	29.3
12% fat (USDA)	2½-oz. slice (⅛ of qt. brick)	147	14.6
12% fat (USDA)	Small container (3½ fl. oz.)	128	12.8
16% fat (USDA)	1 cup (5.2 oz.)	329	26.6
Deluxe (Carnation)	1 pt.	536	64.5
Dietetic (Carnation)	1 pt.	480	D.N.A.

ICE CREAM BAR, chocolate-coated:

(Popsicle Industries)	3 fl. oz.	180	D.N.A.
(Rosedale)	3 oz.	180	D.N.A.
(Sealtest)	1 bar (2½ fl. oz.)	149	12.1

ICE CREAM CONE, cone only:

(USDA)	1 piece (5 grams)	19	3.9
(Comet)	1 piece (4 grams)	19	3.9
Assorted colors (Comet)	1 piece (4 grams)	19	3.9
Rolled sugar (Comet), any color	1 piece (.4 oz.)	49	10.2

ICE CREAM CUP, cup only:

(Comet), any color	1 piece (5 grams)	20	4.1
Pilot (Comet)	1 piece (4 grams)	19	3.9

ICE CREAM SANDWICH

(Sealtest)	1 sandwich (3 fl. oz.)	173	26.1

ICE MILK:

Hardened (USDA)	1 cup (4.6 oz.)	199	29.3

Food and Description	Measure or Quantity	Calories	Carbo-hydrates (grams)
Soft-serve (USDA)	1 cup (6.2 oz.)	266	39.2
Any flavor (Borden) *Lite Line*	¼ pt.	99	16.0
ICE MILK BAR, chocolate-coated:			
(Popsicle Industries)	3 fl. oz.	133	D.N.A.
(Rosedale)	2½ oz.	130	D.N.A.
(Sealtest)	1 bar (2½ fl. oz.)	132	13.6
ICE STICK, twin pop (Sealtest)	3 fl. oz.	70	17.9
ICES (See **LIME ICE**)			
ICING (See **CAKE ICING**)			
INCONNU or SHEEFISH, raw:			
Whole (USDA)	1 lb. (weighed whole)	417	0.
Meat only (USDA)	4 oz.	166	0.
INDIAN PUDDING, New England (B & M)	½ cup (4 oz.)	120	27.1
INSTANT BREAKFAST (See individual brand name or company listings)			
IRISH WHISKEY (See **DISTILLED LIQUOR**)			
ITALIAN DINNER, frozen:			
(Banquet)	11-oz. dinner	414	44.0
(Swanson)	13½-oz. dinner	448	54.1

(USDA): United States Department of Agriculture
DNA: Data Not Available
* Prepared as Package Directs

Food and Description	Measure or Quantity	Calories	Carbo-hydrates (grams)

J

JACKFRUIT, fresh (USDA):
Whole	1 lb. (weighed with seeds & skin)	124	32.3
Flesh only	4 oz.	111	28.8

JACK MACKEREL, raw, meat
only (USDA) | 4 oz. | 162 | 0. |

JACK ROSE MIX (Bar-Tender's) | 1 serving (⅝ oz.) | 70 | 17.2 |

JALAPENO BEAN DIP
(Frito-Lay) | 1 oz. | 37 | 4.1 |

JAM, sweetened (See also
individual listings by flavor):
(USDA)	1 oz.	77	19.8
(USDA)	1 T. (.7 oz.)	54	14.0

**JAPANESE-STYLE
VEGETABLES**, frozen
(Birds Eye) | ⅓ pkg. (3⅓ oz.) | 105 | 5.8 |

JELLY, sweetened (See also
individual listings by flavor):
(USDA)	1 oz.	77	20.0
(USDA)	1 T. (.6 oz.)	49	12.7
All flavors (Crosse & Blackwell)	1 T. (.7 oz.)	51	12.8
All flavors (Kraft)	1 oz.	74	18.4
All flavors (Polaner)	1 T.	54	13.5
All flavors (Smucker's)	1 T. (.7 oz.)	49	12.4

JELLY ROLL (Van de
Kamp's):
Lemon	9-oz. cake	879	D.N.A.
Raspberry	9-oz. cake	589	D.N.A.

Food and Description	Measure or Quantity	Calories	Carbo-hydrates (grams)
JERUSALEM ARTICHOKE (USDA):			
Unpared	1 lb. (weighed with skin)	207	52.3
Pared	4 oz.	75	18.9
JOHANNISBERGER RIESLING WINE:			
(Deinhard) 11% alcohol	3 fl. oz.	72	4.5
(Louis M. Martini) 12.5% alcohol	3 fl. oz.	90	.2
JORDAN ALMOND (See **CANDY**)			
JUICE (See individual flavors)			
JUJUBE or CHINESE DATE (USDA):			
Fresh, whole	1 lb. (weighed with seeds)	443	116.4
Fresh, flesh only	4 oz.	119	31.3
Dried, whole	1 lb. (weighed with seeds)	1159	297.1
Dried, flesh only	4 oz.	325	83.5
JUNIOR FOOD (See **BABY FOOD**)			
JUNIORS (Tastykake):			
Chocolate	1 pkg. (2¾ oz.)	397	70.8
Chocolate devil food	1 pkg. (2¾ oz.)	284	45.2
Coconut	1 pkg. (2¾ oz.)	415	83.5
Coconut devil food	1 pkg. (2¾ oz.)	318	60.4
Jelly square	1 pkg. (3¼ oz.)	429	91.7
Koffee Kake	1 pkg. (2½ oz.)	395	59.7
Lemon	1 pkg. (2¾ oz.)	422	84.8
JUNKET (See individual flavors)			

(USDA): United States Department of Agriculture
DNA: Data Not Available
* Prepared as Package Directs

Food and Description	Measure or Quantity	Calories	Carbo-hydrates (grams)

K

KABOOM, cereal	1 oz.	109	24.6
KAFE VIN (Lejon) 19.7% alcohol	3 fl. oz.	183	22.8
KALE:			
Raw, leaves only (USDA)	1 lb. (weighed untrimmed)	154	26.1
Boiled, leaves including stems (USDA)	½ cup (1.9 oz.)	15	2.2
Frozen:			
Not thawed (USDA)	4 oz.	36	6.2
Boiled, drained (USDA)	½ cup (3.2 oz.)	29	5.0
Chopped (Birds Eye)	½ cup (3.3 oz.)	29	4.2
KARO, syrup:			
Dark corn	1 T. (.7 oz.)	59	14.7
Imitation maple	1 T. (.7 oz.)	57	14.3
Light corn	1 T. (.7 oz.)	58	14.6
Pancake & waffle	1 T. (.7 oz.)	58	14.6
KETCHUP (See **CATSUP**)			
KIDNEY (USDA):			
Beef, raw	4 oz.	147	1.0
Beef, braised	4 oz.	286	.9
Calf, raw	4 oz.	128	.1
Hog, raw	4 oz.	120	1.2
Lamb, raw	4 oz.	119	1.0
KIELBASA (Oscar Mayer)	6-oz. link	530	10.0
KINGFISH, raw (USDA):			
Whole	1 lb. (weighed whole)	210	0.
Meat only	4 oz.	119	0.
KIPPERS (See **HERRING**)			
KIRSCH LIQUEUR (Garnier) 96 proof	1 fl. oz.	83	8.8

Food and Description	Measure or Quantity	Calories	Carbo-hydrates (grams)
KIRSCHWASSER (Leroux)			
96 proof	1 fl. oz.	80	0.
KIX, cereal	1½ cup (1 oz.)	112	23.9
KNOCKWURST (USDA)	1 oz.	79	.6
KOHLRABI (USDA):			
Raw, whole	1 lb. (weighed with skin, without leaves)	96	21.9
Raw, diced	1 cup (4.8 oz.)	40	9.1
Boiled, drained	4 oz.	27	6.0
Boiled, drained	1 cup (5.5 oz.)	37	8.2
KOOL-AID, regular (General Foods)	1 cup (9.3 oz.)	98	25.0
KOOL-POPS (General Foods)	1 bar (1.5 oz.)	32	8.1
KOTTBULLAR (Hormel)	1 oz. (1-lb. can)	48	.9
KRIMPETS (Tastykake):			
Apple spice	1 cake (.9 oz.)	135	25.2
Butterscotch	1 cake (.9 oz.)	123	22.9
Chocolate	1 cake (.9 oz.)	119	21.6
Jelly	1 cake (.9 oz.)	103	21.0
Lemon	1 cake (.9 oz.)	113	21.4
Orange	1 cake (.9 oz.)	114	21.5
KUMMEL LIQUEUR:			
(Garnier) 70 proof	1 fl. oz.	75	4.3
(Hiram Walker) 70 proof	1 fl. oz.	71	3.2
(Leroux) 70 proof	1 fl. oz.	75	4.1
(Old Mr. Boston) 70 proof	1 fl. oz.	78	2.0
KUMQUAT, fresh (USDA):			
Whole	1 lb. (weighed with seeds)	274	72.1
Flesh & skin	4 oz.	74	19.4
Flesh only	5–6 med. kumquats	65	17.1

(USDA): United States Department of Agriculture
DNA: Data Not Available
* Prepared as Package Directs

Food and Description	Measure or Quantity	Calories	Carbo-hydrates (grams)

L

LAKE COUNTRY WINE
(Taylor):
White dinner, 12.5% alcohol	3 fl. oz.	78	2.2
Red dinner, 12.5% alcohol	3 fl. oz.	81	2.9

LAKE HERRING, raw
(USDA):
Whole	1 lb.	226	0.
Meat only	4 oz.	109	0.

LAKE TROUT, raw (USDA):
Drawn	1 lb. (weighed with head, fins & bones)	282	0.
Meat only	4 oz.	191	0.

LAKE TROUT or SISCOWET,
raw (USDA):
Less than 6.5 lb. whole	1 lb. (weighed whole)	404	0.
Less than 6.5 lb. whole	4 oz. (meat only)	273	0.
More than 6.5 lb. whole	1 lb. (weighed whole)	856	0.
More than 6.5 lb. whole	4 oz. (meat only)	594	0.

LAMB, choice grade (USDA):
Chop, broiled:
  Loin. One 5-oz. chop
    (weighed before
    cooking with bone)
    will give you:
Lean & fat	2.8 oz.	280	0.
Lean only	2.3 oz.	122	0.
  Rib. One 5-oz. chop
    (weighed before
    cooking with bone)
    will give you:
Lean & fat	2.9 oz.	334	0.
Lean only	2 oz.	118	0.
Fat, separable, cooked	1 oz.	201	0.

Food and Description	Measure or Quantity	Calories	Carbo-hydrates (grams)
Leg:			
Raw, lean & fat	1 lb. (weighed with bone)	845	0.
Roasted, lean & fat	4 oz.	316	0.
Roasted, lean only	4 oz.	211	0.
Shoulder:			
Raw, lean & fat	1 lb. (weighed with bone)	1082	0.
Roasted, lean & fat	4 oz.	383	0.
Roasted, lean only	4 oz.	232	0.
LAMB KABOB, frozen (Colonial)	6-oz. kabob	365	D.N.A.
LAMB'S-QUARTERS (USDA):			
Raw, trimmed	1 lb.	195	33.1
Boiled, drained	4 oz.	36	5.7
LAMB STEW, canned (B & M)	1 cup (8.1 oz.)	192	11.4
LARD:			
(USDA)	1 lb.	4091	0.
(USDA)	1 cup (7.2 oz.)	1849	0.
(USDA)	1 T. (.5 oz.)	117	0.
LASAGNE:			
Canned (Chef Boy-Ar-Dee)	8 oz. (⅕ of 40-oz. can)	279	29.7
Canned (Nalley's)	8 oz.	227	27.2
Frozen, with meat sauce (Buitoni)	½ of 15-oz. pkg.	255	24.9
*Mix, dinner (Chef Boy-Ar-Dee)	8¾-oz. pkg.	273	37.7
Mix, *Skillet* (Hunt's)	1-lb. 1-oz. pkg.	812	114.6
LEEKS, raw (USDA):			
Whole	1 lb. (weighed untrimmed)	123	26.4
Trimmed	4 oz.	59	12.7

(USDA): United States Department of Agriculture
DNA: Data Not Available
* Prepared as Package Directs

Food and Description	Measure or Quantity	Calories	Carbo-hydrates (grams)
LEMON, fresh, peeled			
(USDA)	1 med. (2⅛" dia.)	20	6.1
LEMONADE:			
Chilled (Sealtest)	½ cup (4.4 oz.)	55	13.4
Frozen, concentrate, sweetened:			
(USDA)	6-fl.-oz. can	427	112.0
*Diluted with 4⅓ parts water (USDA)	½ cup (4.4 oz.)	55	14.1
*(Minute Maid)	½ cup (4.2 oz.)	49	13.1
*(Seneca)	½ cup (4.3 oz.)	56	14.0
*(7L)	½ cup	55	14.0
*(Snow Crop)	½ cup (4.2 oz.)	49	13.1
*Pink (Treesweet)	½ cup	50	D.N.A.
Mix:			
*(Salada)	6 fl. oz.	79	19.2
*(Wyler's)	6 fl. oz.	64	15.8
*(Wyler's) pink	6 fl. oz.	64	15.8
LEMON CAKE MIX:			
*(Betty Crocker) *Sunkist*	1/12 of cake	202	36.1
*(Duncan Hines)	1/12 of cake	202	35.0
*Chiffon (Betty Crocker)	1/16 of cake	151	26.8
Coconut (Betty Crocker)	1 oz.	121	22.3
Cream moist cake (Pillsbury)	1 oz.	122	21.8
*Pudding cake (Betty Crocker)	⅛ of cake	227	45.4
LEMON EXTRACT, pure (Ehlers)	1 tsp.	14	D.N.A.
LEMON FLAVORING, imitation (Ehlers)	1 tsp.	3	D.N.A.
LEMON JUICE:			
Fresh:			
(USDA)	1 cup (8.6 oz.)	61	19.5
(USDA)	1 T. (.5 oz.)	4	1.2
(Sunkist)	1 lemon (3.9 oz.)	11	4.0
(Sunkist)	1 T. (.5 oz.)	4	1.0
Canned, unsweetened (USDA)	1 cup (8.6 oz.)	56	18.6

Food and Description	Measure or Quantity	Calories	Carbohydrates (grams)
Canned, unsweetened			
(USDA)	1 T. (.5 oz.)	3	1.1
Plastic container (USDA)	¼ cup (2 oz.)	13	4.3
Plastic container, *ReaLemon*	1 T. (.5 oz.)	3	1.2
Frozen, unsweetened:			
Concentrate (USDA)	½ cup (5.1 oz.)	169	54.6
Single strength (USDA)	½ cup (4.3 oz.)	27	8.8
Full strength, already reconstituted (Minute Maid)	½ cup (4.2 oz.)	27	8.8
Full strength, already reconstituted (Snow Crop)	½ cup (4.2 oz.)	27	8.8
LEMON-LIMEADE, sweetened, concentrate, frozen:			
*(Minute Maid)	½ cup	50	13.1
*(Snow Crop)	½ cup	50	13.1
LEMON-LIME SOFT DRINK:			
Sweetened:			
Green (Canada Dry)	6 fl. oz.	90	23.4
Rickey (Canada Dry)	6 fl. oz.	71	18.4
(Dr. Brown's)	6 fl. oz.	74	18.4
(Dr. Pepper)	6 fl. oz.	72	18.0
(Key Food)	6 fl. oz.	74	18.4
(Kirsch)	6 fl. oz.	70	17.5
(Shasta)	6 fl. oz.	73	18.4
(Waldbaum)	6 fl. oz.	74	18.4
(White Rock)	6 fl. oz.	77	D.N.A.
Low calorie (Shasta)	6 fl. oz.	<1	<.1
LEMON PEEL, CANDIED:			
(USDA)	1 oz.	90	22.9
(Liberty)	1 oz.	93	22.6
LEMON PIE:			
(Tastykake)	4-oz. pie	366	52.0
(Hostess)	4½-oz. pie	357	53.9

(USDA): United States Department of Agriculture
DNA: Data Not Available
* Prepared as Package Directs

Food and Description	Measure or Quantity	Calories	Carbo- hydrates (grams)
Chiffon, home recipe (USDA)	1/8 of 9" pie (3.8 oz.)	338	47.3
Cream, frozen (Banquet)	2½ oz.	179	25.5
Cream, frozen (Mrs. Smith's)	1/8 of 8" pie (2.3 oz.)	203	22.7
Meringue, home recipe (USDA)	1/6 of 9" pie (4.9 oz.)	357	52.8
Meringue, frozen (Mrs. Smith's)	1/8 of 8" pie (3.7 oz.)	288	41.1
LEMON PIE FILLING (Lucky Leaf)	8 oz.	412	95.4
LEMON PIE FILLING MIX (See **LEMON PUDDING MIX**)			
LEMON PUDDING:			
Canned (Betty Crocker)	½ cup	198	40.1
Canned (Hunt's)	5-oz. can	175	35.3
LEMON PUDDING or PIE FILLING MIX:			
Regular:			
*(Jell-O)	½ cup (5.1 oz.)	178	38.8
*(My-T-Fine)	½ cup (5 oz.)	179	31.7
*(Royal)	1/8 of 9" pie (including crust) 4.2 oz.	308	45.2
Instant:			
*(Jell-O)	½ cup (5.3 oz.)	178	30.5
*(Royal)	½ cup (5.1 oz.)	184	31.9
*Dietetic with skim milk (Dia-Mel)	4 oz.	53	8.2
LEMON RENNET CUSTARD MIX:			
Powder:			
(Junket)	1 oz.	116	28.1
*(Junket)	4 oz.	109	14.7

Food and Description	Measure or Quantity	Calories	Carbo-hydrates (grams)
Tablet:			
(Junket)	1 tablet	1	.2
*With sugar (Junket)	4 oz.	101	13.5
LEMON SOFT DRINK:			
Sweetened:			
(Canada Dry)	6 fl. oz.	88	19.2
(Dr. Brown's) *Tune-Up*	6 fl. oz.	75	18.8
(Hoffman)	6 fl. oz.	81	20.2
(Kirsch)	6 fl. oz.	64	16.1
Low calorie:			
(Dr. Brown's) *Slim-Ray*	6 fl. oz	3	.8
(Hoffman)	6 fl. oz	3	.8
(No-Cal)	6 fl. oz.	2	0.
(Shasta)	6 fl. oz.	<1	<.1
LEMON TURNOVER, frozen			
(Pepperidge Farm)	1 turnover (3.3 oz.)	341	33.1
LENTIL:			
Whole:			
Dry:			
(USDA)	½ lb.	771	136.3
(USDA)	1 cup (6.7 oz.)	649	114.8
(Sinsheimer)	1 oz.	95	17.0
Cooked, drained (USDA)	½ cup (3.6 oz.)	107	19.5
Split, dry (USDA)	½ lb.	782	140.2
LENTIL SOUP, canned:			
With ham (Crosse & Blackwell)	6½ oz. (½ can)	123	17.0
*(Manischewitz)	8 oz. (by wt.)	166	29.3
LETTUCE (USDA):			
Bibb, untrimmed	1 lb. (weighed untrimmed)	47	8.4
Bibb, untrimmed	7.8-oz. head (4″ dia.)	23	4.1

(USDA): United States Department of Agriculture
DNA: Data Not Available
* Prepared as Package Directs

Food and Description	Measure or Quantity	Calories	Carbo-hydrates (grams)
Boston, untrimmed	1 lb. (weighed untrimmed)	47	8.4
Boston, untrimmed	7.8-oz. head (4″ dia.)	23	4.1
Butterhead varieties (See Bibb & Boston)			
Cos (See Romaine)			
Dark green (See Romaine)			
Grand Rapids	1 lb. (weighed untrimmed)	52	10.2
Grand Rapids	2 large leaves (1.8 oz.)	9	1.8
Great Lakes	1 lb. (weighed untrimmed)	56	12.5
Great Lakes, trimmed	1-lb. head (4¾″ dia.)	59	13.2
Iceberg:			
Untrimmed	1 lb. (weighed untrimmed)	56	12.5
Trimmed	1-lb. head (4¾″ dia.)	59	13.2
Leaves	1 cup (2.3 oz.)	9	1.9
Chopped	1 cup (2 oz.)	8	1.7
Chunks	1 cup (2.6 oz.)	10	2.1
Looseleaf varieties (See Salad Bowl)			
New York	1 lb. (weighed untrimmed)	56	12.5
New York	1-lb. head (4¾″dia.)	59	13.2
Romaine:			
Untrimmed	1 lb. (weighed untrimmed)	52	10.2
Trimmed, shredded & broken into pieces	½ cup (.8 oz.)	4	.8
Salad Bowl	1 lb. (weighed untrimmed)	52	10.2
Salad Bowl	2 large leaves (1.8 oz.)	9	1.8
Simpson	1 lb. (weighed untrimmed)	52	10.2
Simpson	2 large leaves (1.8 oz.)	9	1.8
White Paris (See Romaine)			

Food and Description	Measure or Quantity	Calories	Carbo-hydrates (grams)
LIEBFRAUMILCH WINE:			
(Anheuser) 10% alcohol	3 fl. oz.	63	.9
(Deinhard) 11% alcohol	3 fl. oz.	60	3.6
(Deinhard) *Hans Christof,* 11% alcohol	3 fl. oz.	60	3.6
(Julius Kayser) Glockenspiel, 10% alcohol	3 fl. oz.	57	1.8
LIFE, cereal (Quaker)	1 cup (1.5 oz.)	160	29.8
LIKE, soft drink, low calorie (Seven-Up)	6 fl. oz.	1	.3
LIMA BEAN (See **BEAN, LIMA**)			
LIME, fresh, whole:			
(USDA)	1 lb. (weighed with skin & seeds)	107	36.2
(USDA)	1 med. (2" dia., 2.4 oz.)	15	4.9
LIMEADE, concentrate, sweetened, frozen:			
(USDA)	6-fl.-oz. can	408	107.9
*Diluted with 4⅓ parts water (USDA)	½ cup (4.4 oz.)	51	13.6
*(Minute Maid)	½ cup (4.2 oz.)	50	13.4
*(7L)	½ cup	52	13.5
*(Snow Crop)	½ cup (4.2 oz.)	50	13.4
***LIMEADE MIX** (Wyler's)	6 fl. oz.	64	15.8
LIME ICE, home recipe (USDA)	8 oz. (by wt.)	177	73.9
LIME JUICE:			
Fresh (USDA)	1 cup (8.7 oz.)	64	22.1
Canned or bottled, unsweetened:			
(USDA)	1 cup (8.7 oz.)	64	22.1
(USDA)	1 fl. oz. (1.1 oz.)	8	2.8

(USDA): United States Department of Agriculture
DNA: Data Not Available
* Prepared as Package Directs

Food and Description	Measure or Quantity	Calories	Carbo-hydrates (grams)
(Calavo)	1 fl. oz.	8	2.8
Plastic container *ReaLime*	1 T. (.6 oz.)	4	1.5
LIME PIE, Key lime, cream, frozen (Banquet)	2½ oz.	204	27.5
*LIME PIE FILLING MIX, Key lime (Royal)	⅛ of 9″ pie (including crust)	301	43.4
LIME SHERBET or FRUIT ICE MIX (Junket)	6 serving pkg. (4 oz.)	388	108.8
LIME SOFT DRINK (Yukon Club)	6 fl. oz.	64	16.1
LINGCOD, raw (USDA):			
Whole	1 lb. (weighed whole)	130	0.
Meat only	4 oz.	95	0.
LIQUEUR (See individual kinds)			
LITCHI NUT (USDA):			
Fresh:			
Whole	4 oz. (weighed in shell, with seeds)	44	11.2
Flesh only	4 oz.	73	18.6
Dried:			
Whole	4 oz. (weighed in shell, with seeds)	145	36.9
Flesh only	2 oz.	157	40.1
LIVER (USDA):			
Beef, raw	1 lb.	635	24.0
Beef, fried	4 oz.	260	6.0
Calf, raw	1 lb.	635	18.6
Calf, fried	4 oz.	296	4.5
Chicken, raw	1 lb.	585	13.2
Chicken, simmered	4 oz.	187	3.5

Food and Description	Measure or Quantity	Calories	Carbo-hydrates (grams)
Goose, raw	1 lb.	826	24.5
Hog, raw	1 lb.	594	11.8
Hog, fried	4 oz.	273	2.8
Lamb, raw	1 lb.	617	13.2
Lamb, broiled	4 oz.	296	3.2
Turkey, raw	1 lb.	626	13.2
Turkey, simmered	4 oz.	197	3.5

LIVER PATE (See **PATE**)

LIVER SAUSAGE or LIVER-WURST (USDA):
Fresh	1 oz.	87	.5
Smoked	1 oz.	90	.7

LOBSTER:
Raw:
Whole (USDA)	1 lb. (weighed whole)	107	.6
Meat only (USDA)	4 oz.	103	.6
Northern, meat only (Booth)	4 oz.	103	.6
Cooked, meat only (USDA)	4 oz.	108	.3
Canned, meat only (USDA)	4 oz.	108	.3

LOBSTER NEWBURG:
Home recipe (USDA)	4 oz.	220	5.8
Frozen (Stouffer's)	11½-oz. pkg.	671	16.0

LOBSTER PASTE, canned (USDA)
	1 oz.	51	.4

LOBSTER SALAD, home recipe (USDA)
	4 oz.	125	2.6

LOBSTER SOUP, canned:
Bisque (Crosse & Blackwell)	6½ oz. (½ can)	88	6.6
Cream of (Crosse & Blackwell)	6½ oz. (½ can)	92	6.5

(USDA): United States Department of Agriculture
DNA: Data Not Available
* Prepared as Package Directs

Food and Description	Measure or Quantity	Calories	Carbo-hydrates (grams)
LOCHON ORA, Scottish liqueur (Leroux) 70 proof	1 fl. oz.	89	7.4
LOGANBERRY (USDA):			
Fresh:			
Untrimmed	1 lb. (weighed with caps)	267	64.2
Trimmed	1 cup (5.1 oz.)	89	21.5
Canned, solids & liq.:			
Water pack	4 oz.	45	10.7
Juice pack	4 oz.	61	14.4
Light syrup	4 oz.	79	19.5
Heavy syrup	4 oz.	101	25.2
Extra heavy syrup	4 oz.	122	30.8
LOG CABIN, syrup:			
Buttered	1 T. (.7 oz.)	52	12.7
Maple-honey	1 T.	54	14.0
LONGAN (USDA):			
Fresh:			
Whole	1 lb. (weighed with shell & seeds)	147	38.0
Flesh only	4 oz.	69	17.9
Dried:			
Whole	1 lb. (weighed with shell & seeds)	467	120.8
Flesh only	4 oz.	324	83.9
LOOK FIT, any flavor (A&P)	1 can	225	19.0
LOQUAT, fresh (USDA):			
Whole	1 lb. (weighed with seeds)	168	43.3
Flesh only	4 oz.	54	14.1
LUCKY CHARMS, cereal	1 cup (1 oz.)	110	23.6
LUMBERJACK, syrup (Nalley's)	1 oz.	78	19.6

Food and Description	Measure or Quantity	Calories	Carbo-hydrates (grams)
LUNCHEON MEAT (See also individual listings, e.g. **BOLOGNA**):			
Meat loaf (USDA)	1 oz.	57	.9
(Eckrich):			
Beef, chopped, *Slender Sliced*	1 oz.	38	D.N.A.
Chicken, chipped, *Slender Sliced*	1 oz.	77	D.N.A.
Ham, chipped, smoked, *Slender Sliced*	1 oz.	45	D.N.A.
Loaves:			
Chicken breast	1 oz.	32	D.N.A.
Gourmet	1 oz.	28	D.N.A.
Honey style	1 oz.	42	D.N.A.
Peppered	1 oz.	38	D.N.A.
Pressed luncheon	1 oz.	40	D.N.A.
Pork loin, chipped, smoked, *Slender Sliced*	1 oz.	40	D.N.A.
Turkey, chipped, smoked, *Slender Sliced*	1 oz.	38	D.N.A.
(Sugardale)	1- oz. slice	77	Tr.
Old-fashioned loaf (Sugardale)	1-oz. slice	76	Tr.
Pickle & pimento:			
(Hormel)	1 oz. (6-lb. can)	81	.3
(Sugardale)	1-oz. slice	78	Tr.
Spiced (Hormel)	1 oz. (6-lb. can)	101	.3
LUNG, raw (USDA):			
Beef	1 lb.	435	0.
Calf	1 lb.	481	0.
Lamb	1 lb.	467	0.

(USDA): United States Department of Agriculture
DNA: Data Not Available
* Prepared as Package Directs

Food and Description	Measure or Quantity	Calories	Carbohydrates (grams)

M

MACADAMIA NUT (USDA):

Whole	1 lb. (weighed in shell)	972	22.4
Shelled	4 oz.	784	18.0

MACARONI. Plain macaroni products are essentially the same in caloric value and carbohydrate content on the same weight basis. The longer they are cooked, the more water is absorbed and this affects the nutritive values.

Dry:

Elbow-type (USDA)	1 cup (4.8 oz.)	502	102.3
1-inch pieces (USDA)	1 cup (3.8 oz.)	406	82.7
2-inch pieces (USDA)	1 cup (3 oz.)	317	64.7
(USDA)	1 oz.	105	21.3

Cooked (USDA):

8–10 minutes, firm	1 cup (4.6 oz.)	192	39.1
8–10 minutes, firm	4 oz.	168	34.1
14–20 minutes, tender	1 cup (4.9 oz.)	155	32.2
14–20 minutes, tender	4 oz.	126	26.1

MACARONI & BEEF:

(Morton House)	12¾-oz. can	745	D.N.A.
In tomato sauce, canned (Franco-American)	1 cup	225	25.0
With tomatoes, frozen (Stouffer's)	11½-oz. pkg.	410	39.0

MACARONI & CHEESE:

Home recipe, baked (USDA)	1 cup (7.1 oz.)	430	40.2
Canned:			
(USDA)	1 cup	228	25.7
(Franco-American)	1 cup	219	25.0
(Heinz)	8¼-oz. can	231	27.0
MacaroniO's (Franco-American)	1 cup	171	22.3

Food and Description	Measure or Quantity	Calories	Carbo-hydrates (grams)
Frozen:			
(Banquet)	20-oz. pkg.	742	82.0
(Banquet) cookin' bag	8 oz.	280	36.0
(Kraft)	12½-oz. pkg.	612	54.2
(Morton) casserole	8-oz. pkg.	297	31.5
(Stouffer's)	12-oz. pkg.	477	52.1
(Swanson)	8-oz. pkg.	328	29.2
(Van de Kamp's)	1 pkg.	495	D.N.A.

MACARONI & CHEESE MIX:

Dry (USDA)	1 oz.	113	17.8
*Cheddar sauce (Betty Crocker)	¾ cup	244	36.7
*Stir 'n Serv, instant (Golden Grain)	4 oz.	197	25.4

MACARONI & CHILI SAUCE MIX:

*Mac-A-Roni Fiesta (Golden Grain)	½ cup (3.5 oz.)	156	25.0
Mexi Casserole (Betty Crocker)	6-oz. pkg.	564	120.6

MACARONI CREOLE

(Heinz)	7¾-oz. can	143	24.4

MACARONI DINNER:

& beef, frozen:			
(Morton)	11-oz. dinner	365	56.3
(Swanson)	11¼-oz. dinner	302	35.0
& cheese:			
*(Chef Boy-Ar-Dee)	4½-oz. pkg.	201	33.8
*(Kraft)	4 oz.	203	26.1
*(Kraft) deluxe	4 oz.	202	27.9
Frozen (Banquet)	12-oz. dinner	342	47.0
Frozen (Morton)	12¾-oz. dinner	317	38.5
Frozen (Swanson)	12¾-oz. dinner	367	48.4
*Italian-style (Kraft)	4 oz.	119	20.5
*Mexican-style (Kraft)	4 oz.	126	22.6

(USDA): United States Department of Agriculture
DNA: Data Not Available
* Prepared as Package Directs

Food and Description	Measure or Quantity	Calories	Carbo-hydrates (grams)
*Monte Bello with sauce mix (Betty Crocker)	1 cup	350	38.9
MACARONI SALAD, canned (Nalley's)	4 oz.	181	13.9
MACKEREL (USDA):			
Atlantic:			
Raw:			
Whole	1 lb. (weighed whole)	468	0.
Meat only	4 oz.	217	0.
Broiled with butter	4 oz.	268	0.
Canned, solids & liq.	4 oz.	208	0.
Pacific:			
Raw:			
Dressed	1 lb. (weighed with bones & skin)	519	0.
Meat only	4 oz.	180	0.
Canned, solids & liq.	4 oz.	204	0.
Salted	4 oz.	346	0.
Smoked	4 oz.	248	0.
MACKEREL, JACK (See **JACK MACKEREL**)			
MADEIRA WINE:			
(Leacock) 19% alcohol	3 fl. oz.	120	6.3
(Leacock) *St. John,* 19% alcohol	3 fl. oz.	120	6.3
MAGGI, seasoning	1 T.	22	.1
MAI TAI COCKTAIL, 48 proof (Lemon Hart)	3 fl. oz.	180	15.6
MAI TAI MIX (Bar-Tender's)	1 serving (⅝ oz.)	69	17.0
MALT, dry (USDA)	1 oz.	104	21.9
MALTED MILK MIX:			
Dry powder (USDA)	1 oz.	116	20.1

Food and Description	Measure or Quantity	Calories	Carbo-hydrates (grams)
*Prepared with whole milk (USDA)	1 cup (8.3 oz.)	244	27.5
Instant (Borden)	2 heaping tsp. (.7 oz.)	77	16.0
(Horlicks)	1 oz.	118	19.8
Instant, chocolate (Borden)	2 heaping tsp. (.7 oz.)	77	16.0
MALTED TABLETS (Horlicks)	1 tablet (1 gram)	6	.9
MALTEX, cereal	1 oz.	109	22.7
MALT EXTRACT, dried (USDA)	1 oz.	104	25.3
MALT LIQUOR:			
Big Cat	12 fl. oz.	155	D.N.A.
Country Club, 6.8% alcohol	12 fl. oz.	183	2.8
MALT-O-MEAL, cereal	¾ cup (1 oz. dry)	102	22.1
MAMEY or MAMMEE APPLE, fresh (USDA)	1 lb. (weighed with skin & seeds)	143	35.2
MANDARIN ORANGE, CANNED, solids & liq.:			
Light syrup (Del Monte)	½ cup (4.5 oz.)	77	20.6
Low calorie (Diet Delight)	½ cup (4.3 oz.)	31	7.4
MANDARIN ORANGE, FRESH (See **TANGERINE**)			
MANGO, fresh (USDA):			
Whole	1 lb. (weighed with seeds & skin)	201	51.1

(USDA): United States Department of Agriculture
DNA: Data Not Available
* Prepared as Package Directs

Food and Description	Measure or Quantity	Calories	Carbohydrates (grams)
Whole	1 med. (7 oz.)	88	22.5
Flesh only, diced or sliced	½ cup (2.9 oz.)	54	13.8
MANHATTAN COCKTAIL:			
(Calvert) 60 proof	3 fl. oz.	161	2.0
(Hiram Walker) 55 proof	3 fl. oz.	147	3.0
MANHATTAN MIX			
(Bar-Tender's)	1 serving (⅕ oz.)	24	5.6
MANICOTTI, without sauce, frozen (Buitoni)	4 oz.	218	19.9
MAPLE FLAVORING, imitation maple (Ehlers)	1 tsp.	8	D.N.A.
MAPLE RENNET CUSTARD MIX:			
Powder:			
(Junket)	1 oz.	117	27.9
*(Junket)	4 oz.	109	14.7
Tablet:			
(Junket)	1 tablet	1	.2
*& sugar (Junket)	4 oz.	101	13.5
MAPLE SYRUP (See also individual brand names):			
(USDA)	1 T. (.7 oz.)	50	13.0
Dietetic (Dia-Mel)	1 T.	22	5.5
MARASCHINO LIQUEUR:			
(Garnier) 60 proof	1 fl. oz.	94	11.1
(Leroux) 60 proof	1 fl. oz.	88	9.7
MARBLE CAKE MIX:			
Dry (USDA)	1 oz.	120	21.4
*With boiled white icing (USDA)	4 oz.	375	70.3
*(Betty Crocker)	½₁₂ of cake	206	37.2
MARGARINE, salted or unsalted:			
(USDA)	1 lb.	3266	1.8
(USDA)	1 cup (8 oz.)	1633	.9

Food and Description	Measure or Quantity	Calories	Carbo-hydrates (grams)
(USDA)	4 oz. (1 stick)	816	.5
(USDA)	1 T. (.5 oz.)	101	<.1
(Blue Bonnet) regular or soft	1 T. (.5 oz.)	102	<.1
(Borden) Danish flavor	1 T. (.5 oz.)	101	<.1
(Fleischmann's) regular or soft	1 T.	102	<.1
(Golden Glow)	1 cup	1426	1.6
(Golden Glow)	1 T. (.4 oz.)	89	.1
(Good Luck) soft	1 T. (.4 oz.)	89	.1
(Good Luck) stick	1 T. (.5 oz.)	102	.1
(Imperial) stick	1 T. (.5 oz.)	102	.1
(Imperial) *Sof-Spread*	1 T. (.4 oz.)	89	.1
(Mazola) polyunsaturated	1 T. (.5 oz.)	102	.1
(Nucoa) polyunsaturated	1 T. (.5 oz.)	102	.1
(Nucoa) soft	1 T. (.4 oz.)	91	.1
(Parkay) regular	1 T. (.5 oz.)	101	.1
(Parkay) soft	1 T. (.5 oz.)	95	.1
(Parkay) corn oil, soft	1 T. (.5 oz.)	95	.1
(Parkay) safflower oil, soft	1 T. (.5 oz.)	95	.1
(Saffola) regular or soft	1 T. (.5 oz.)	101	<.1
MARGARINE, IMITATION, diet:			
(Fleischmann's)	1 T. (.5 oz.)	50	.1
(Imperial)	1 T. (.5 oz.)	48	0.
(Mazola)	1 cup	804	0.
(Mazola)	1 T. (.5 oz.)	50	0.
(Nucoa)	1 T.	50	Tr.
(Parkay) soft	1 T.	55	0.
MARGARINE, WHIPPED:			
(Blue Bonnet)	1 T. (8 grams)	58	<.1
(Miracle)	1 T. (9 grams)	67	<.1
(Nucoa)	1 T.	70	.1
(Parkay) cup	1 T.	67	<.1
MARGARITA COCKTAIL, (Calvert) 45 proof	3 fl. oz.	176	9.5
MARGARITA MIX (Bar-Tender's)	1 serving (⅝ oz.)	70	17.3

(USDA): United States Department of Agriculture
DNA: Data Not Available
* Prepared as Package Directs

Food and Description	Measure or Quantity	Calories	Carbo-hydrates (grams)
MARGAUX, French red Bordeaux (Barton & Guestier) 12% alcohol	3 fl. oz.	62	.4
MARINADE MIX:			
(Adolph's) instant	1 pkg. (.8 oz.)	39	8.5
(Lawry's) lemon pepper	1 pkg. (2.7 oz.)	159	29.7
MARMALADE:			
Sweetened:			
(USDA)	1 oz.	73	19.9
(USDA)	1 T. (.7 oz.)	51	14.0
(Crosse & Blackwell)	1 T. (.6 oz.)	60	14.9
(King Kelly)	1 T.	48	D.N.A.
(Kraft)	1 oz.	78	19.3
Dietetic or low calorie:			
(Dia-Mel)	1 T.	22	5.4
(Kraft)	1 oz.	35	8.6
(S and W) *Nutradiet*	1 T. (.5 oz.)	11	2.6
(Slenderella)	1 T. (.6 oz.)	22	5.6
MARMALADE PLUM (USDA):			
Fresh, whole	1 lb. (with skin & seeds)	431	108.9
Fresh, flesh only	4 oz.	142	35.8
MARSALA WINE (Italian Swiss Colony-Private Stock) 19.7% alcohol	3 fl. oz.	124	7.1
MARTINI COCKTAIL:			
Gin:			
(Calvert) 60 proof	3 fl. oz.	176	Tr.
(Hiram Walker) 67.5 proof	3 fl. oz.	168	.6
Vodka (Hiram Walker) 60 proof	3 fl. oz.	147	Tr.
*MASA HARINA (Quaker)	2 tortillas (6″ dia.)	139	27.9
*MASA TRIGO (Quaker)	2 tortillas (6″ dia.)	149	24.6

Food and Description	Measure or Quantity	Calories	Carbo-hydrates (grams)
MATZO:			
Regular (Manischewitz)	1 matzo (1.1 oz.)	114	28.1
American (Manischewitz)	1 matzo (1 oz.)	121	22.6
Diet-10's (Goodman's)	1 sq.	109	23.0
Diet-10's (Goodman's)	1 cracker	12	2.5
Diet-thins (Manischewitz)	1 matzo (1 oz.)	113	24.5
Egg (Manischewitz)	1 matzo (1.2 oz.)	133	26.6
Egg 'n Onion (Manischewitz)	1 matzo (1 oz.)	116	24.6
Midgetea (Goodman's)	1 matzo (.4 oz.)	40	7.4
Onion Tams (Manischewitz)	1 piece (3 grams)	13	1.9
Round tea (Goodman's)	1 matzo (.6 oz.)	70	12.9
Tam Tams (Manischewitz)	1 piece (3 grams)	14	1.7
Tasteas (Manischewitz)	1 matzo (1 oz.)	119	24.2
Thin tea (Manischewitz)	1 matzo (1 oz.)	114	24.8
Unsalted (Goodman's)	1 matzo (1 oz.)	109	23.0
Unsalted (Horowitz-Margareten)	1 matzo (1.2 oz.)	135	28.2
Whole wheat (Manischewitz)	1 matzo (1.2 oz.)	124	24.2
MATZO MEAL			
(Manischewitz)	1 cup (4.1 oz.)	438	96.2
MAYONNAISE:			
(USDA)	1 cup (7.8 oz.)	1587	4.9
(USDA)	1 T. (.5 oz.)	101	.3
(Hellmann's-Best Foods) *Real*	1 cup (7.7 oz.)	1572	3.3
(Hellmann's-Best Foods) *Real*	1 T. (.5 oz.)	101	.2
(Kraft)	1 T. (.5 oz.)	102	.1
(Kraft) *Salad Bowl*	1 T. (.5 oz.)	102	.2
(Nalley's)	1 oz.	204	.9
(Saffola)	1 T. (.5 oz.)	92	2.9
(Wesson)	1 T.	110	Tr.
Sugar-free (Chelten House)	1 T.	108	D.N.A.
MAYPO, cereal, dry, any flavor:			
Instant	1 oz.	105	19.8
1-minute	1 oz.	107	19.8

(USDA): United States Department of Agriculture
DNA: Data Not Available
* Prepared as Package Directs

Food and Description	Measure or Quantity	Calories	Carbohydrates (grams)
MAY WINE (Deinhard) 11% alcohol	3 fluid oz.	60	1.0
MEAL (See **CORNMEAL** or **CRACKER MEAL** or **MATZO MEAL**)			
MEATBALL:			
Cocktail (Cresca)	1 meatball	10	D.N.A.
Dinner, with Kluski noodles, frozen (Tom Thumb)	3-lb. 8-oz. tray	2362	140.5
In sauce, canned (Prince)	1 can (3.7 oz.)	171	8.1
Stew, canned (Chef Boy-Ar-Dee)	7½ oz. (¼ of 30-oz. can)	179	11.7
Stew (Morton House)	24-oz. can	1240	D.N.A.
With gravy, canned (Chef Boy-Ar-Dee)	3⅘ oz. (¼ of 15¼-oz. can)	118	4.6
MEAT LOAF DINNER, frozen:			
With tomato sauce, mashed potato & peas (USDA)	12 oz.	445	33.3
(Banquet)	11-oz. dinner	420	28.8
(Morton)	11-oz. dinner	398	27.7
(Swanson)	10-oz. dinner	419	42.2
(Swanson) 3-course	16½-oz. dinner	544	52.8
MEAT LOAF SEASONING MIX (Lawry's)	1 pkg. (3½ oz.)	333	65.2
MEAT, POTTED:			
(Armour Star)	3-oz. can	181	0.
(Hormel)	3-oz. can	158	1.0
(Van Camp)	½ cup (3.9 oz.)	272	D.N.A.
MEAT TENDERIZER (Adolph's)			
Unseasoned	1 tsp. (5 grams)	2	.5
Seasoned	1 tsp. (5 grams)	2	.4
MEDOC WINE (Cruse) 12% alcohol	3 fl. oz.	72	D.N.A.

Food and Description	Measure or Quantity	Calories	Carbohydrates (grams)
MELBA TOAST:			
Garlic (Keebler)	1 piece (2 grams)	9	1.5
Garlic, rounds (Old London)	1 piece (2 grams)	8	1.4
Onion, rounds (Old London)	1 piece (2 grams)	8	1.4
Plain (Keebler)	1 piece (2 grams)	9	1.5
Pumpernickel (Old London)	1 piece (4 grams)	15	3.0
Rye:			
(Keebler)	1 piece (2 grams)	8	1.7
(Old London)	1 piece (4 grams)	14	3.1
Unsalted (Old London)	1 piece (4 grams)	15	3.3
Sesame (Keebler)	1 piece (2 grams)	11	1.4
Sesame, rounds (Old London)	1 piece (2 grams)	9	1.2
Wheat (Old London)	1 piece (4 grams)	15	3.1
Wheat, unsalted (Old London)	1 piece (4 grams)	15	3.2
White:			
(Keebler)	1 piece (4 grams)	16	3.3
(Old London)	1 piece (4 grams)	15	3.1
Rounds (Old London)	1 piece (2 grams)	9	1.6
Unsalted (Old London)	1 piece (4 grams)	15	3.2
MELON (See individual listings, e.g. **CANTALOUPE, WATERMELON,** etc.)			
MELON BALL, cantaloupe & honeydew, in syrup, frozen (USDA)	½ cup (4.1 oz.)	72	18.2
MELON BALL CRISPS, dehydrated snack (Epicure)	1 oz.	87	22.0
MENHADEN, Atlantic, canned, solids & liq. (USDA)	4 oz.	195	0.
METRECAL DINNER, any kind	9-oz. can	225	23.5
MEXICAN DINNER:			
Combination, frozen:			
(Patio)	12-oz. dinner	683	63.8

(USDA): United States Department of Agriculture
DNA: Data Not Available
* Prepared as Package Directs

Food and Description	Measure or Quantity	Calories	Carbohydrates (grams)
(Rosarita)	12-oz. dinner	518	D.N.A.
Mexican style, frozen:			
(Banquet)	16¼-oz. dinner	568	74.0
(Patio)	15-oz. dinner	723	83.3
(Rosarita)	15-oz. dinner	530	D.N.A.
(Swanson)	16¼-oz. dinner	658	67.3
Skillet Mexicana (Hunt's)	1-lb. 2-oz. pkg.	730	130.1
MEXICAN-STYLE VEGETABLES, frozen (Birds Eye)	⅓ pkg. (3⅓ oz.)	144	17.0
MILK AMPLIFIER, syrup (Hershey's)	1 oz.	78	18.6
MILK CONDENSED, sweetened, canned:			
(USDA)	1 cup (10.8 oz.)	982	166.2
Dime Brand	1 fl. oz.	125	21.1
Eagle Brand	1 fl. oz.	125	21.1
Magnolia Brand	1 fl. oz.	125	21.1
(Nestlé's) *Lion's Brand*	1 oz.	96	12.8
(Sealtest)	1 cup	982	166.8
(Sealtest)	1 T.	64	10.9
MILK, DRY:			
Whole (USDA) packed cup	1 cup (5.1 oz.)	728	55.4
Nonfat, instant:			
(USDA) ⅞ cup makes 1 qt.	⅞ cup (3.2 oz.)	330	47.6
*(Carnation)	1 cup (8.6 oz.)	81	12.4
*(Pet)	1 cup	81	11.8
*(Sanalac)	1 cup	82	11.6
(Weight Watchers)	1 packet (3 grams)	10	1.4
Buttermilk, cultured, dried (USDA)	1 cup (4.2 oz.)	464	60.0
MILK, EVAPORATED, canned:			
Regular:			
Unsweetened (USDA)	1 cup (8.9 oz.)	345	24.4
(Carnation)	1 cup (8.9 oz.)	348	25.0
(Pet)	1 cup	352	24.0

Food and Description	Measure or Quantity	Calories	Carbohydrates (grams)
Skimmed:			
(Pet)	1 cup	176	26.4
(Sunshine)	1 cup (8.9 oz.)	200	28.8
MILK, FRESH:			
Whole:			
3.5% fat (USDA)	1 cup (8.6 oz.)	159	12.0
3.7% fat (USDA)	1 cup (8.5 oz.)	159	11.8
3.25% fat (Borden) homogenized	1 cup (8.6 oz.)	152	11.8
3.25% fat (Sealtest)	1 cup (8.6 oz.)	144	10.8
3.5% fat (Sealtest)	1 cup (8.6 oz.)	151	11.0
3.7% fat (Sealtest)	1 cup (8.6 oz.)	157	11.1
Multivitamin (Sealtest)	1 cup (8.6 oz.)	151	11.0
Skim:			
(USDA)	1 cup (8.6 oz.)	88	12.5
Partially skimmed with 2% nonfat milk solids added			
(USDA)	1 cup (8.6 oz.)	145	14.8
(Sealtest)	1 cup (8.6 oz.)	79	11.3
Diet (Sealtest)	1 cup (8.6 oz.)	103	13.8
Light n' Lively (Sealtest)	1 cup (8.6 oz.)	114	13.6
Lite Line (Borden)	1 cup (8.6 oz.)	119	14.2
Vita Lure (Sealtest) 2% fat	1 cup (8.6 oz.)	137	13.6
Buttermilk, cultured, fresh:			
(USDA)	1 cup (8.6 oz.)	88	12.5
0.1% fat (Borden)	1 cup (8.6 oz.)	88	12.4
1.0% fat (Borden)	1 cup (8.6 oz.)	107	12.4
3.5% fat (Borden)	1 cup (8.6 oz.)	159	12.0
Light n' Lively (Sealtest)	1 cup (8.6 oz.)	95	10.5
Skim milk (Sealtest)	1 cup (8.6 oz.)	71	9.3
Chocolate milk drink, fresh:			
With whole milk:			
(USDA)	1 cup (8.8 oz.)	212	27.5
Dutch chocolate (Borden)	1 cup	210	26.1
2% fat (Sealtest)	1 cup (8.6 oz.)	178	26.1
3.4% fat (Sealtest)	1 cup (8.6 oz.)	207	25.9

(USDA): United States Department of Agriculture
DNA: Data Not Available
* Prepared as Package Directs

Food and Description	Measure or Quantity	Calories	Carbo-hydrates (grams)
With skim milk:			
(USDA)	1 cup (8.8 oz.)	190	27.2
.5% fat (Sealtest)	1 cup (8.6 oz.)	146	26.2
1% fat (Sealtest)	1 cup (8.6 oz.)	158	26.2
MILK, GOAT, whole (USDA)	1 cup (8.6 oz.)	163	11.2
MILK, HUMAN (USDA)	1 oz. (by wt.)	22	2.7
MILK, REINDEER (USDA)	1 oz. (by wt.)	66	1.2
MILK SHAKE MIX, any flavor, *Great Shakes:*			
*With whole milk	1 cup (9.6 oz.)	259	37.0
*With nonfat milk	1 cup (9.7 oz.)	189	38.0
MILLET, whole-grain (USDA)	1 lb.	1483	330.7
MINCEMEAT:			
(Crosse & Blackwell)	1 T. (.7 oz.)	60	14.3
Condensed (None Such)	9-oz. block	997	211.4
Ready-to-use (None Such)	1 cup (10.3 oz.)	655	151.6
MINCE PIE:			
Home recipe, 2-crust (USDA)	⅛ of 9″ pie (5.6 oz.)	428	65.1
Frozen:			
(Banquet)	5 oz.	401	62.8
(Morton)	⅛ of 20-oz. pie	247	35.8
(Mrs. Smith's)	⅛ of 8″ pie (4.2 oz.)	335	48.2
MINESTRONE SOUP:			
Condensed (USDA)	8 oz. (by wt.)	197	26.3
*Prepared with equal volume water (USDA)	1 cup (8.6 oz.)	105	14.2
*(Campbell)	1 cup	82	10.5
(Crosse & Blackwell)	6½ oz. (½ can)	107	17.0
*Mix (Golden Grain)	1 cup	69	11.2
MISO, cereal & soybeans (USDA)	4 oz.	194	26.6

Food and Description	Measure or Quantity	Calories	Carbo-hydrates (grams)
MOCHA EXTRACT (Ehlers)	1 tsp.	2	D.N.A.
***MOCHA NUT PUDDING MIX**, instant (Royal)	½ cup (5.1 oz.)	194	31.0
MOLASSES:			
Barbados (USDA)	½ cup (5.4 oz.)	417	108.0
Barbados (USDA)	1 T. (.7 oz.)	51	13.3
Blackstrap (USDA)	½ cup (5.4 oz.)	328	85.0
Blackstrap (USDA)	1 T. (.7 oz.)	40	10.4
Light (USDA)	½ cup (5.4 oz.)	388	100.1
Light (USDA)	1 T. (.7 oz.)	48	12.4
Medium (USDA)	½ cup (5.4 oz.)	357	92.4
Medium (USDA)	1 T. (.7 oz.)	44	11.4
(Brer Rabbit) Gold Label	1 T.	60	14.6
(Brer Rabbit) Green Label	1 T.	53	13.3
Unsulphured (Grandma's)	1 T. (.7 oz.)	57	13.7
MOR (Wilson) canned luncheon meat	3 oz.	266	1.6
MORTADELLA, sausage (USDA)	1 oz.	89	.2
MOSELMAID, German Moselle wine (Deinhard) 11% alcohol	3 fl. oz.	60	1.0
MOUNTAIN WINE (Louis M. Martini) 12.5% alcohol, red, Riesling, vin rosé or white	3 fl. oz.	90	.2
MOXIE, soft drink	6 fl. oz.	89	22.2
MR. PiBB, soft drink	6 fl. oz.	70	18.6
MRS. BUTTERWORTH'S SYRUP	1 T. (.7 oz.)	53	13.0
MUFFIN:			
Blueberry, home recipe (USDA)	1.4-oz. muffin (3″ dia.)	112	16.8

(USDA): United States Department of Agriculture
DNA: Data Not Available
* Prepared as Package Directs

Food and Description	Measure or Quantity	Calories	Carbohydrates (grams)
Bran:			
Home recipe (USDA)	1.4-oz. muffin (3″ dia.)	104	17.2
With raisins (Thomas')	1 muffin (1.9 oz.)	170	26.7
Corn:			
Home recipe, prepared with whole-ground cornmeal (USDA)	1.4-oz. muffin (2⅜″ dia.)	115	17.0
Home recipe, prepared with degermed cornmeal (USDA)	1.4-oz. muffin (2⅜″ dia.)	126	19.2
(Thomas')	1 muffin (2 oz.)	194	26.8
English:			
(Arnold)	1 muffin (2.2 oz.)	145	26.7
(Di Carlo)	1 muffin	145	28.0
(Hostess)	1 muffin	145	28.0
(Newly Weds)	1 muffin (2.5 oz.)	167	33.2
(Thomas')	1 muffin (2.1 oz.)	140	28.4
(Wonder)	1 muffin (2 oz.)	137	26.7
Golden Egg Toasting (Arnold)	1 muffin (2.5 oz.)	162	26.8
Plain, home recipe (USDA)	1.4-oz. muffin (2⅜″ dia.)	118	16.9
Scone (Wonder)	1 scone (2 oz.)	137	27.9
MUFFIN MIX:			
*Apple cinnamon (Betty Crocker)	2¾″ muffin	159	26.4
*Banana nut (Betty Crocker)	2¾″ muffin	167	24.6
Blueberry:			
*Wild (Betty Crocker)	2¾″ muffin	118	19.3
*(Duncan Hines)	1 muffin (1.2 oz.)	89	15.6
*Butter pecan (Betty Crocker)	2¾″ muffin	159	21.3
Corn:			
With enriched flour (USDA)	1 oz.	118	20.4
*Prepared with egg & milk (USDA)	1.4-oz. muffin (2⅜″ dia.)	119	20.8

Food and Description	Measure or Quantity	Calories	Carbo- hydrates (grams)
With cake flour & nonfat dry milk (USDA)	1 oz.	116	20.3
*Prepared with egg & water (USDA)	1.4-oz. muffin (2⅜" dia.)	119	20.8
*(Betty Crocker)	2¾" muffin	156	24.8
*(Dromedary)	1.4-oz. muffin	144	20.5
*(Flako)	1.3-oz. muffin (1/12 of pkg.)	131	20.4
(Pillsbury) golden	1 oz.	112	18.8
*Date nut (Betty Crocker)	2¾" muffin	152	21.8
*Honey bran (Betty Crocker)	2¾" muffin	154	26.2
*Oatmeal (Betty Crocker)	2¾" muffin	166	23.8
*Orange (Betty Crocker) *Sunkist*	2¾" muffin	153	26.6
*Spice (Betty Crocker)	2¾" muffin	151	23.4
MULLET, raw (USDA):			
Whole	1 lb. (weighed whole)	351	0.
Meat only	4 oz.	166	0.
MUNG BEAN SPROUT (See **BEAN SPROUT**)			
MUSCATEL WINE:			
(Gallo) 14% alcohol	3 fl. oz.	86	7.8
(Gallo) 16% alcohol	3 fl. oz.	101	7.2
(Gallo) 20% alcohol	3 fl. oz.	111	8.4
(Gold Seal) 19% alcohol	3 fl. oz.	158	9.4
(Italian Swiss Colony-Gold Medal) 19.7% alcohol	3 fl. oz.	130	9.0
(Italian Swiss Colony-Private Stock) golden, 19.7% alcohol	3 fl. oz.	138	10.8
(Taylor) 19.5% alcohol	3 fl. oz.	147	11.1
MUSHROOM:			
Raw (USDA):			
Whole	½ lb. (weighed untrimmed)	62	9.7

(USDA): United States Department of Agriculture
DNA: Data Not Available
* Prepared as Package Directs

Food and Description	Measure or Quantity	Calories	Carbohydrates (grams)
Trimmed, slices	½ cup (1.2 oz.)	10	1.5
Canned, solids & liq.:			
(USDA)	½ cup (4.3 oz.)	21	2.9
(USDA)	4 oz.	19	2.7
Sliced, chopped or whole, broiled in butter (B in B)	6-oz. can	50	4.1
Sliced (Green Giant)	4-oz. can	27	4.5
Stems & pieces (Green Giant)	4-oz. can	23	4.0
Whole (Green Giant)	4-oz. can	31	5.1
(Oxford Royal)	4 oz.	17	2.4
Frozen:			
Whole (Birds Eye)	⅓ pkg. (1.5 oz.)	11	1.9
Whole, in butter sauce (Green Giant)	6-oz. pkg.	92	5.1
MUSHROOM SOUP:			
*Barley (Manischewitz)	1 cup	72	12.2
Bisque (Crosse & Blackwell)	6½ oz. (½ can)	103	8.3
Cream of:			
Condensed (USDA)	8 oz. (by wt.)	252	19.1
*Prepared with equal volume water (USDA)	1 cup (8.5 oz.)	134	10.1
*Prepared with equal volume milk (USDA)	1 cup (8.6 oz.)	216	16.2
*(Campbell)	1 cup	131	8.5
(Heinz) *Great American*	1 cup (8¾ oz.)	131	12.4
*(Heinz)	1 cup (8½ oz.)	124	10.4
*Dietetic (Claybourne)	8 oz. (by wt.)	79	10.7
Low sodium (Campbell)	7¼-oz. can	121	8.9
*Golden (Campbell)	1 cup	80	7.7
MUSHROOM SOUP MIX:			
*(Golden Grain)	1 cup	121	16.0
(Lipton)	1 pkg. (1¼ oz.)	125	20.5
*(Wyler's)	6 fl. oz.	113	7.0
MUSKELLUNGE, raw (USDA):			
Whole	1 lb. (weighed whole)	242	0.
Meat only	4 oz.	124	0.

Food and Description	Measure or Quantity	Calories	Carbo-hydrates (grams)
MUSKMELON (See CANTA-LOUPE, CASABA or HONEYDEW)			
MUSKRAT, roasted (USDA)	4 oz.	174	0.
MUSSEL (USDA):			
Atlantic & Pacific, raw, in shell	1 lb. (weighed in shell)	153	7.2
Atlantic & Pacific, raw, meat only	4 oz.	108	3.7
Pacific, canned, drained	4 oz.	129	1.7
MUSTARD, prepared:			
Brown:			
(USDA)	1 tsp. (9 grams)	8	.5
(Gulden's)	¼-oz. packet (1 scant tsp.)	6	.4
(Heinz)	1 tsp.	8	.5
German style (Kraft)	1 oz.	30	1.7
Horseradish (Kraft)	1 oz.	29	1.6
Salad (Kraft)	1 oz.	23	1.7
Yellow:			
(USDA)	1 tsp. (9 grams)	7	.6
(Gulden's)	¼-oz. packet (1 scant tsp.)	5	.4
(Heinz)	1 tsp.	5	.5
(Kraft)	1 oz.	23	1.7
MUSTARD GREENS:			
Raw, whole (USDA)	1 lb. (weighed untrimmed)	98	17.8
Boiled, drained (USDA)	1 cup (7.8 oz.)	51	8.8
Frozen:			
Not thawed (USDA)	4 oz.	23	3.6
Boiled, drained (USDA)	½ cup (3.8 oz.)	21	3.3
Chopped (Birds Eye)	½ cup (3.3 oz.)	19	2.2
MUSTARD SPINACH (USDA):			
Raw	1 lb.	100	17.7
Boiled, drained solids	4 oz.	18	3.2

(USDA): United States Department of Agriculture
DNA: Data Not Available
* Prepared as Package Directs

Food and Description	Measure or Quantity	Calories	Carbohydrates (grams)

N

NASSAU DRY WINE (Gallo)
20% alcohol | 3 fl. oz. | 106 | 7.5

NATTO, fermented soybean (USDA) | 4 oz. | 189 | 13.0

NEAR BEER (See **BEER, NEAR**)

NEAPOLITAN CREAM PIE,
frozen:
(Banquet) | 2½ oz. | 188 | 27.2
(Mrs. Smith's) | ⅛ of 8″ pie (2.3 oz.) | 221 | 25.5

NECTARINE, fresh (USDA):
Whole | 1 lb. (weighed with pits) | 267 | 71.4
Flesh only | 4 oz. | 73 | 19.4

NEW ZEALAND SPINACH (USDA):
Raw | 1 lb. | 86 | 14.1
Boiled, drained solids | 4 oz. | 15 | 2.4

NIERSTEINER, German Rhine wine (Julius Kayser) 10% alcohol | 3 fl. oz. | 54 | .9

NOODLE. Plain noodle products are essentially the same in caloric value and carbohydrate content on the same weight basis. The longer they are cooked, the more water is absorbed and this affects the nutritive values. (USDA):
Dry, 1½″ strips | 1 cup (2.6 oz.) | 283 | 52.6
Dry | 1 oz. | 110 | 20.4
Cooked | 1 cup (5.6 oz.) | 200 | 37.3
Cooked | 1 oz. | 35 | 6.6

Food and Description	Measure or Quantity	Calories	Carbo- hydrates (grams)
NOODLE & BEEF, canned:			
(Heinz)	8½-oz. can	171	18.1
(Nalley's)	8 oz.	318	11.8
With gravy (College Inn)	4 oz.	318	59.1
With tomato sauce (College Inn)	4 oz.	319	47.4
NOODLE, CHOW MEIN, canned:			
(USDA)	1 cup (1.6 oz.)	220	26.1
(Chun King)	1 cup	211	23.2
(Hung's)	1 oz.	148	16.1
NOODLE DINNER:			
*Canton, mix (Betty Crocker)	1 cup	403	33.1
*With cheese, mix (Kraft)	4 oz.	204	21.7
*With chicken, canned (Lynden)	14 oz.	421	33.0
*With chicken, mix (Kraft)	4 oz.	122	18.9
With chicken & vegetables, canned (Lynden)	15 oz.	550	50.0
With chicken, frozen (Swanson)	10¾-oz. dinner	370	46.0
*Romanoff, mix (Kraft)	4 oz.	215	20.0
*Stroganoff, mix (Betty Crocker)	1 cup	500	41.6
With turkey, canned (Lynden)	15 oz.	369	28.0
NOODLE MIX:			
*Almondine (Betty Crocker)	½ cup	213	26.2
*Almondine *Noodle-Roni*	4 oz.	143	21.7
*Au gratin *Noodle-Roni*	4 oz.	129	22.2
*Italiano (Betty Crocker)	½ cup	207	27.6
*Parmesano *Noodle-Roni*	4 oz.	156	25.5
*Romanoff (Betty Crocker)	½ cup	241	26.4
*Romanoff *Noodle-Roni*	4 oz.	179	22.5
Scallop-A-Roni	½ cup	88	13.4
Twist-A-Roni	½ cup (3.5 oz.)	120	18.0

(USDA): United States Department of Agriculture
DNA: Data Not Available
* Prepared as Package Directs

Food and Description	Measure or Quantity	Calories	Carbo-hydrates (grams)
NOODLE SOUP:			
Beef (See **BEEF SOUP**)			
Chicken (See **CHICKEN SOUP**)			
*With ground beef, canned (Campbell)	1 cup	91	9.2
N-RICH, cream substitute	⅛ oz.	10	1.7
NUITS ST. GEORGE, French red Burgundy (Barton & Guestier) 13.5% alcohol	3 fl. oz.	70	.5
NUT, mixed (See also individual kinds):			
Dry roasted:			
(Planters)	1 oz.	176	6.2
(Skippy)	1 oz.	181	6.4
Oil roasted:			
With peanuts (Planters)	1 oz.	176	6.2
Without peanuts (Planters)	1 oz.	178	6.0
(Skippy)	1 oz.	185	6.0
NUT LOAF (See **BREAD, CANNED**)			
NUTMEG (Ehlers)	1 tsp.	12	D.N.A.
NUTRAMENT (Drackett):			
Liquid:			
Cherry	1 can (12½ fl. oz.)	423	56.0
Chocolate or chocolate marshmallow	1 can (12½ fl. oz.)	399	50.0
Dutch chocolate	1 can (12½ fl. oz.)	422	56.0
Strawberry	1 can (12½ fl. oz.)	375	44.0
Vanilla	1 can (12½ fl. oz.)	387	47.0
Powder:			
Chocolate or chocolate malt	1 packet (2 oz.)	214	37.3
Strawberry or vanilla	1 packet (2 oz.)	214	38.3

Food and Description	Measure or Quantity	Calories	Carbo-hydrates (grams)

OAT FLAKES, cereal:

(USDA)	1 cup (1.4 oz.)	162	29.0
(Post) fortified	⅔ cup (1 oz.)	107	19.0

OATMEAL:
Instant:
  Dry:

(H-O)	1 cup (2.3 oz.)	251	44.3
(H-O)	1 T. (4 grams)	15	2.7
(Quaker)	1-oz. packet (¾ cup cooked)	107	19.0
(3 Minute)	1 oz.	109	19.3
With apple & cinnamon (Quaker)	1⅛-oz. packet (¾ cup cooked)	119	23.9
With maple & brown sugar (Quaker)	1⅝-oz. packet (¾ cup cooked)	177	35.9
With raisins & spice (Quaker)	1.5-oz. packet (¾ cup cooked)	154	31.9
*Cooked (3 Minute)	1 cup	175	31.0

Quick:
  Dry:

(H-O)	1 cup (2.3 oz.)	251	44.3
(H-O)	1 T. (4 grams)	15	2.7
(Ralston Oats)	5 T. (1 oz.)	109	18.3

  Cooked:

*(USDA)	1 cup (8.3 oz.)	130	22.9
*(Albers)	1 cup	148	26.0
*(Quaker)	⅔ cup (1 oz. dry)	107	18.7
*(Ralston Oats)	1 cup	160	27.5

Regular:
  Dry:

(USDA)	1 cup (2.5 oz.)	281	49.1
(USDA)	1 T. (4 grams)	18	3.1

(USDA): United States Department of Agriculture
DNA: Data Not Available
* Prepared as Package Directs

Food and Description	Measure or Quantity	Calories	Carbo-hydrates (grams)
Old fashioned (H-O)	1 cup (2.3 oz.)	251	44.3
Old fashioned (H-O)	1 T. (4 grams)	15	2.7
*(Ralston Oats)	3⅓ T. (1 oz.)	103	20.3
Cooked:			
*(USDA)	1 cup (8.5 oz.)	132	23.3
*Old fashioned (Albers)	1 cup	148	26.0
*Old fashioned (Quaker)	⅔ cup (1 oz. dry)	107	18.7
*(Ralston Oats)	1 cup	160	27.5
OCEAN PERCH (USDA):			
Atlantic:			
Raw, whole	1 lb. (weighed whole)	124	0.
Fried	4 oz.	257	7.7
Frozen, breaded, fried, reheated	4 oz.	362	18.7
Pacific, raw:			
Whole	1 lb. (weighed whole)	116	0.
Meat only	4 oz.	108	0.
OCEAN PERCH MEAL,			
frozen:			
(Banquet)	9-oz. dinner	472	49.2
(Weight Watchers)	16-oz. dinner	313	23.7
OCTOPUS, raw, meat only			
(USDA)	4 oz.	83	0.
OESTRICHLER LENCHEN RIESLING, German Rhine wine (Deinhard) 11% alcohol	3 fl. oz.	72	4.5
OIL, salad or cooking:			
(USDA) including olive	½ cup (3.9 oz.)	972	0.
(USDA) including olive	1 T. (.5 oz.)	124	0.
Buttery flavor (Wesson)	1 T.	125	0.
Corn (Mazola)	1 cup (7.7 oz.)	1962	0.
Corn (Mazola)	1 T. (.5 oz.)	126	0.
Cottonseed winterized (Kraft)	1 oz.	257	0.
Peanut (Planters)	1 T. (.5 oz.)	126	0.
Safflower (Kraft)	1 oz.	251	0.
Safflower (Saff-o-life)	1 T.	124	0.

Food and Description	Measure or Quantity	Calories	Carbo- hydrates (grams)
(Saffola)	1 T. (.5 oz.)	124	0.
(Wesson)	1 T.	125	0.
OKRA:			
Raw, whole (USDA)	1 lb. (weighed untrimmed)	140	29.6
Boiled, drained (USDA):			
Whole	½ cup (3.1 oz.)	26	5.3
Pods	8 pods (3″ x ⅝″, 3 oz.)	25	5.1
Slices	½ cup (2.8 oz.)	23	4.8
Canned, with tomatoes (King Pharr)	½ cup	26	5.0
Frozen:			
Cut & pods, not thawed (USDA)	4 oz.	44	10.2
Cut, boiled, drained (USDA)	½ cup (3.2 oz.)	35	8.1
Whole, boiled, drained (USDA)	½ cup (2.4 oz.)	26	6.1
Cut (Birds Eye)	½ cup (2.5 oz.)	27	5.7
OKS, cereal (Kellogg's)	1 cup (¾ oz.)	73	14.9
OLD FASHIONED COCKTAIL (Hiram Walker) 62 proof	3 fl. oz.	165	3.0
OLD FASHIONED MIX (Bar-Tender's)	1 serving (⅛ oz.)	20	4.7
OLD MANSE SYRUP	1 T. (.7 oz.)	53	13.2
OLEOMARGARINE (See **MARGARINE**)			
OLIVE:			
Greek style, with pits, drained (USDA)	1 oz.	308	7.9
Green, pitted & drained: (USDA)	1 oz.	33	.4

(USDA): United States Department of Agriculture
DNA: Data Not Available
* Prepared as Package Directs

Food and Description	Measure or Quantity	Calories	Carbohydrates (grams)
(USDA)	4 med. or 3 extra large or 2 giant	19	.2
(USDA)	1 olive (13⁄16″ x 11⁄16″)	6	<.1
(La Manna, Azema & Farnan)	1 med.-size manzanilla	4	.1
(La Manna, Azema & Farnan)	1 queen size	5	.1
Ripe, by variety:			
Ascolano, any size (USDA)	1 oz.	37	.7
Manzanilla, any size (USDA)	1 oz.	37	.7
Mission, any size (USDA)	1 oz.	52	.9
Mission (USDA)	3 small or 2 large	18	.3
Mission, slices (USDA)	½ cup (2.2 oz.)	114	2.0
Sevillano, any size (USDA)	1 oz.	26	.8
Ripe, by size:			
Select (Lindsay)	1 olive	3	.1
Medium (Lindsay)	1 olive	4	.1
Large (Lindsay)	1 olive	5	.1
Extra large (Lindsay)	1 olive	5	.1
Mammoth (Lindsay)	1 olive	6	.1
Giant (Lindsay)	1 olive	8	.2
Jumbo (Lindsay)	1 olive	10	.2
Colossal (Lindsay)	1 olive	13	.3
Supercolossal (Lindsay)	1 olive	16	.3
Super supreme (Lindsay)	1 olive	18	.3
ONION:			
Raw (USDA):			
Whole	1 lb. (weighed untrimmed)	157	35.9
Whole	3.9-oz. onion (2½″ dia.)	38	8.7
Chopped	½ cup (3 oz.)	33	7.5
Chopped	1 T. (.4 oz.)	4	1.0
Grated	1 T. (.5 oz.)	5	1.2
Slices	½ cup (2 oz.)	21	4.9
Boiled, drained (USDA):			
Whole	½ cup (3.7 oz.)	30	6.8
Halves or pieces	½ cup (3.2 oz.)	26	5.8

Food and Description	Measure or Quantity	Calories	Carbohydrates (grams)
Cream sauce:			
Canned (Durkee) *O & C*	15½-oz. can	352	36.6
Frozen (Birds Eye)	⅛ pkg. (3 oz.)	132	12.7
Dehydrated, flakes (USDA)	1 cup (2.3 oz.)	224	52.5
Frozen:			
Chopped (Birds Eye)	¼ cup	11	2.5
Whole, small (Birds Eye)	½ cup (4 oz.)	51	12.0
French-fried rings:			
(Durkee) *O & C*	2 cups (3½-oz. can)	618	44.5
Frozen (Birds Eye)	2 oz.	168	17.1
Frozen (Commodore)	1 oz.	55	2.9
Frozen (Mrs. Paul's)	5-oz. pkg.	418	41.3
Pickled, cocktail (Crosse & Blackwell)	1 T. (.5 oz.)	1	.3
Pickled, sweet Dutch (Smucker's)	1 onion	4	1.0
ONION BOUILLON:			
Cube (Herb-Ox)	1 cube (4 grams)	10	1.4
Cube (Wyler's)	1 cube (4 grams)	10	1.2
Instant (Herb-Ox)	1 packet (5 grams)	15	2.0
ONION, GREEN, raw (USDA):			
Whole	1 lb. (weighed untrimmed)	157	35.7
Bulb & entire top	1 oz.	10	2.3
Bulb without green top	3 small onions (.9 oz.)	11	2.6
Slices, bulb & white portion of top	½ cup (1.8 oz.)	22	5.2
Tops only	1 oz.	8	1.6
ONION JUICE (McCormick)	1 tsp.	<1	D.N.A.
ONION SOUP:			
Condensed (USDA)	8 oz. (by wt.)	122	9.8
*Prepared with equal volume water (USDA)	1 cup (8.5 oz.)	65	5.3
*(Campbell)	1 cup	41	3.3

(USDA): United States Department of Agriculture
DNA: Data Not Available
* Prepared as Package Directs

Food and Description	Measure or Quantity	Calories	Carbo- hydrates (grams)
(Crosse & Blackwell)	6½ oz. (½ can)	46	4.8
(Hormel)	15-oz. can	144	5.5
ONION SOUP MIX:			
Dry (USDA)	1½-oz. pkg.	151	23.2
*Prepared (USDA)	1 cup (8.1 oz.)	34	5.2
*(Golden Grain)	1 cup	41	7.0
*(Lipton)	1 cup	35	5.5
*(Wyler's)	6 fl. oz.	28	5.3
ONION, WELCH, raw (USDA):			
Whole	1 lb. (weighed untrimmed)	100	19.2
Trimmed	4 oz.	39	7.4
OPOSSUM, roasted, meat only (USDA)	4 oz.	251	0.
ORANGE, fresh:			
All varieties:			
Orange, whole, medium	5.5-oz. orange (3″ dia.)	77	19.0
Sections (USDA)	1 cup (8.5 oz.)	118	29.4
Sections, sweetened, chilled, bottled (Kraft)	4 oz.	61	14.1
California Navel:			
Whole (USDA)	1 lb. (weighed with rind & seeds)	157	39.2
Whole (USDA)	6.3-oz. orange (2⅜″ dia.)	62	15.5
Sections (USDA)	1 cup (8.5 oz.)	123	30.6
Wedge, unpeeled (Sunkist)	⅛ orange	10	4.0
Cut, bite-size (Sunkist)	½ cup	62	16.0
California Valencia (USDA):			
Whole	1 lb. (weighed with rind & seeds)	174	42.2
Fruit including peel	6.3-oz. orange (2⅝″ dia.)	72	27.9
Sections	1 cup (8.5 oz.)	123	29.9
Florida, all varieties (USDA):			
Whole	1 lb. (weighed with rind & seeds)	158	40.3
Whole	7.4-oz. orange (3″ dia.)	73	18.6
Sections	1 cup (8.5 oz.)	113	28.9

Food and Description	Measure or Quantity	Calories	Carbo-hydrates (grams)
ORANGEADE:			
Chilled (Sealtest)	½ cup (4.4 oz.)	64	15.6
Frozen, sweetened:			
*(Minute Maid)	½ cup (4.2 oz.)	63	15.1
*(Snow Crop)	½ cup (4.2 oz.)	63	15.1
*Mix (Salada)	6 fl. oz.	80	19.4
ORANGE-APRICOT JUICE DRINK, canned:			
(USDA) 40% fruit juices	1 cup (8.8 oz.)	124	31.6
(BC)	1 cup	120	D.N.A.
(Del Monte)	1 cup (8.6 oz.)	115	31.8
ORANGE-BANANA JUICE DRINK, canned (BC)	1 cup	120	D.N.A.
ORANGE CAKE MIX:			
*(Betty Crocker)	1/12 of cake	201	36.8
*Chiffon (Betty Crocker)	1/16 of cake	135	27.1
*(Duncan Hines)	1/12 of cake (2.7 oz.)	201	35.0
(Pillsbury)	1 oz.	120	21.9
ORANGE DRINK:			
Canned (Hi-C)	6 fl. oz. (16.3 oz.)	89	22.2
Chilled (Sealtest)	6 fl. oz.	87	21.3
*Mix (Wyler's)	6 fl. oz.	64	15.8
ORANGE EXTRACT (Ehlers)	1 tsp.	14	D.N.A.
ORANGE-GRAPEFRUIT JUICE:			
Canned, unsweetened (USDA)	1 cup (8.7 oz.)	106	24.8
Canned, sweetened (Del Monte)	½ cup (4.3 oz.)	55	14.0
Canned (Treesweet)	½ cup	62	D.N.A.
Frozen, concentrate:			
Unsweetened (USDA)	6-fl.-oz. can	330	77.9

(USDA): United States Department of Agriculture
DNA: Data Not Available
* Prepared as Package Directs

Food and Description	Measure or Quantity	Calories	Carbo-hydrates (grams)
*Unsweetened, diluted with 3 parts water (USDA)	½ cup (4.4 oz.)	55	13.0
*(7L)	½ cup	55	13.0
*(Treesweet)	½ cup	62	D.N.A.
*Unsweetened (Minute Maid)	½ cup (4.2 oz.)	51	12.7
*Unsweetened (Snow Crop)	½ cup (4.2 oz.)	51	12.7
ORANGE-GRAPEFRUIT JUICE DRINK, canned (BC)	6 fl. oz.	90	D.N.A.
ORANGE ICE (Sealtest)	¼ pt. (3.2 oz.)	130	32.6
ORANGE JUICE:			
Fresh:			
All varieties (USDA)	½ cup (4.4 oz.)	56	12.9
California Navel (USDA)	½ cup (4.4 oz.)	60	14.0
California Valencia (USDA)	½ cup (4.4 oz.)	58	13.0
Florida, early or midseason (USDA)	½ cup (4.4 oz.)	50	11.5
Florida Temple (USDA)	½ cup (4.4 oz.)	67	16.0
Florida Valencia (USDA)	½ cup (4.4 oz.)	56	13.0
(Sunkist)	½ cup (4.4 oz.)	52	13.0
Canned, sweetened:			
(USDA)	½ cup (4.4 oz.)	66	15.4
(Del Monte)	½ cup (4.3 oz.)	59	14.9
(Heinz)	5½-fl.-oz. can	91	21.0
(Treesweet)	½ cup (4.4 oz.)	65	15.3
Canned, unsweetened:			
(USDA)	½ cup (4.4 oz.)	60	13.9
(Del Monte)	½ cup (4.3 oz.)	46	11.7
(Heinz)	5½-fl.-oz. can	71	16.5
Chilled, fresh (Kraft)	½ cup (4.4 oz.)	60	13.8
Chilled, fresh (Sealtest)	½ cup (4.3 oz.)	64	14.4
Dehydrated, crystals:			
(USDA)	4-oz. can	431	100.8
*Reconstituted (USDA)	½ cup (4.4 oz.)	57	13.4
Frozen, concentrate:			
(USDA)	6-fl.-oz. can	337	80.9
*Diluted with 3 parts water (USDA)	½ cup (4.4 oz.)	56	13.3

Food and Description	Measure or Quantity	Calories	Carbo-hydrates (grams)
*(Birds Eye)	½ cup (4 oz.)	51	13.3
*Orange Plus (Birds Eye)	½ cup (4 oz.)	67	16.6
*(Lake Hamilton)	½ cup (4.4 oz.)	58	13.3
*(Minute Maid)	½ cup	60	13.7
*(Seald-Sweet)	½ cup	56	13.3
*(7L)	½ cup	55	13.5
*(Snow Crop)	½ cup	60	13.7
*(Treesweet)	½ cup	62	D.N.A.

ORANGE, MANDARIN (See MANDARIN ORANGE & TANGERINE)

ORANGE PEEL, CANDIED:

(USDA)	1 oz.	90	22.9
(Liberty)	1 oz.	93	22.6

ORANGE-PINEAPPLE DRINK, canned:

Juice drink (BC)	6 fl. oz.	96	D.N.A.
(Hi-C)	6 fl. oz.	88	21.8

ORANGE-PINEAPPLE PIE

(Tastykake)	4-oz. pie	374	56.2

ORANGE RENNET CUSTARD MIX:
Powder:

(Junket)	1 oz.	116	27.7
*(Junket)	4 oz.	108	14.6

Tablet:

(Junket)	1 tablet (<1 gram)	1	.2
*With sugar (Junket)	4 oz.	101	13.5

ORANGE SHERBET (See SHERBET)

ORANGE SOFT DRINK:
Sweetened:

(Canada Dry)	6 fl. oz.	94	24.6
(Clicquot Club)	6 fl. oz.	103	25.0

(USDA): United States Department of Agriculture
DNA: Data Not Available
* Prepared as Package Directs

Food and Description	Measure or Quantity	Calories	Carbo-hydrates (grams)
(Cott)	6 fl. oz.	103	25.0
(Dr. Brown's)	6 fl. oz.	91	22.6
(Dr. Pepper)	6 fl. oz.	102	25.2
(Fanta)	6 fl. oz.	92	23.8
(Hoffman)	6 fl. oz.	93	23.2
(Key Food)	6 fl. oz.	86	21.5
(Kirsch)	6 fl. oz.	88	21.9
(Mission)	6 fl. oz.	103	25.0
(Nedick's)	6 fl. oz.	91	22.6
Orangette	6 fl. oz.	94	24.3
(Shasta)	6 fl. oz.	95	24.0
(Waldbaum)	6 fl. oz.	91	22.6
(White Rock)	6 fl. oz.	89	D.N.A.
(Yoo-Hoo)	6 fl. oz.	90	18.0
High-protein (Yoo-Hoo)	6 fl. oz.	114	24.6
(Yukon Club)	6 fl. oz.	95	23.8
Low calorie:			
(Dr. Brown's)	6 fl. oz.	1	.2
(Hoffman)	6 fl. oz.	1	.2
(No-Cal)	6 fl. oz.	2	0.
(Shasta)	6 fl. oz.	<1	<.1
ORGEAT SYRUP (Julius Wile)	1 fl. oz.	103	26.0
ORVIETO WINE, Italian white:			
(Antinori) 12% alcohol	3 fl. oz.	84	6.3
(Antinori) *Castello La Scala,* 12½% alcohol	3 fl. oz.	87	6.3
OVALTINE, dry:			
Malt	1 oz.	110	23.0
Swiss chocolate	1 oz.	111	24.0
OXTAIL CONSOMME MIX, instant (Knorr Swiss)	1 tsp.	11	D.N.A.
OXTAIL SOUP (Crosse & Blackwell)	6½ oz. (½ can)	136	7.5
OYSTER: Raw: Eastern, meat only: (USDA)	13–19 med. oysters (1 cup, 8.5 oz.)	158	8.2

Food and Description	Measure or Quantity	Calories	Carbo-hydrates (grams)
(USDA)	4 oz.	75	3.9
(Epicure)	1 cup	220	13.0
Pacific & Western, meat only (USDA)	4 oz.	103	7.3
Canned, solids & liq. (USDA)	4 oz.	86	5.6
Fried (USDA)	4 oz.	271	21.1
Smoked, Japanese baby (Cresca)	3⅔-oz. can	222	D.N.A.

OYSTER CRACKER (See **CRACKER**)

OYSTER STEW:
Home recipe (USDA):			
1 part oysters to 1 part milk by volume	1 cup (8.5 oz., 6–8 oysters)	245	14.2
1 part oysters to 2 parts milk by volume	1 cup (8.5 oz.)	233	10.8
1 part oysters to 3 parts milk by volume	1 cup (8.5 oz.)	206	11.3
*Canned (Campbell)	1 cup	142	11.6
Frozen, commercial:			
Condensed (USDA)	8 oz. (by wt.)	231	15.6
*Prepared with equal volume water (USDA)	1 cup (8.5 oz.)	122	8.2
*Prepared with equal volume milk (USDA)	1 cup (8.5 oz.)	202	14.2

Food and Description	Measure or Quantity	Calories	Carbohydrates (grams)

P

Food and Description	Measure or Quantity	Calories	Carbohydrates (grams)
PAGAN PINK WINE (Gallo) 11% alcohol	3 fl. oz.	81	6.8
PAISANO WINE (Gallo) 13% alcohol	3 fl. oz.	53	1.3
PANCAKE, home recipe (USDA)	4″ pancake (1 oz.)	62	9.2
PANCAKE & WAFFLE MIX (See also **PANCAKE & WAFFLE MIX, DIETETIC**):			
Blueberry (Pillsbury)	1 oz.	98	20.6
Buckwheat:			
(USDA)	1 cup (4.8 oz.)	443	94.9
(USDA)	1 oz.	93	19.9
*Prepared with egg & milk (USDA)	4″ pancake (1 oz.)	54	6.4
*(Aunt Jemima)	4″ pancake (1.2 oz.)	61	8.0
Hungry Jack (Pillsbury)	1 oz.	95	20.2
Buttermilk:			
(USDA)	1 cup (4.8 oz.)	481	102.2
(USDA)	1 oz.	101	21.5
*Prepared with milk (USDA)	4″ pancake (1 oz.)	55	8.6
*Prepared with milk & egg (USDA)	4″ pancake (1 oz.)	61	8.7
*(Aunt Jemima)	4″ pancake (1 oz.)	83	11.3
(Betty Crocker)	1 oz.	99	21.7
Complete (Betty Crocker)	1 oz.	106	21.2
*(Duncan Hines)	4″ pancake (2 oz.)	109	19.4
Hungry Jack (Pillsbury)	1 oz.	98	20.5
Plain:			
(USDA)	1 cup (4.8 oz.)	480	102.2
(USDA)	1 oz.	101	21.5
*Prepared with milk (USDA)	1 pancake (1 oz.)	57	9.0
*Prepared with milk & egg (USDA)	1 pancake (1 oz.)	64	9.2

Food and Description	Measure or Quantity	Calories	Carbo-hydrates (grams)
(Aunt Jemima) complete	4" pancake (1.2 oz.)	59	11.4
*(Aunt Jemima) original	4" pancake (1 oz.)	59	7.8
*(Aunt Jemima) *Easy Pour*	4" pancake (1.2 oz.)	78	10.9
(Albers)	1 cup	459	99.2
(Golden Mix)	1 cup	459	80.8
*(Golden Mix)	4" pancake	106	12.5
Hungry Jack (Pillsbury)	1 oz.	97	19.9
Hungry Jack, extra light (Pillsbury)	1 oz.	97	20.2
Sweet cream (Pillsbury)	1 oz.	101	20.2

PANCAKE & WAFFLE MIX, DIETETIC:

*Buttermilk (Tillie Lewis)	4" pancake (1.2 oz.)	42	8.0
*Plain (Tillie Lewis)	4" pancake (1.2 oz.)	42	8.0

PANCAKE & WAFFLE SYRUP:

Cane & Maple (USDA)	1 T. (.7 oz.)	50	13.0
Chiefly corn, light & dark (USDA)	1 T. (.7 oz.)	58	15.0
Sweetened (Polaner)	1 T.	54	13.5
Dietetic or low calorie:			
(Dia-Mel)	1 T.	22	5.5
(Diet Delight)	1 T. (.6 oz.)	12	3.1
(Tillie Lewis)	1 T.	13	3.0

PANCREAS, raw (USDA):

Beef, lean only	4 oz.	160	0.
Beef, medium-fat	4 oz.	321	0.
Calf	4 oz.	183	0.
Hog or hog sweetbread	4 oz.	274	0.

PAPAW, fresh (USDA):

Whole	1 lb. (weighed with rind & seeds)	289	57.2
Flesh only	4 oz.	96	19.1

(USDA): United States Department of Agriculture
DNA: Data Not Available
* Prepared as Package Directs

Food and Description	Measure or Quantity	Calories	Carbo-hydrates (grams)
PAPAYA:			
Fresh (USDA):			
Whole	1 lb. (weighed with skin & seeds)	119	30.4
Flesh only	4 oz.	44	11.3
Cubed	1 cup (6.4 oz., ½″ cubes)	71	18.2
Concentrate (Karika):			
*3 to 1 blend	6 fl. oz.	14	D.N.A.
*4 to 1 blend	6 fl. oz.	11	D.N.A.
*5 to 1 blend	6 fl. oz.	9	D.N.A.
PARSLEY, fresh (USDA):			
Whole	½ lb.	100	19.3
Chopped	1 T. (4 grams)	2	.3
PARSNIP (USDA):			
Raw, whole	1 lb. (weighed unpared)	293	67.5
Boiled, drained, cut in pieces	½ cup (3.7 oz.)	70	15.8
PARTY FRUIT, soft drink (Kirsch)	6 fl. oz.	88	22.1
PARTY PUNCH, undiluted (Mogen David) 12% alcohol	3 fl. oz.	156	21.3
PASHA TURKISH COFFEE, Turkish liqueur (Leroux) 53 proof	1 fl. oz.	97	13.3
PASSION FRUIT, fresh (USDA):			
Whole	1 lb. (weighed with shell)	212	50.0
Pulp & seeds	4 oz.	102	24.0
PASTINAS, dry (USDA):			
Carrot	1 oz.	105	21.5
Egg	1 oz.	109	20.4
Spinach	1 oz.	104	21.2
PASTRAMI (Vienna)	1 oz.	57	.4

Food and Description	Measure or Quantity	Calories	Carbo-hydrates (grams)
PASTRY SHELL (See also **PIE CRUST**):			
Home recipe, baked (USDA)	1 shell (1.5 oz.)	212	18.6
Frozen (Pepperidge Farm)	1 shell (1.8 oz.)	232	14.5
Pot pie, bland (Stella D'oro)	1 shell (1.6 oz.)	205	22.8
Pot pie, bland (Keebler)	4″ shell (1.7 oz.)	236	29.6
Tart, sweet (Keebler)	3″ shell (1. oz.)	158	16.6
PATE, canned:			
De foie gras (USDA)	1 oz.	131	1.4
De foie gras (USDA)	1 T. (.5 oz.)	69	.7
Liver (Hormel)	1 oz.	78	1.1
Liver (Sell's)	1 T. (.5 oz.)	45	.5
Swiss Parfait with herbs or truffles (Cresca)	1 oz.	73	D.N.A.
PEA, GREEN:			
Raw (USDA):			
In pod	1 lb. (weighed in pod)	145	24.8
Shelled	1 lb.	381	65.3
Shelled	½ cup (2.4 oz.)	58	9.9
Boiled, drained (USDA)	½ cup (2.9 oz.)	58	9.9
Canned, regular pack:			
Alaska, Early or June, solids & liq. (USDA)	½ cup (4.4 oz.)	82	15.5
Alaska, Early or June, drained solids (USDA)	½ cup (3 oz.)	76	14.4
Alaska, Early or June, drained liq. (USDA)	4 oz.	29	5.9
Alaska, drained solids (Butter Kernel)	½ cup (4.1 oz.)	69	12.8
Early (Le Sueur), solids & liq.	½ of 8.5-oz. can	58	11.8
Early June, drained solids (Cannon)	4 oz.	100	19.1
Early June, drained solids (Fall River)	½ cup	69	12.8
Sweet, drained solids (Butter Kernel)	½ cup	60	10.4

(USDA): United States Department of Agriculture
DNA: Data Not Available
* Prepared as Package Directs

Food and Description	Measure or Quantity	Calories	Carbohydrates (grams)
Sweet, drained solids (Cannon)	4 oz.	91	17.0
Sweet, drained solids (Fall River)	½ cup	60	10.4
Sweet, solids & liq. (Green Giant)	½ of 8.5-oz. can	54	10.7
(King Pharr)	½ cup	98	17.0
Canned, dietetic pack:			
Alaska, Early or June, solids & liq. (USDA)	4 oz.	62	11.1
Drained solids (USDA)	4 oz.	88	16.2
Drained liq. (USDA)	4 oz.	25	4.6
Solids & liq. (Blue Boy)	4 oz.	49	8.0
Solids & liq. (Diet Delight)	½ cup (4.4 oz.)	52	9.0
(S and W) *Nutradiet*	4 oz.	40	7.6
(Tillie Lewis)	½ cup (4.4 oz.)	54	8.6
Frozen:			
Not thawed (USDA)	½ cup (2.5 oz.)	53	9.2
Boiled, drained (USDA)	½ cup (3 oz.)	57	9.9
(Blue Goose)	4 oz.	76	12.4
Sweet (Birds Eye)	½ cup (3.3 oz.)	70	12.2
Tender tiny (Birds Eye)	½ cup (3.3 oz.)	70	12.0
In butter sauce, baby peas (Green Giant) *Le Sueur*	⅛ of 10-oz. pkg.	74	11.0
In butter sauce, sweet (Green Giant)	⅛ of 10-oz. pkg.	78	10.6
With cream sauce (Birds Eye)	½ cup (2.7 oz.)	125	13.6
With cream sauce (Green Giant)	⅛ of 10-oz. pkg.	63	10.7
PEA, MATURE SEED, dry:			
Raw:			
Whole (USDA)	1 lb.	1542	273.5
Whole (USDA)	1 cup (7.1 oz.)	680	120.6
Split:			
(USDA)	1 lb.	1579	284.4
(USDA)	1 cup (7.2 oz.)	706	127.3
(Sinsheimer)	1 oz.	99	17.5
Cooked, split, drained solids (USDA)	½ cup (3.4 oz.)	112	20.2

PEA POD, edible-podded or Chinese:

Food and Description	Measure or Quantity	Calories	Carbo-hydrates (grams)
Raw (USDA)	1 lb. (weighed untrimmed)	228	51.7
Boiled, drained solids (USDA)	4 oz.	49	10.8
PEA & CARROT:			
Canned, regular pack, solids & liq. (Del Monte)	½ cup (4 oz.)	46	8.9
Canned, dietetic pack, solids & liq.:			
(Blue Boy)	4 oz.	26	5.9
(Diet Delight)	½ cup (4.2 oz.)	47	8.4
(S and W) *Nutradiet*	4 oz.	36	7.4
Frozen:			
Not thawed (USDA)	4 oz.	62	11.8
Boiled, drained solids (USDA)	½ cup (3.1 oz.)	46	8.8
(Birds Eye)	½ cup (3.3 oz.)	55	8.7
(Blue Goose)	4 oz.	57	10.0
In cream sauce (Green Giant)	⅛ of 10-oz. pkg.	56	9.7
PEA & CELERY, frozen (Birds Eye)	½ cup (3.3 oz.)	55	9.8
PEA & ONION, frozen (Birds Eye)	½ cup (3.3 oz.)	67	12.3
PEA & POTATO, with cream sauce, frozen (Birds Eye)	½ cup (2.7 oz.)	131	14.9
PEA with SAUTEED MUSHROOM, frozen (Birds Eye)	½ cup (3.3 oz.)	67	11.7
PEA SOUP, GREEN:			
Canned, low sodium (Campbell)	7½-oz. can (by wt.)	140	22.2
Canned, regular pack:			
Condensed (USDA)	8 oz. (by wt.)	240	41.7

(USDA): United States Department of Agriculture
DNA: Data Not Available
* Prepared as Package Directs

Food and Description	Measure or Quantity	Calories	Carbohydrates (grams)
*Prepared with equal volume water (USDA)	1 cup (8.6 oz.)	130	22.5
*Prepared with equal volume milk (USDA)	1 cup (8.6 oz.)	208	28.7
*(Campbell)	1 cup	131	21.0
Dry mix:			
(USDA)	1 oz.	103	17.5
*(USDA)	1 cup (8.5 oz.)	121	20.3
*(Golden Grain)	1 cup	76	10.5
(Lipton)	1 pkg. (4 oz.)	422	69.3
Frozen, condensed:			
With ham (USDA)	8 oz. (by wt.)	256	36.3
*With ham, prepared with equal volume water (USDA)	8 oz. (by wt.)	129	18.1
PEA SOUP, SPLIT:			
Canned, regular pack:			
Condensed (USDA)	8 oz. (by wt.)	268	38.6
*Prepared with equal volume water (USDA)	1 cup (8.6 oz.)	145	20.6
*With ham (Campbell)	1 cup	160	21.7
*(Manischewitz)	8 oz. (by wt.)	133	22.6
*With ham (Heinz)	1 cup (8¾ oz.)	153	23.0
With smoked ham (Heinz) *Great American*	1 cup (9 oz.)	186	24.0
Canned, dietetic (Tillie Lewis)	1 cup	152	26.1
PEACH:			
Fresh:			
Whole, without skin (USDA)	1 lb. (weighed unpeeled)	150	38.3
Whole (USDA)	4-oz. peach (2″ dia.)	38	9.6
Diced (USDA)	½ cup (4.7 oz.)	51	12.9
Sliced (USDA)	½ cup (3 oz.)	32	8.2
Chilled, bottled (Kraft)	4 oz.	66	17.2
Canned, regular pack, solids & liq.:			
Juice pack (USDA)	4 oz.	51	13.2
Light syrup (USDA)	4 oz.	66	17.1

Food and Description	Measure or Quantity	Calories	Carbo-hydrates (grams)
Heavy syrup (USDA)	2 med. halves & 2 T. syrup	91	23.5
Heavy syrup, halves (USDA)	½ cup (4.1 oz.)	100	25.7
Heavy syrup, sliced (USDA)	½ cup (4.4 oz.)	98	25.3
Extra heavy syrup (USDA)	4 oz.	110	28.4
(Hunt's)	½ cup (4.5 oz.)	96	25.7
(Stokely-Van Camp)	½ cup (4 oz.)	89	23.1
(White House)	½ cup (4.5 oz.)	100	25.6
Canned, dietetic or unsweetened pack:			
Water pack, solids & liq. (USDA)	½ cup (4.3 oz.)	38	9.9
(Blue Boy) sliced, solids & liq.	4 oz.	32	7.4
(Diet Delight) cling, halves	½ cup (4.4 oz.)	61	15.0
(Diet Delight) freestone, halves	½ cup (4.4 oz.)	64	15.1
(Libby's) halves or slices	4 oz.	34	9.2
(Naturmade)	4 oz.	32	7.8
(S and W) *Nutradiet*, cling, halves, unsweetened	2 halves (3.5 oz.)	28	6.6
(Yes Madame) Elberta, halves & slices	4 oz.	34	8.1
Dehydrated:			
Uncooked (USDA)	1 oz.	96	24.9
Cooked, with added sugar, solids & liq. (USDA)	½ cup (5.4 oz.)	184	47.6
Slices (Vacu-Dry)	1 oz.	96	24.9
Dried:			
Uncooked (USDA)	1 lb.	1188	309.8
Uncooked (USDA)	½ cup (3.1 oz.)	231	60.1
Cooked, unsweetened (USDA)	½ cup (5–6 halves & 3 T. liq., 4.8 oz.)	111	28.9

(USDA): United States Department of Agriculture
DNA: Data Not Available
* Prepared as Package Directs

Food and Description	Measure or Quantity	Calories	Carbohydrates (grams)
Cooked, with added sugar (USDA)	½ cup (5–6 halves & 3 T. liq., 5.4 oz.)	181	46.8
Uncooked (Del Monte)	½ cup (3.1 oz.)	204	52.4
Frozen:			
Not thawed, slices, sweetened (USDA)	12-oz. pkg.	299	76.8
Not thawed, slices, sweetened (USDA)	16-oz. can	400	102.6
Quick thaw (Birds Eye)	½ cup (5 oz.)	87	22.3
(Spiegl)	½ cup	88	22.5
PEACH LIQUEUR:			
(Bols) 60 proof	1 fl. oz.	96	8.9
(Hiram Walker) 60 proof	1 fl. oz.	81	8.0
(Leroux) 60 proof	1 fl. oz.	85	8.9
PEACH NECTAR, canned:			
(USDA)	1 cup (8.8 oz.)	120	31.0
(Del Monte)	1 cup (8.7 oz.)	140	38.1
PEACH PIE:			
Home recipe (USDA)	⅙ of 9″ pie (5.6 oz.)	403	60.4
(Tastykake)	4-oz. pie	360	52.8
Frozen (Banquet)	5 oz.	320	45.5
Frozen (Mrs. Smith's)	⅙ of 8″ pie (4.2 oz.)	299	42.0
PEACH PIE FILLING:			
(Lucky Leaf)	8 oz.	300	74.0
(Musselman's)	1 cup	292	D.N.A.
PEACH PRESERVE, dietetic or low calorie:			
(Dia-Mel)	1 T.	22	5.4
(Kraft)	1 oz.	35	8.6
(Tillie Lewis)	1 T. (.5 oz.)	10	2.4
PEACH TURNOVER, frozen (Pepperidge Farm)	1 turnover (3.3 oz.)	323	33.4

Food and Description	Measure or Quantity	Calories	Carbohydrates (grams)
PEANUT:			
Raw (USDA):			
In shell	1 lb. (weighed in shell)	1868	61.6
With skins	1 oz.	160	5.3
Without skins	1 oz.	161	5.0
Roasted:			
Whole (USDA)	1 lb. (weighed in shell)	1769	62.6
Shelled, with skins (USDA)	1 oz.	165	5.8
Salted (USDA)	1 oz.	166	5.3
Halves, salted (USDA)	½ cup (2.5 oz.)	421	13.5
Chopped (USDA)	½ cup (2.4 oz.)	404	13.0
Chopped, salted (USDA)	1 T. (9 grams)	53	1.7
Dry (Franklin)	1 oz.	163	5.4
Dry (Frito-Lay)	1 oz.	180	3.3
Dry (Planters)	1 oz. (jar)	170	5.4
Dry (Skippy)	1 oz.	175	5.4
Oil (Planters) cocktail	¾-oz. bag	133	3.7
Oil (Planters) cocktail	1 oz. (can)	179	5.0
Oil (Skippy)	1 oz.	178	5.2
(Nab)	1 packet (1¼ oz.)	223	6.7
Spanish, dry roasted (Planters)	1 oz. (jar)	175	3.4
Spanish, oil roasted (Planters)	1 oz. (can)	182	3.4
PEANUT BUTTER:			
(USDA)	½ cup (4.4 oz.)	732	21.7
(USDA)	1 T. (.6 oz.)	93	2.8
(The Peanut Kids)	1 oz.	165	5.5
(Peter Pan)	1 T. (.5 oz.)	100	3.9
(Planters)	1 T. (.5 oz.)	93	2.9
(Skippy) chunky or creamy	1 T. (.6 oz.)	102	2.3
(Smucker's) creamy or crunchy	1 T. (.5 oz.)	85	2.4
Diet spread (Peter Pan)	1 T. (.5 oz.)	100	2.0

(USDA): United States Department of Agriculture
DNA: Data Not Available
* Prepared as Package Directs

Food and Description	Measure or Quantity	Calories	Carbo-hydrates (grams)
PEAR:			
Fresh (USDA):			
Whole	1 lb. (weighed with stems & core)	252	63.2
Whole	6.4-oz. pear (3″ x 2½″ dia.)	101	25.4
Quartered	1 cup (6.8 oz.)	117	29.4
Slices	½ cup (6.8 oz.)	50	12.5
Canned, regular pack, solids & liq.:			
Juice pack (USDA)	4 oz.	52	13.4
Light syrup (USDA)	4 oz.	69	17.7
Heavy syrup, halves or slices (USDA)	½ cup (with syrup, 4 oz.)	87	22.3
Heavy syrup (USDA)	2 med. halves & 2 T. syrup (4.1 oz.)	89	22.9
Extra heavy syrup (USDA)	4 oz.	104	26.8
(Hunt's)	½ cup (4.5 oz.)	99	23.9
Canned, unsweetened or low calorie:			
Water pack, solids & liq. (USDA)	½ cup (4.3 oz.)	39	10.1
Solids & liq. (Blue Boy) Bartlett	4 oz.	33	9.6
Solids and liq. (Diet Delight)	½ cup (4.4 oz.)	66	16.1
(Dole)	½ cup & 2 T. liq.	38	D.N.A.
(Libby's) halves	4 oz.	31	9.4
(S and W) *Nutradiet*, quartered	4 oz.	31	7.9
(Yes Madame) Bartlett, halves	½ cup	32	8.6
Dried:			
Uncooked (USDA)	1 lb.	1216	305.3
Cooked, without added sugar, solids & liq. (USDA)	4 oz.	143	36.0
Cooked, with added sugar, solids & liq. (USDA)	4 oz.	171	43.1
PEAR, CANDIED (USDA)	1 oz.	86	21.5

Food and Description	Measure or Quantity	Calories	Carbohydrates (grams)
PEAR NECTAR, sweetened:			
(USDA)	1 cup (8.5 oz.)	125	31.7
(Del Monte)	1 cup (8.7 oz.)	140	38.4
PECAN:			
In shell (USDA)	1 lb. (weighed in shell)	1652	35.1
Shelled (USDA):			
Whole	1 lb.	3116	66.2
Halves	12–14 (.5 oz.)	96	2.0
Halves	½ cup (1.9 oz.)	371	7.9
Chopped	½ cup (1.8 oz.)	357	7.6
Chopped	1 T. (7 grams)	48	1.0
Dry roasted (Planters)	1 oz.	206	3.5
PECAN PIE:			
Home recipe (USDA)	⅙ of 9" pie (4.9 oz.)	577	70.8
Frozen (Mrs. Smith's)	⅛ of 8" pie (4. oz.)	422	52.0
PEPPER, BLACK:			
(USDA)	¼ tsp.	1	.3
(Lawry's) seasoned	1 tsp. (2 grams)	8	1.6
PEPPER, HOT CHILI:			
Green (USDA):			
Raw, whole	4 oz.	31	7.5
Raw, without seeds	4 oz.	42	10.3
Canned, chili sauce	1 oz.	6	1.4
Canned pods, without seeds, solids & liq.	4 oz.	28	6.9
Red:			
Raw, whole (USDA)	4 oz. (weighed with seeds)	105	20.5
Raw, trimmed, pods only (USDA)	4 oz.	54	13.1
Canned, chili sauce (USDA)	1 oz.	6	1.1

(USDA): United States Department of Agriculture
DNA: Data Not Available
* Prepared as Package Directs

Food and Description	Measure or Quantity	Calories	Carbohydrates (grams)
Canned, pods, without seeds, solids & liq. (USDA)	⅛ cup	7	1.8
Dried:			
Pods (USDA)	1 oz.	91	17.0
Pods (Chili Products)	1 oz.	88	16.9
Powder with added seasoning (USDA)	1 oz.	96	16.0
Powder with added seasoning (USDA)	1 T. (.5 oz.)	51	8.5
*PEPPER POT SOUP (Campbell's)	1 cup	94	8.6
PEPPER, SWEET:			
Green:			
Raw:			
Whole (USDA)	1 lb. (weighed untrimmed)	82	17.9
Without stem & seeds (USDA)	1 med. pepper (2.6 oz.)	13	2.9
Chopped (USDA)	½ cup (2.6 oz.)	16	3.6
Slices (USDA)	½ cup (1.4 oz.)	9	2.0
Strips (USDA)	½ cup (1.7 oz.)	11	2.4
Boiled, strips, drained (USDA)	½ cup (2.4 oz.)	12	2.6
Boiled, drained (USDA)	1 med. pepper (2.6 oz.)	13	2.8
Canned, halves (Cannon)	4 oz.	20	D.N.A.
Red:			
Raw, whole (USDA)	1 lb. (weighed with stems & seeds)	112	25.8
Raw, without stem & seeds (USDA)	1 med. pepper (2.2 oz.)	19	2.4
Canned, diced (Cannon)	4 oz.	31	D.N.A.
PEPPER, STUFFED:			
Home recipe, with beef & crumbs (USDA)	2¾" x 2½" pepper with 1⅛ cups stuffing (6.5 oz.)	314	31.1

Food and Description	Measure or Quantity	Calories	Carbo-hydrates (grams)
Frozen, with beef, in creole sauce (Holloway House)	1 pepper (7 oz.)	279	58.0
PEPPERMINT EXTRACT (Ehlers)	1 tsp.	12	D.N.A.
PEPPERMINT SCHNAPPS (See **SCHNAPPS**)			
PEP WHEAT FLAKES, cereal (Kellogg's)	1 cup (1 oz.)	108	23.0
PERCH, raw (USDA):			
White, whole	1 lb. (weighed whole)	193	0.
White, meat only	4 oz.	134	0.
Yellow, whole	1 lb. (weighed whole)	161	0.
Yellow, meat only	4 oz.	103	0.
PERNOD (Julius Wile)	1 fl. oz.	79	1.1
PERSIMMON (USDA):			
Japanese or Kaki, fresh:			
With seeds	1 lb. (weighed with skin, calyx & seeds)	286	78.3
With seeds	4.4-oz. persimmon	79	20.1
Seedless	1 lb. (weighed with skin & calyx)	293	75.1
Seedless	4.4-oz. persimmon (2½" dia.)	81	20.7
Native, fresh, whole	1 lb. (weighed with seeds & calyx)	472	124.6
Native, fresh, flesh only	4 oz.	144	38.0
PERX, cream substitute	1 tsp.	5	.6
PETITE MARMITE SOUP, canned (Crosse & Blackwell)	6½ oz. (½ can)	33	3.7

(USDA): United States Department of Agriculture
DNA: Data Not Available
* Prepared as Package Directs

Food and Description	Measure or Quantity	Calories	Carbo- hydrates (grams)
PETTIJOHNS, rolled whole wheat, cooked (Quaker)	⅔ cup (1 oz. dry)	97	20.4
PHEASANT, raw (USDA):			
Ready-to-cook	1 lb. (weighed ready-to-cook)	596	0.
Meat & skin	4 oz.	172	0.
Meat only	4 oz.	184	0.
PICKEREL, chain, raw (USDA):			
Whole	1 lb. (weighed whole)	194	0.
Meat only	4 oz.	95	0.
PICKLE:			
Chowchow (See **CHOWCHOW**)			
Cucumber, fresh or bread & butter:			
(USDA)	½ cup (3 oz.)	62	15.2
(USDA)	3 slices (¼" x 1½")	15	3.8
(Durkee)	½ cup	59	D.N.A.
(Durkee)	3 slices (¼" x 1½")	15	D.N.A.
(Fanning's)	2 fl. oz.	31	7.3
(Heinz)	3 slices	20	4.7
Dill:			
(USDA)	4.8-oz. pickle (4" x 1¾")	15	3.0
(USDA)	1 oz.	3	.6
(Albro)	1 oz.	3	.5
(Durkee)	1 pickle (4" x 1¾")	15	D.N.A.
(Heinz)	1 pickle (4")	7	1.1
Processed (Heinz)	1 pickle (3")	1	.1
(Smucker's)	1 pickle (2¾")	3	.6
Dill, candied sticks (Smucker's)	.8-oz. pickle	46	11.2
Dill, hamburger (Heinz)	3 slices	1	.1
Dill, hamburger (Smucker's)	3 slices (.4 oz.)	2	.3
Kosher dill (Smucker's)	3½" pickle (1.8 oz.)	8	1.4

Food and Description	Measure or Quantity	Calories	Carbo-hydrates (grams)
Sour:			
Cucumber (USDA)	4.8-oz. pickle (1¾" x 4")	14	2.7
Cucumber (USDA)	1 oz.	3	.6
(Albro)	1 oz.	3	.5
(Durkee)	1 pickle (¾" x 4")	15	D.N.A.
(Heinz)	1 pickle (2")	1	.2
Sweet:			
Cucumber (USDA):			
Whole	1 oz.	41	10.3
Whole, gherkin	.5-oz. pickle (2½" x ¾")	22	5.5
Chopped	½ cup (2.6 oz.)	108	27.0
Chopped	1 T. (9 grams)	13	3.3
(Albro)	1 oz.	24	5.9
(Durkee)	1 pickle (2¾" x ¾")	20	D.N.A.
(Smucker's)	2½" pickle (.4 oz.)	17	4.2
Candied, midgets (Smucker's)	2" pickle (9 grams)	14	3.5
Chips, fresh pack (Smucker's)	1 piece (5 grams)	10	2.5
Chopped (Durkee)	½ cup	112	D.N.A.
Chopped (Durkee)	1 T.	14	D.N.A.
Gherkin (Heinz)	1 pickle (2")	16	3.9
Mixed (Durkee)	1 pickle (1¾" x 4")	15	D.N.A.
Mixed (Heinz)	3 slices	23	5.6
Mixed (Smucker's)	1 piece (8 grams)	12	2.9
Mixed, chopped (Durkee)	½ cup	112	D.N.A.
Mixed, chopped (Durkee)	1 T.	14	D.N.A.
Mustard (Heinz)	1 T.	30	6.8
Relish (See **RELISH**)			
Sticks, fresh pack (Smucker's)	4" stick (1.1 oz.)	29	7.1

PIE (See individual kinds)

(USDA): United States Department of Agriculture
DNA: Data Not Available
* Prepared as Package Directs

Food and Description	Measure or Quantity	Calories	Carbo-hydrates (grams)
PIECRUST (See also **PASTRY SHELL**):			
Home recipe, baked, 9″ pie (USDA)	1 crust (6.3 oz.)	900	78.8
Home recipe, baked, 9″ pie (USDA)	2 crusts (12.7 oz.)	1800	157.7
Frozen:			
(Mrs. Smith's)	8″ shell (5 oz.)	760	62.4
(Mrs. Smith's)	9″ shell (7 oz.)	1100	90.7
(Mrs. Smith's)	10″ shell (8 oz.)	1240	102.1
PIECRUST MIX:			
Dry (USDA)	10-oz. pkg. (2 crusts)	1482	140.6
*Prepared with water (USDA)	4 oz.	526	49.9
*Double crust (Betty Crocker)	⅛ of 2 crusts	302	24.1
*Graham cracker (Betty Crocker)	⅛ of crust	159	22.3
*(Flako)	⅛ of 9″ shell (.8 oz. dry)	121	12.0
PIE FILLING (See individual kinds)			
PIESPORTER RIESLING, German Moselle wine (Julius Kayser) 10% alcohol	3 fl. oz.	57	1.7
PIGEON (See **SQUAB**)			
PIGEONPEA (USDA):			
Raw, immature seeds in pods	1 lb.	207	37.7
Dry seeds	1 lb.	1551	288.9
PIGNOLIA (See **PINE NUT**)			
PIGS FEET, pickled:			
(USDA)	4 oz.	226	0.
(Hormel)	1-pt. can	442	.2
PIKE, raw (USDA)			
Blue, whole	1 lb. (weighed whole)	180	0.

Food and Description	Measure or Quantity	Calories	Carbo-hydrates (grams)
Blue, meat only	4 oz.	102	0.
Northern, whole	1 lb. (weighed whole)	104	0.
Northern, meat only	4 oz.	100	0.
Walleye, whole	1 lb. (weighed whole)	240	0.
Walleye, meat only	4 oz.	105	0.
PILI NUT (USDA):			
In shell	1 lb. (weighed in shell)	546	6.9
Shelled	4 oz.	759	9.5
PILLSBURY INSTANT BREAKFAST:			
Chocolate	1 oz.	101	19.0
Chocolate malt	1 oz.	101	18.8
Strawberry	1 oz.	104	19.2
Vanilla	1 oz.	101	17.9
PIMIENTO, canned:			
Solids & liq. (USDA)	1 med. pod (1.3 oz.)	10	2.2
Solids & liq. (USDA)	4 oz.	31	6.6
Diced, solids & liq. (Cannon)	4 oz.	31	6.6
Pieces, pods, slices (Dromedary)	4 oz.	31	4.6
PIMM'S CUP-SLINGS (Julius Wile):			
#1-Gin	1 fl. oz.	69	3.3
#2-Scotch or #3-Brandy	1 fl. oz.	68	3.0
#4-Rum & brandy	1 fl. oz.	59	.9
#5-Canadian rye	1 fl. oz.	60	1.0
#6-Vodka	1 fl. oz.	63	1.8
PINEAPPLE:			
Fresh:			
Whole (USDA)	1 lb. (weighed untrimmed)	123	32.3

(USDA): United States Department of Agriculture
DNA: Data Not Available
* Prepared as Package Directs

Food and Description	Measure or Quantity	Calories	Carbo-hydrates (grams)
Diced (USDA)	½ cup (2.8 oz.)	41	10.7
Slices (USDA)	3-oz. slice (¾" x 3½")	44	11.5
Diced (Calavo)	½ cup	38	9.5
Canned, regular pack:			
Juice pack:			
Solids & liq. (USDA)	4 oz.	66	17.1
Solids & liq. (Del Monte)	½ cup (4.9 oz.)	79	20.7
Chunks or crushed (Dole)	½ cup (includes 2 T. juice)	64	D.N.A.
Sliced (Dole)	2 slices & 2 T. juice	64	D.N.A.
Light syrup, solids & liq. (USDA)	4 oz.	67	17.5
Heavy syrup:			
Chunks (Dole)	½ cup (includes 2 T. syrup)	84	D.N.A.
Crushed, solids & liq. (USDA)	½ cup (4.6 oz.)	97	25.4
Crushed (Dole)	½ cup (includes 2 T. syrup)	94	D.N.A.
Slices, solids & liq. (USDA)	½ cup (4.9 oz.)	103	27.0
Slices, solids & liq. (USDA)	4 oz.	84	22.0
Slices (USDA)	2 small or 1 large slice & 2 T. syrup	90	23.7
Slices (Dole)	1 large slice & 2 T. syrup	76	D.N.A.
Slices (Dole)	2 med. slices & 2 T. syrup	84	D.N.A.
Spears (Dole)	2 spears & 2 T. syrup	52	D.N.A.
Tidbits, solids & liq. (USDA)	½ cup (4.6 oz.)	95	25.0
Tidbits (Dole)	½ cup (includes 2 T. syrup)	94	D.N.A.
Extra heavy syrup, solids & liq. (USDA)	4 oz.	102	26.5
Canned, unsweetened, low calorie or dietetic:			
Water pack, except crushed			

Food and Description	Measure or Quantity	Calories	Carbo-hydrates (grams)
(USDA)	4 oz.	44	11.6
Chunks, low calorie (Diet Delight)	½ cup (4.4 oz.)	65	15.6
Chunks, low calorie (Dole)	½ cup (includes 2 T. liq.)	54	D.N.A.
Crushed, solids & liq. (Diet Delight)	½ cup (4.4 oz.)	77	18.5
Slices:			
Solids & liq. (Diet Delight)	½ cup (4.3 oz.)	44	8.6
(Dole)	2 slices & 2 T. liq.	54	D.N.A.
In pineapple juice (Dole)	2 slices & 2 T. juice	56	D.N.A.
(Libby's)	4 oz.	48	11.6
(S and W) *Nutradiet*	2½ slices (3.5 oz.)	69	17.1
(White Rose)	4 oz.	67	16.2
Tidbits:			
(Diet Delight)	½ cup (4.4 oz.)	65	15.6
In pineapple juice (Dole)	½ cup (includes 2 T. juice)	77	D.N.A.
(S and W) *Nutradiet*	4 oz.	78	19.2
Frozen:			
Chunks, sweetened, not thawed (USDA)	½ cup (4.3 oz.)	105	27.3
Chunks in heavy syrup (Dole)	½ cup (includes 2 T. syrup)	92	D.N.A.
PINEAPPLE & APRICOT JUICE DRINK			
(Del Monte)	1 cup (8.6 oz.)	132	32.6
PINEAPPLE CAKE MIX:			
*(Betty Crocker) *Dole*	1/12 of cake	199	36.1
*Upside down (Betty Crocker) *Dole*	1/9 of cake	270	42.3
*(Duncan Hines)	1/12 of cake (2.7 oz.)	201	35.0
(Pillsbury)	1 oz.	122	21.8

(USDA): United States Department of Agriculture
DNA: Data Not Available
* Prepared as Package Directs

Food and Description	Measure or Quantity	Calories	Carbohydrates (grams)
PINEAPPLE, CANDIED:			
(USDA)	1 oz.	90	22.6
(Liberty)	1 oz.	93	22.6
PINEAPPLE FLAVORING,			
imitation (Ehlers)	1 tsp.	12	D.N.A.
PINEAPPLE & GRAPEFRUIT JUICE DRINK, canned:			
(USDA) 40% fruit juices	½ cup (4.4 oz.)	68	17.0
(Del Monte)	½ cup (4.3 oz.)	62	15.6
Pink (Del Monte)	½ cup (4.3 oz.)	64	16.1
(Dole)	½ cup	62	D.N.A.
(Hi-C)	½ cup (4.2 oz.)	63	15.7
Ping (Stokely-Van Camp)	½ cup	61	D.N.A.
Pink grapefruit (Dole)	½ cup	62	D.N.A.
*PINEAPPLE & GRAPEFRUIT JUICE, unsweetened, frozen (Dole)	½ cup	51	D.N.A.
PINEAPPLE JUICE:			
Canned, unsweetened:			
(USDA)	½ cup (4.4 oz.)	68	16.7
(Del Monte)	½ cup (4.3 oz.)	65	16.1
(Dole)	½ cup	74	D.N.A.
(Heinz)	5½-fl.-oz. can	101	23.5
(S and W) *Nutradiet*	4 oz.	67	16.2
(Stokely-Van Camp)	½ cup (3.7 oz.)	63	17.0
Frozen, concentrate:			
Unsweetened, undiluted (USDA)	6-fl.-oz. can	387	95.7
*Unsweetened, diluted with 3 parts water (USDA)	½ cup (4.4 oz.)	64	15.9
*Unsweetened, diluted (Dole)	½ cup	67	D.N.A.
PINEAPPLE & ORANGE JUICE DRINK, canned:			
(USDA) 40% fruit juices	½ cup (4.4 oz.)	67	16.7
(Del Monte)	½ cup (4.3 oz.)	62	15.7
PINEAPPLE & ORANGE JUICE:			
(Kraft)	½ cup	56	12.6
*Unsweetened, frozen (Dole)	½ cup	51	D.N.A.

Food and Description	Measure or Quantity	Calories	Carbo- hydrates (grams)
PINEAPPLE-PAPAYA FRUIT SPREAD (Vita)	1 T.	9	D.N.A.
PINEAPPLE PIE:			
Home recipe:			
(USDA)	⅛ of 9″ pie (5.6 oz.)	400	60.2
Chiffon (USDA)	⅛ of 9″ pie (3.8 oz.)	311	42.2
Custard (USDA)	⅛ of 9″ pie (5.4 oz.)	334	48.8
(Tastykake)	4-oz. pie	389	57.8
With cheese (Tastykake)	4-oz. pie	436	59.4
Frozen (Morton)	⅛ of 46-oz. pie	399	60.6
PINEAPPLE PIE FILLING			
(Lucky Leaf)	8 oz.	240	59.0
PINEAPPLE PRESERVE, low calorie:			
(Dia-Mel)	1 T.	22	5.4
(Tillie Lewis)	1 T. (.5 oz.)	10	2.4
PINEAPPLE SOFT DRINK:			
(Hoffman)	6 fl. oz.	89	22.3
(Kirsch)	6 fl. oz.	89	22.3
(Nedick's)	6 fl. oz.	89	22.3
(Yoo-Hoo)	6 fl. oz.	90	18.0
High-protein (Yoo-Hoo)	6 fl. oz.	114	24.6
PINE NUT (USDA):			
Pignolias, shelled	4 oz.	626	13.2
Piñon, whole	4 oz. (weighed in shell)	418	13.5
Piñon, shelled	4 oz.	720	23.2
PINOT CHARDONNAY WINE (Louis M. Martini) 12.5% alcohol	3 fl. oz.	90	.2

(USDA): United States Department of Agriculture
DNA: Data Not Available
* Prepared as Package Directs

Food and Description	Measure or Quantity	Calories	Carbo- hydrates (grams)
PINOT NOIR WINE (Louis M. Martini) 12.5% alcohol	3 fl. oz.	90	.2
PISTACHIO NUT:			
In shell (USDA)	4 oz. (weighed in shell)	337	10.8
Shelled (USDA)	½ cup (2.2 oz.)	368	11.8
Shelled (USDA)	1 T. (8 grams)	46	1.5
***PISTACHIO NUT PUDDING MIX,** instant (Royal)	½ cup (5.1 oz.)	186	31.2
PITANGA, fresh (USDA):			
Whole	1 lb. (weighed whole)	187	45.9
Flesh only	4 oz.	58	14.2
PIZZA PIE:			
Home recipe, with cheese topping (USDA)	4 oz.	268	32.1
Home recipe, with sausage topping (USDA)	4 oz.	265	33.6
Chilled, partially baked (USDA)	4 oz.	236	35.0
Chilled, baked (USDA)	4 oz.	278	41.2
Frozen:			
Partially baked (USDA)	4 oz.	260	37.5
Baked (USDA)	4 oz.	278	40.1
Baked (USDA)	⅛ of 14″ pie (2.6 oz.)	184	26.6
Little, with cheese (Chef Boy-Ar-Dee)	1 pie (2½ oz.)	162	22.7
With cheese (Buitoni)	4 oz.	270	36.6
With cheese (Chef Boy-Ar-Dee)	⅛ of 12½-oz. pie	131	18.0
With pepperoni (Chef Boy-Ar-Dee)	⅛ of 14-oz. pie	150	18.1
Little, with sausage (Chef Boy-Ar-Dee)	1 pie (2½ oz.)	168	22.3
With sausage (Chef Boy-Ar-Dee)	⅛ of 13¼-oz. pie	141	17.9

Food and Description	Measure or Quantity	Calories	Carbo- hydrates (grams)
PIZZA PIE MIX:			
*With cheese (Chef Boy-Ar-Dee)	⅛ of 15½-oz. pie	187	26.5
*With cheese (Kraft)	4 oz.	265	26.1
*With sausage (Chef Boy-Ar-Dee)	⅛ of 17-oz. pie	222	27.0
PIZZA SAUCE, canned:			
(Buitoni)	4 oz.	76	10.0
(Chef Boy-Ar-Dee)	5¼ oz. (½ of 10½-oz. can)	116	7.0
(Contadina)	1 cup (8 oz.)	144	23.2
PLANTAIN, raw (USDA):			
Whole	1 lb. (weighed with skin)	389	101.9
Flesh only	4 oz.	135	35.4
PLUM:			
Damson, fresh (USDA):			
Whole	1 lb. (weighed with pits)	272	73.5
Flesh only	4 oz.	75	20.2
Japanese and hybrid, fresh (USDA):			
Whole	1 lb. (weighed with pits)	205	52.4
Whole	2.1-oz. plum (2″ dia.)	27	6.9
Diced	½ cup (2.9 oz.)	39	10.1
Halves	½ cup (3.1 oz.)	42	10.8
Slices	½ cup (3 oz.)	40	10.3
Prune-type, fresh (USDA):			
Whole	1 lb. (weighed with pits)	320	84.0
Halves	½ cup (2.8 oz.)	60	15.8
Canned, purple, regular pack, solids & liq.:			
Light syrup (USDA)	4 oz.	71	18.8

(USDA): United States Department of Agriculture
DNA: Data Not Available
* Prepared as Package Directs

Food and Description	Measure or Quantity	Calories	Carbo-hydrates (grams)
Heavy syrup:			
(USDA) with pits	½ cup (4.5 oz.)	106	27.6
(USDA) without pits	½ cup (4.2 oz.)	100	25.9
(USDA)	3 plums & 2 T. syrup	101	26.4
(Del Monte)	½ cup (4.1 oz.)	112	30.4
Extra heavy syrup (USDA)	4 oz.	116	30.3
Canned, unsweetened or low calorie:			
Greengage, water pack	4 oz.	37	9.8
Purple:			
Water pack, solids & liq. (USDA)	4 oz.	52	13.5
Solids & liq. (Diet Delight)	½ cup (4.4 oz.)	80	19.7
Whole (Yes Madame)	½ cup	52	12.4
PLUM PIE (Tastykake)	4-oz. pie	364	53.8
PLUM PRESERVE, DAMSON, low calorie (Polaner)	1 T.	6	.3
PLUM PUDDING (Crosse & Blackwell)	4 oz.	340	62.4
POHA (See **GROUND-CHERRY**)			
POKE SHOOTS (USDA):			
Raw	1 lb.	104	16.8
Boiled, drained solids	4 oz.	23	3.5
POLISH-STYLE SAUSAGE:			
(USDA)	3 oz.	258	1.0
(Wilson)	3 oz.	245	1.0
POLLOCK (USDA):			
Raw, drawn	1 lb. (weighed with head, tail, fins & bones)	194	0.
Cooked, creamed	4 oz.	145	4.5
POMEGRANATE, raw (USDA):			
Whole	1 lb. (weighed whole)	160	41.7
Pulp only	4 oz.	71	18.6

Food and Description	Measure or Quantity	Calories	Carbohydrates (grams)
POMMARD WINE, French red Burgundy:			
(Barton & Guestier) 13% alcohol	3 fl. oz.	67	.4
(Chanson) *St. Vincent,* 11½% alcohol	3 fl. oz.	60	6.3
(Cruse) 12% alcohol	3 fl. oz.	72	D.N.A.
POMPANO, raw (USDA):			
Whole	1 lb. (weighed whole)	422	0.
Meat only	4 oz.	188	0.
POPCORN:			
Unpopped (USDA)	1 oz.	103	20.4
Popped (USDA):			
Plain	1 oz.	109	21.7
Plain, large kernel	1 cup (6 grams)	23	4.6
Oil & salt added	1 oz.	129	16.8
Oil & salt added	1 cup (9 grams)	41	5.3
Sugar-coated	1 oz.	109	24.2
(Jiffy Pop)	2½ oz. (½ pkg.)	332	29.8
Balls (Pophitt)	1 oz.	91	D.N.A.
Buttered (Wise)	½ cup (4 grams)	21	2.9
Butter flavor (Jiffy Pop)	2½ oz. (½ pkg.)	247	29.4
Caramel-coated:			
Peanut (Wise)	½ cup (.6 oz.)	64	13.5
Pixies with peanuts (Wise)	1 oz.	103	23.0
(Old London)	1 oz.	117	22.2
(Wise)	½ cup (.6 oz.)	53	14.8
Cheese-flavored (Old London)	¾-oz. bag	110	12.2
Cheese-flavored (Wise)	⅝-oz. bag	90	9.6
Cracker Jack, regular-size pack	1⅜-oz. pkg. (approx. 1 cup)	193	32.4
Cracker Jack, pass around pack	6-oz. pkg. (approx. 4 cups)	750	131.0
Fiddle Faddle (Ovaltine)	1 oz.	125	23.0

(USDA): United States Department of Agriculture
DNA: Data Not Available
* Prepared as Package Directs

Food and Description	Measure or Quantity	Calories	Carbo-hydrates (grams)
POPOVER, home recipe (USDA)	1 average popover (2 oz.)	128	14.7
*POPOVER MIX (Flako)	2.3-oz. popover (⅙ of pkg.)	161	22.5
POPSICLE (Popsicle Industries):			
All flavors, except chocolate	3 fl. oz. (3.4 oz.)	70	17.5
Chocolate	3 fl. oz.	106	D.N.A.
POP-UP (See **TOASTER CAKE**)			
PORGY, raw (USDA):			
Whole	1 lb. (weighed whole)	208	0.
Meat only	4 oz.	127	0.
PORK, medium-fat:			
Fresh (USDA):			
Boston butt:			
Raw	1 lb. (weighed with bone & skin)	1220	0.
Roasted, lean & fat	4 oz.	400	0.
Roasted, lean only	4 oz.	277	0.
Chop:			
Broiled, lean & fat	1 chop (4 oz., weighed with bone)	295	0.
Broiled, lean & fat	1 chop (3 oz., weighed without bone)	332	0.
Broiled, lean only	1 chop (3 oz., weighed without bone)	230	0.
Fat, separable, cooked	1 oz.	219	0.
Ham (See also **HAM**):			
Raw	1 lb. (weighed with bone & skin)	1188	0.
Roasted, lean & fat	4 oz.	424	0.

Food and Description	Measure or Quantity	Calories	Carbo-hydrates (grams)
Roasted, lean only	4 oz.	246	0.
Loin:			
Raw	1 lb. (weighed with bone)	1065	0.
Roasted, lean & fat	4 oz.	411	0.
Roasted, lean only	4 oz.	288	0.
Picnic:			
Raw	1 lb. (weighed with bone & skin)	1083	0.
Simmered, lean & fat	4 oz.	424	0.
Simmered, lean only	4 oz.	240	0.
Spareribs:			
Raw, with bone	1 lb. (weighed with bone)	976	0.
Braised, lean & fat	4 oz.	499	0.
Cured, light commercial cure:			
Bacon (See **BACON**)			
Boston butt (USDA):			
Raw	1 lb. (weighed with bone & skin)	1227	0.
Roasted, lean & fat	4 oz.	374	0.
Roasted, lean only	4 oz.	276	0.
Ham (See also **HAM**):			
Raw (USDA)	1 lb. (weighed with bone & skin)	1100	0.
Roasted, lean & fat (USDA)	4 oz.	328	0.
Roasted, lean only (USDA)	4 oz.	212	0.
Fully cooked, boneless:			
Parti-Style (Armour Star)	3 oz.	125	<.1
(Wilson)	3 oz.	166	0.
Picnic:			
Raw (USDA)	1 lb. (weighed with bone & skin)	1060	0.

(USDA): United States Department of Agriculture
DNA: Data Not Available
* Prepared as Package Directs

Food and Description	Measure or Quantity	Calories	Carbo-hydrates (grams)
Raw (Wilson) smoked	3 oz.	209	0.
Roasted, lean & fat (USDA)	4 oz.	366	0.
Roasted, lean only (USDA)	4 oz.	239	0.
PORK & BEANS (See **BEANS, BAKED**)			
PORK & BEEF, luncheon meat (USDA)	1 oz.	95	0.
PORK, CANNED, chopped luncheon meat:			
(USDA)	1 oz.	83	.4
Chopped (USDA)	1 cup (4.8 oz.)	400	1.8
Diced (USDA)	1 cup (5 oz.)	415	1.8
(Hormel)	1 oz.	70	.3
PORK DINNER, loin of pork, frozen (Swanson)	10-oz. dinner	460	40.5
PORK & GRAVY, canned (USDA)	4 oz.	290	7.1
PORK KABOB, frozen (Colonial Beef)	6-oz. kabob	500	D.N.A.
PORK RINDS, fried, *Baken·ets* (See also other brand names)	1 oz.	147	D.N.A.
PORK SAUSAGE:			
Uncooked, links or bulk (USDA)	1 oz.	141	Tr.
(Armour Star)	1-oz. sausage	133	0.
Little Friers (Oscar Mayer)	1 link (1 oz.)	129	.2
(Wilson)	1 oz.	135	0.
Cooked, links or bulk (USDA)	1 oz.	135	Tr.
Cooked, links, 16 raw per lb. (USDA)	2 links (.9 oz.)	124	Tr.
Canned, solids & liq. (USDA)	1 oz.	118	.7
Canned, drained (USDA)	1 oz.	108	.5

Food and Description	Measure or Quantity	Calories	Carbo-hydrates (grams)
PORK, SWEET & SOUR, frozen (Chun King)	1 cup	338	27.5
PORT WINE			
(Gallo) 16% alcohol	3 fl. oz.	94	7.8
(Gallo) ruby, 20% alcohol	3 fl. oz.	112	8.7
(Gallo) tawny, Old Decanter, 20% alcohol	3 fl. oz.	112	8.4
(Gallo) white, 20% alcohol	3 fl. oz.	111	8.4
(Gold Seal) 19% alcohol	3 fl. oz.	158	9.4
(Great Western) Solera, 19% alcohol	3 fl. oz.	155	11.8
(Great Western) Solera, tawny, 19% alcohol	3 fl. oz.	152	11.0
(Great Western) white, 19% alcohol	3 fl. oz.	156	12.3
(Italian Swiss Colony-Gold Medal) 19.7% alcohol	3 fl. oz.	130	8.7
(Italian Swiss Colony-Gold Medal) white, 19.7% alcohol	3 fl. oz.	132	9.3
(Italian Swiss Colony-Private Stock) 19.7% alcohol	3 fl. oz.	138	10.8
(Italian Swiss Colony-Private Stock) tawny, 19.7% alcohol	3 fl. oz.	137	10.5
Louis M. Martini) 19½% alcohol	3 fl. oz.	165	2.0
(Louis M. Martini) tawny, 19½% alcohol	3 fl. oz.	165	2.0
(Robertson's) ruby, 20% alcohol	3 fl. oz.	138	9.9
(Robertson's) tawny, *Dry Humour,* 21% alcohol	3 fl. oz.	145	9.9
(Robertson's) tawny, *Game Bird,* 21% alcohol	3 fl. oz.	145	9.9
(Robertson's) *Rebello Valente,* 20½% alcohol	3 fl. oz.	141	9.9
(Taylor) 19.5% alcohol	3 fl. oz.	150	10.9

(USDA): United States Department of Agriculture
DNA: Data Not Available
* Prepared as Package Directs

Food and Description	Measure or Quantity	Calories	Carbo-hydrates (grams)
(Taylor) tawny, 19.5% alcohol	3 fl. oz.	144	10.0
POST TOASTIES, cereal	1 cup (1 oz.)	108	24.0
*POSTUM, instant	1 cup	16	3.7
POTATO:			
Raw, whole (USDA)	1 lb. (weighed unpared)	279	62.8
Cooked (USDA):			
Au gratin, with cheese (USDA)	4 oz.	164	15.4
Au gratin, without cheese	4 oz.	118	16.7
Baked, peeled after baking	2½″ dia. potato (3 raw to 1 lb.)	92	20.9
Boiled, peeled after boiling	1 med. (3 raw to 1 lb.)	103	23.3
Boiled, peeled before boiling	1 med. (3 raw to 1 lb.)	79	17.7
French-fried in deep fat	10 pieces (2″ x ½″ x ½″, 2 oz.)	156	20.5
Hash-browned, after holding overnight	½ cup (3.4 oz.)	223	28.4
Mashed, milk added	½ cup (3.5 oz.)	64	12.7
Mashed, milk & butter added	½ cup (3.5 oz.)	92	12.1
Pan-fried from raw	½ cup (3 oz.)	228	27.7
Scalloped (see **AU GRATIN**)			
Canned:			
Solids & liq. (USDA)	1 cup (8.8 oz.)	110	24.5
Solids & liq. (USDA)	4 oz.	50	11.1
Solids & liq. (Del Monte)	1 cup (5.3 oz.)	46	10.3
White (Butter Kernel)	3–4 small potatoes	96	22.0
Whole, new (Hunt's)	4 oz.	50	11.1
& ham (Morton House)	12¾-oz. can	660	D.N.A.
Dehydrated, mashed:			
Flakes, without milk (USDA):			
Dry	½ cup (.8 oz.)	84	19.3
*Prepared with water, milk & fat	½ cup (3.8 oz.)	100	15.5

Food and Description	Measure or Quantity	Calories	Carbo-hydrates (grams)
Granules, without milk (USDA):			
Dry	½ cup (3.5 oz.)	352	80.4
*Prepared with water, milk & fat	½ cup (3.7 oz.)	101	15.1
Granules, with milk (USDA):			
Dry	½ cup (3.5 oz.)	358	77.7
*Prepared with water & fat	½ cup (3.7 oz.)	83	13.8
Frozen:			
Au gratin (Stouffer's)	11½-oz. pkg.	304	35.6
Au gratin (Swanson)	8-oz. pkg.	241	16.8
Diced for hash-browning, not thawed (USDA)	4 oz.	83	19.7
Diced, hash-browned (USDA)	4 oz.	254	32.9
French-fried:			
Not thawed (USDA)	9-oz. pkg.	434	66.6
Heated (USDA)	10 pieces (2" x ½" x ½", 2 oz.)	125	19.2
(Birds Eye)	17 pieces (3 oz.)	144	22.0
Crinkle-cut (Birds Eye)	17 pieces (3 oz.)	144	22.0
Fanci-fries (Birds Eye)	¼ pkg. (3 oz.)	173	21.0
(Mrs. Paul's)	4 oz.	250	38.8
Mashed, not thawed (USDA)	4 oz.	85	19.4
Mashed, heated (USDA)	4 oz.	105	17.8
Potato puffs, French-fried (Birds Eye)	⅓ pkg. (2.7 oz.)	149	14.6
Scalloped (Swanson)	8-oz. pkg.	257	12.9
Shredded for hash-browns (Birds Eye)	⅓ pkg. (3 oz.)	63	14.7
Stuffed, baked, with cheese topping (Holloway House)	1 potato (6 oz.)	251	28.0
Stuffed, baked, with sour cream & chives (Holloway House)	1 potato (6 oz.)	256	27.4
Tiny Taters (Birds Eye)	⅙ pkg. (2.7 oz.)	109	11.6

(USDA): United States Department of Agriculture
DNA: Data Not Available
* Prepared as Package Directs

Food and Description	Measure or Quantity	Calories	Carbohydrates (grams)
POTATO CHIP:			
(USDA)	1 oz.	161	14.2
(USDA)	10 chips (2″ dia., 2 oz.)	114	10.0
(Lay's)	1 oz.	158	14.1
(Nalley's)	1 oz.	154	13.9
(Ruffles)	1 oz.	158	14.1
(Wise)	1 oz.	156	14.8
Barbecue flavored (Wise)	1 oz.	152	15.0
Onion-garlic chips (Wise)	1 oz.	155	14.8
Ridgies (Wise)	1 oz.	155	14.7
POTATO MIX:			
*Au gratin (Betty Crocker)	½ cup	160	20.8
Au gratin (French's)	5.5-oz. pkg.	672	95.0
*Au gratin (French's)	½ cup	112	16.0
*Buds, instant (Betty Crocker)	½ cup	134	17.1
Mashed, country style (French's)	1⅓ cups (2⅔-oz. pkg.)	267	60.0
*Mashed, country style (French's)	½ cup	137	16.5
Mashed, instant (French's)	3.5-oz. pkg.	352	73.0
*Mashed, instant (French's)	½ cup	114	16.0
*Scalloped (Betty Crocker)	½ cup	150	22.2
Scalloped (French's)	5⅝-oz. pkg.	552	117.0
*Scalloped (French's)	½ cup	109	20.0
Scalloped (Pillsbury)	1 oz.	97	20.2
POTATO PANCAKE MIX:			
(French's)	3-oz. pkg.	284	62.0
*(French's)	¼ pkg. (3 small pancakes)	90	15.5
POTATO SALAD:			
Home recipe, with cooked salad dressing, seasonings (USDA)	4 oz.	112	18.5
Home recipe, with mayonnaise & French dressing, hard-cooked eggs, seasonings (USDA)	4 oz.	164	15.2
Canned (Nalley's)	4 oz.	159	20.3

Food and Description	Measure or Quantity	Calories	Carbohydrates (grams)
POTATO SOUP, Cream of:			
*Canned (Campbell)	1 cup	105	13.1
Frozen:			
Condensed (USDA)	8 oz. (by wt.)	197	22.7
*Prepared with equal volume water (USDA)	1 cup (8.5 oz.)	106	11.8
*Prepared with equal volume milk (USDA)	1 cup (8.6 oz.)	186	18.4
POTATO SOUP MIX:			
*(Lipton)	1 cup	100	19.1
*With leek (Wyler's)	6 fl. oz.	116	6.4
POTATO STICK:			
(USDA)	1 oz.	154	14.4
O & C (Durkee)	1½ cups (1¾-oz. can)	282	24.8
O & C (Durkee)	1 oz.	161	14.2
Julienne (Wise)	1-oz. bag	151	15.6
POUILLY-FUISSE WINE, French white Burgundy:			
(Barton & Guestier) 12½% alcohol	3 fl. oz.	64	.3
(Chanson) *St. Vincent,* 12% alcohol	3 fl. oz.	84	6.3
(Cruse) 12% alcohol	3 fl. oz.	72	D.N.A.
POUILLY-FUME, French white Loire Valley (Barton & Guestier) 12% alcohol	3 fl. oz.	60	.1
POUND CAKE:			
Home recipe, old fashioned (USDA)	1.1-oz. slice (3½" x 3" x ½")	142	14.1
Marble (Drake's)	1 slice	186	31.2
Plain (Drake's)	1 slice (1½ oz.)	171	27.8
Plain (Sara Lee)	1 oz.	110	13.0
Raisin (Drake's)	1 slice (1½ oz.)	210	34.0
Frozen (Morton)	1 oz.	117	14.8

(USDA): United States Department of Agriculture
DNA: Data Not Available
* Prepared as Package Directs

Food and Description	Measure or Quantity	Calories	Carbo-hydrates (grams)
POUND CAKE MIX:			
*(Betty Crocker)	⅟₁₂ of cake	210	28.0
*(Dromedary)	1″ slice (2.9 oz.)	313	40.7
PREAM, cream substitute	1 tsp.	11	1.1
PRESERVE (See also individual listings by flavor):			
(USDA)	1 oz.	77	19.8
(USDA)	1 T. (.7 oz.)	54	14.0
(Crosse & Blackwell)	1 T. (.8 oz.)	59	14.8
(Kraft)	1 oz.	78	19.3
(Polaner)	1 T.	54	13.5
(Smucker's)	1 T.	52	12.9
PRETZEL:			
(USDA)	1 oz.	111	21.5
(USDA)	1 small stick (1 gram)	4	.8
(Keebler) Log	1 piece (4 grams)	16	3.4
(Keebler) Stix	1 piece (<1 gram)	2	.4
(Keebler) Twist	1 piece (6 grams)	23	4.3
(Nab) Pretzelette	1 packet (1¼ oz.)	132	26.5
(Nab) *Very-Thin* Sticks	1 packet (¾ oz.)	79	16.7
(Nabisco) Pretzelette	1 piece (2 grams)	6	1.3
(Nabisco) *Mister Salty* Dutch	1 piece (.4 oz.)	51	11.2
(Nabisco) *Mister Salty* 3-ring	1 piece (3 grams)	12	2.3
(Nabisco) *Mister Salty* *Veri-Thin*	1 piece (5 grams)	20	4.1
(Nabisco) *Mister Salty* *Veri-Thin* Stick	1 piece (<1 gram)	1	.2
(Old London) nuggets	2-oz. bag	211	44.1
(Quinlan)	5 pieces (1 oz.)	100	D.N.A.
(Quinlan) Rods	2 pieces (1 oz.)	100	D.N.A.
(Quinlan) Sticks	35 pieces (1 oz.)	100	D.N.A.
(Quinlan) Thick, beer-type	3 pieces (1 oz.)	100	D.N.A.
(Quinlan) Thin	6 pieces (1 oz.)	100	D.N.A.
(Rold Gold)	1 pkg. (1 oz.)	105	21.5
(Sunshine) Extra thin	1 piece (5 grams)	20	4.0
PRICKLY PEAR, fresh			
(USDA)	1 lb. (weighed with rind & seeds)	84	21.8

Food and Description	Measure or Quantity	Calories	Carbo-hydrates (grams)
PRINCE BLANC WINE, French white Bordeaux (Barton & Guestier) 12% alcohol	3 fl. oz.	62	.6
PRINCE NOIR WINE, French red Bordeaux (Barton & Guestier) 12% alcohol	3 fl. oz.	61	.4
PRODUCT 19, cereal (Kellogg's)	1 cup (1 oz.)	105	23.1
PRUNE:			
Dried, "softenized":			
Small, uncooked (USDA)	1 prune (5 grams)	11	3.0
Medium, whole, with pits	1 cup (6.6 oz.)	405	107.2
Medium	1 prune (7 grams)	15	4.0
Large	1 prune (9 grams)	20	5.2
Dried, "softenized," cooked:			
Unsweetened (USDA)	1 cup (17–18 med. with ⅓ cup liq.)	295	77.9
With sugar (USDA)	1 cup (16–18 prunes with ⅓ cup liq., 11.1 oz.)	504	132.1
Canned, diet (Dia-Mel)	4 prunes	54	13.1
Dehydrated:			
Nugget-type & pieces (USDA)	4 oz.	390	103.5
Nugget-type & pieces, cooked with sugar, solids & liq. (USDA)	½ cup (4.4 oz.)	227	59.3
Pitted (Vacu-Dry)	1 oz.	98	25.9
PRUNE JUICE, canned:			
(USDA)	½ cup (4.5 oz.)	99	24.3
(Heinz)	5½-fl.-oz. can	119	28.3
RealPrune	½ cup (4.5 oz.)	98	24.1
(Santa Clara)	4 oz.	100	24.0

(USDA): United States Department of Agriculture
DNA: Data Not Available
* Prepared as Package Directs

Food and Description	Measure or Quantity	Calories	Carbo-hydrates (grams)
PRUNE WHIP, home recipe (USDA)	1 cup (4.8 oz.)	211	49.8
PUDDING or PUDDING MIX (See individual kinds)			
PUFF (See **CRACKER** or individual kinds of hors d'oeuvres, such as *CHICKEN PUFF*)			
PUFFA PUFFA RICE, cereal (Kellogg's)	1 cup (1 oz.)	124	23.8
PUFFED OAT CEREAL (USDA):			
Added nutrients	1 oz.	113	21.3
Sugar-coated, added nutrients	1 oz.	112	24.3
PUFFED RICE CEREAL (See **RICE, PUFFED**)			
PULIGNY MONTRACHET WINE, French white Burgundy: (Barton & Guestier) 12% alcohol	3 fl. oz.	61	.3
(Chanson) 12% alcohol	3 fl. oz.	84	6.3
PUMPKIN:			
Fresh, whole (USDA)	1 lb. (weighed with rind & seeds)	83	20.6
Fresh, flesh only (USDA)	4 oz.	29	7.4
Canned (USDA)	½ cup (4.3 oz.)	40	9.6
Canned (Stokely-Van Camp)	½ cup (4.1 oz.)	38	9.0
PUMPKIN PIE:			
Home recipe (USDA)	⅛ of 9″ pie (5.4 oz.)	321	37.2
(Tastykake)	4-oz. pie	368	50.5
Frozen (Banquet)	5 oz.	306	46.5
Frozen (Mrs. Smith's)	⅛ of 8″ pie (4 oz.)	229	33.6

Food and Description	Measure or Quantity	Calories	Carbo-hydrates (grams)
PUMPKIN SEED, dry (USDA):			
Whole	4 oz. (weighed in hull)	464	12.6
Hulled	4 oz.	627	17.0
*PUNCH DRINK MIX (Salada)	6 fl. oz.	80	19.4
PURPLE PASSION, soft drink (Canada Dry)	6 fl. oz.	88	22.2
PURSLANE, including stems (USDA):			
Raw	1 lb.	95	17.2
Boiled, drained	4 oz.	17	3.2
PUSSYCAT MIX (Bar-Tender's)	1 serving (⅝ oz.)	75	18.5

(USDA): United States Department of Agriculture
DNA: Data Not Available
* Prepared as Package Directs

Food and Description	Measure or Quantity	Calories	Carbo-hydrates (grams)

Q

QUAIL, raw (USDA):			
Ready-to-cook	1 lb. (weighed with bones)	686	0.
Meat & skin only	4 oz.	195	0.
QUAKE, cereal (Quaker)	1 cup (1 oz.)	119	23.1
QUIK (See individual kinds)			
QUINCE, fresh (USDA):			
Untrimmed	1 lb. (weighed with skin & seeds)	158	42.3
Flesh only	4 oz.	65	17.4
QUININE SOFT DRINK or TONIC WATER:			
Sweetened:			
(Canada Dry)	6 fl. oz.	68	17.6
(Dr. Brown's)	6 fl. oz.	66	16.5
(Fanta)	6 fl. oz.	62	15.7
(Hoffman)	6 fl. oz.	66	16.5
(Schweppes)	6 fl. oz.	66	16.5
(Shasta)	6 fl. oz.	57	14.4
(Yukon Club)	6 fl. oz.	67	16.7
Low calorie (No-Cal)	6 fl. oz.	2	0.
QUISP, cereal (Quaker)	1⅛ cups (1 oz.)	122	23.1

Food and Description	Measure or Quantity	Calories	Carbo-hydrates (grams)

R

RABBIT (USDA):

Domesticated, ready-to-cook | 1 lb. (weighed with bones) | 581 | 0.

Domesticated, stewed, flesh only | 4 oz. | 245 | 0.

Wild, ready-to-cook | 1 lb. (weighed with bones) | 490 | 0.

RACCOON, roasted, meat only (USDA) | 4 oz. | 289 | 0.

RADISH (USDA):

Common, raw:

Without tops | ½ lb. (weighed untrimmed) | 34 | 7.4

Trimmed, whole | 4 small radishes (1.4 oz.) | 7 | 1.4

Trimmed, sliced | ½ cup (2 oz.) | 10 | 2.1

Oriental, raw, without tops | ½ lb. (weighed unpared) | 34 | 7.4

Oriental, raw, trimmed & pared | 4 oz. | 22 | 4.8

RAISIN:

Dried:

Whole (USDA) | 1 small pkg. (.5 oz.) | 40 | 10.8

Whole, pressed down (USDA) | ½ cup (2.9 oz.) | 237 | 63.5

Whole, pressed down (USDA) | 1 T. (.4 oz.) | 29 | 7.7

Chopped (USDA) | ½ cup (2.9 oz.) | 234 | 62.7

Ground (USDA) | ½ cup (4.7 oz.) | 387 | 103.7

Seedless, California Thompson (Sun Maid) | ½ cup (2.8 oz.) | 235 | 62.6

Seedless, California Thompson (Sun Maid) | 1 T. (.4 oz.) | 29 | 7.8

(USDA): United States Department of Agriculture
DNA: Data Not Available
* Prepared as Package Directs

Food and Description	Measure or Quantity	Calories	Carbo-hydrates (grams)
Cooked, added sugar, solids & liq. (USDA)	½ cup (4.3 oz.)	260	68.8
RAISIN PIE:			
Home recipe, 2 crusts (USDA)	⅙ of 9" pie (5.6 oz.)	427	67.9
(Tastykake)	4-oz. pie	391	60.8
Frozen (Mrs. Smith's)	⅙ of 8" pie	315	42.1
RAISIN PIE FILLING (Lucky Leaf)	8 oz.	292	67.8
RAJA FISH (See SKATE)			
RALSTON, cereal, dry:			
Instant	4 T. (1 oz.)	97	20.2
Regular	3⅓ T. (1 oz.)	97	20.2
RASPBERRY:			
Black:			
Fresh:			
(USDA)	½ lb. (weighed with caps & stems)	160	34.6
(USDA) without caps & stems	½ cup (2.4 oz.)	49	10.5
Canned, water pack, unsweetened, solids & liq. (USDA)	4 oz.	58	12.1
Red:			
Fresh:			
(USDA)	½ lb. (weighed with caps & stems)	126	29.9
(USDA) without caps & stems	½ cup (2.5 oz.)	41	9.8
Canned, water pack, unsweetened or low calorie:			
Solids & liq. (USDA)	4 oz.	40	10.0
Solids & liq. (Blue Boy)	4 oz.	48	11.2
Frozen, sweetened:			
Not thawed (USDA)	10-oz. pkg.	278	69.9
Not thawed (USDA)	½ cup (4.4 oz.)	122	30.5
Quick thaw (Birds Eye)	½ cup (5 oz.)	148	37.2

Food and Description	Measure or Quantity	Calories	Carbo-hydrates (grams)
*RASPBERRY DRINK MIX			
(Wyler's)	6 fl. oz.	64	15.8
RASPBERRY LIQUEUR,			
(Leroux) 50 proof	1 fl. oz.	74	8.3
RASPBERRY PRESERVE or JAM, dietetic or low calorie:			
Red (Polaner)	1 T.	6	1.5
Black seedless (Dia-Mel)	1 T.	22	5.4
Black (Kraft)	1 oz.	36	8.8
(S and W) *Nutradiet*	1 T (.5 oz.)	10	2.4
(Slenderella)	1 T (.6 oz.)	22	5.6
RASPBERRY, RED, PIE FILLING (Lucky Leaf)	8 oz.	324	79.0
RASPBERRY RENNET CUSTARD MIX:			
Powder:			
(Junket)	1 oz.	115	28.0
*(Junket)	4 oz.	108	14.7
Tablet:			
(Junket)	1 tablet	1	.2
*With sugar (Junket)	4 oz.	101	13.5
RASPBERRY SHERBET & FRUIT ICE MIX (Junket)	6 serving pkg. (4 oz.)	388	108.8
RASPBERRY SOFT DRINK:			
Sweetened:			
(Canada Dry)	6 fl. oz.	100	26.2
(Hoffman)	6 fl. oz.	90	22.5
(Yukon Club)	6 fl. oz.	90	22.5
Black:			
(Dr. Brown's)	6 fl. oz.	86	21.5
(Key Food)	6 fl. oz.	87	21.9
(Kirsch)	6 fl. oz.	88	22.1
(Waldbaum)	6 fl. oz.	87	21.9

(USDA): United States Department of Agriculture
DNA: Data Not Available
* Prepared as Package Directs

Food and Description	Measure or Quantity	Calories	Carbo-hydrates (grams)
Low calorie (Hoffman) black	6 fl. oz.	2	.4
Low calorie (No-Cal) black	6 fl. oz.	3	<.1
RASPBERRY SYRUP, dietetic:			
(Dia-Mel)	1 T.	22	5.4
(No-Cal)	1 tsp. (5 grams)	<1	0.
RASPBERRY TURNOVER, frozen (Pepperidge Farm)	1 turnover (3.3 oz.)	337	36.9
RAVIOLI:			
Canned:			
Beef or meat:			
(Buitoni)	8 oz.	188	26.9
(Chef Boy-Ar-Dee)	8 oz. (⅕ of 40-oz. can)	211	30.2
(Nalley's)	8 oz.	284	62.4
(Prince)	1 can (3.7 oz.)	136	18.7
Cheese:			
(Buitoni)	8 oz.	218	27.3
(Chef Boy-Ar-Dee)	7½ oz. (½ of 15-oz. can)	262	31.5
(Prince)	1 can (3.7 oz.)	123	18.5
Chicken (Nalley's)	8 oz.	261	82.4
Frozen:			
Beef (Kraft)	12½-oz. pkg.	411	49.9
Cheese (Buitoni)	4 oz.	313	48.6
Cheese (Kraft)	12½-oz. pkg.	407	48.1
Meat, without sauce (Buitoni)	4 oz.	278	41.6
Raviolettes (Buitoni)	4 oz.	324	56.3
READY GRAVY	1 fl. oz.	22	3.7
REDFISH (See **DRUM, RED & OCEAN PERCH**, Atlantic)			
REDHORSE, SILVER, raw (USDA):			
Drawn	1 lb. (weighed eviscerated)	204	0.
Flesh only	4 oz.	111	0.

Food and Description	Measure or Quantity	Calories	Carbo-hydrates (grams)
RED & GRAY SNAPPER,			
raw:			
Whole (USDA)	1 lb. (weighed whole)	219	0.
Meat only (USDA)	4 oz.	105	0.
Meat only (Booth)	4 oz.	105	0.
REINDEER, raw, lean only			
(USDA)	4 oz.	144	0.
RELISH:			
Barbecue (Crosse & Blackwell)	1 T.	22	5.4
Barbecue (Heinz)	1 T.	35	8.5
Corn (Crosse & Blackwell)	1 T. (.6 oz.)	15	3.6
Hamburger (Crosse & Blackwell)	1 T. (.6 oz.)	20	4.7
Hamburger (Heinz)	1 T.	15	3.6
Hot dog (Crosse & Blackwell)	1 T. (.7 oz.)	22	5.4
Hot dog (Heinz)	1 T.	17	3.9
Hot pepper (Crosse & Blackwell)	1 T. (.7 oz.)	22	5.4
India (Crosse & Blackwell)	1 T. (.7 oz.)	26	6.3
India (Heinz)	1 T.	17	3.9
Onion, spicy (Crosse & Blackwell)	1 T.	21	5.0
Piccalilli (Crosse & Blackwell)	1 T. (.7 oz.)	26	6.3
Piccalilli (Heinz)	1 T.	23	5.3
Picnic, tangy (Crosse & Blackwell)	1 T.	24	6.0
Sour (USDA)	1 T. (.5 oz.)	3	.4
Sweet:			
(USDA) finely chopped	1 T. (.5 oz.)	21	5.1
(Crosse & Blackwell)	1 T. (.7 oz.)	26	6.3
(Heinz)	1 T.	28	6.6
(Smucker's)	1 T. (.6 oz.)	23	5.6
RENNIN CUSTARD PRODUCTS			
(See individual flavors)			

(USDA): United States Department of Agriculture
DNA: Data Not Available
* Prepared as Package Directs

Food and Description	Measure or Quantity	Calories	Carbo-hydrates (grams)
RHINESKELLER WINE,			
(Italian Swiss Colony-Gold Medal) 12.4% alcohol	3 fl. oz.	73	3.0
RHINE WINE:			
(Deinhard) Rheinritter, 11% alcohol	3 fl. oz.	60	3.6
(Gallo) 12% alcohol	3 fl. oz.	50	.9
(Gallo) Rhine Garten, 12% alcohol	3 fl. oz.	59	3.0
(Gold Seal) 12% alcohol	3 fl. oz.	82	.4
(Great Western) Dutchess, 12% alcohol	3 fl. oz.	80	2.6
(Italian Swiss Colony-Gold Medal) 11.6% alcohol	3 fl. oz.	59	.6
(Italian Swiss Colony-Private Stock) 12% alcohol	3 fl. oz.	61	.5
(Louis M. Martini) 12.5% alcohol	3 fl. oz.	90	.2
(Taylor) 12.5% alcohol	3 fl. oz.	69	Tr.
RHUBARB:			
Fresh:			
Partly trimmed (USDA)	1 lb. (weighed with part leaves, ends & trimmings)	54	12.6
Trimmed (USDA)	4 oz.	18	4.2
Diced (USDA)	½ cup (2.2 oz.)	10	2.3
Cooked, sweetened, solids & liq. (USDA)	½ cup (4.2 oz.)	169	43.2
Frozen, sweetened:			
Not thawed (USDA)	½ cup (3.9 oz.)	82	20.4
Cooked, added sugar (USDA)	½ cup (4.4 oz.)	177	44.9
(Birds Eye)	½ cup (4 oz.)	84	21.4
RHUBARB PIE, home recipe (USDA)	⅛ of 9" pie (5.6 oz.)	400	60.4
RICE:			
Brown:			
Raw (USDA)	½ cup (3.7 oz.)	374	80.5
Raw (USDA)	1 oz.	102	21.9

Food and Description	Measure or Quantity	Calories	Carbo-hydrates (grams)
Cooked:			
(USDA)	4 oz.	135	28.9
(Carolina)	⅔ cup (3.5 oz.)	119	25.5
(River Brand)	⅔ cup (3.5 oz.)	119	25.5
(Water Maid)	⅔ cup (3.5 oz.)	119	25.5
White:			
Instant or Precooked:			
Dry long-grain (USDA)	½ cup (1.9 oz.)	206	45.4
Cooked:			
Long-grain (USDA)	½ cup (2.5 oz.)	76	16.9
(Carolina)	⅔ cup (3.5 oz.)	109	24.2
(Minute Rice) no butter or salt	⅔ cup (4 oz.)	124	26.5
Long-grain (Uncle Ben's Quick)	½ cup (3.2 oz.)	96	22.0
Parboiled:			
Dry, long-grain (USDA)	1 oz.	105	23.0
Cooked:			
Long-grain (USDA)	½ cup (2.9 oz.)	87	19.1
(Aunt Caroline)	⅔ cup (3.5 oz.)	106	23.1
Long-grain (Uncle Ben's Converted)	½ cup (2.8 oz.)	84	19.0
Regular:			
Raw (USDA)	½ cup (3.5 oz.)	359	79.6
Cooked:			
(USDA)	½ cup (3.6 oz.)	111	24.7
Extra long-grain (Carolina)	⅔ cup (3.5 oz.)	109	24.2
(Mahatma)	⅔ cup (3.5 oz.)	109	24.2
(River Brand) fluffy	⅔ cup (3.5 oz.)	109	24.2
(Water Maid)	⅔ cup (3.5 oz.)	109	24.2
White & wild, frozen (Green Giant)	⅓ of 12-oz. pkg.	107	22.7
RICE BRAN (USDA)	1 oz.	78	14.4
RICE CHEX, cereal (Ralston Purina)	1⅛ cups (1 oz.)	107	24.9

(USDA): United States Department of Agriculture
DNA: Data Not Available
* Prepared as Package Directs

Food and Description	Measure or Quantity	Calories	Carbo-hydrates (grams)
RICE FLAKES, dietetic cereal (Van Brode)	1 oz.	109	25.4
RICE, FRIED, frozen:			
Chicken (Chun King)	1 cup	309	35.4
Shrimp (Temple)	1 cup	297	51.0
RICE HONEYS, cereal (Nabisco)	1 cup (1⅛ oz.)	151	32.7
RICE KRISPIES, cereal (Kellogg's)	1 cup (1 oz.)	109	24.6
RICE MIX:			
Beef:			
Rice-A-Roni	4 oz.	180	30.3
(Uncle Ben's)	½ cup (3.8 oz.)	102	21.3
(Village Inn)	½ cup	125	24.4
*Cheese *Rice-A-Roni*	4 oz.	170	23.2
Chicken:			
Rice-A-Roni	4 oz.	177	29.1
(Uncle Ben's)	½ cup (3.5 oz.)	104	21.2
(Village Inn)	½ cup	125	24.4
*Chinese, fried, *Rice-A-Roni*	4 oz.	226	27.8
*Curry (Uncle Ben's)	½ cup (4.1 oz.)	106	22.9
*Curry (Village Inn)	½ cup	125	24.4
*(Drumstick (Minute Rice)	½ cup (4.1 oz.)	152	22.4
Ham with pineapple, *Rice-A-Roni*	4 oz.	113	15.9
*Herb (Village Inn)	½ cup	125	24.4
*Keriyaki dinner (Betty Crocker)	1 cup	416	39.0
*Long & wild grain (Uncle Ben's)	½ cup (3.8 oz.)	100	21.4
*Long & wild grain (Village Inn)	½ cup	125	24.4
*Milanese (Betty Crocker)	½ cup	172	24.2
*Provence (Betty Crocker)	½ cup	184	28.9
*Rib Roast (Minute Rice)	½ cup (4.1 oz.)	149	24.2
Spanish:			
*(Minute Rice)	½ cup (5.6 oz.)	132	23.0
Rice-A-Roni	4 oz.	132	20.5
*(Uncle Ben's)	½ cup (4.4 oz.)	115	24.0
*(Village Inn)	½ cup	125	24.4

Food and Description	Measure or Quantity	Calories	Carbohydrates (grams)
*Turkey *Rice-A-Roni*	4 oz.	204	29.5
*Wild *Rice-A-Roni*	4 oz.	158	24.0
*Yellow (Village Inn)	½ cup	125	24.4
RICE & PEAS with MUSHROOMS, frozen (Birds Eye)	⅛ pkg. (2.3 oz.)	113	21.9
RICE POLISH (USDA)	1 oz.	75	16.4
RICE, PUFFED, cereal:			
(USDA) added nutrients, unsalted	1 cup (.5 oz.)	60	13.4
(Checker)	½ oz.	56	14.4
(Kellogg's)	1 cup (.5 oz.)	55	12.8
(Quaker)	1¼ cups (.5 oz.)	56	12.5
(Van Brode) dietetic	1 oz.	109	25.2
RICE PUDDING, home recipe, with raisins (USDA)	½ cup (4.7 oz.)	193	35.2
RICE, SPANISH:			
Home recipe (USDA)	4 oz.	99	18.8
Canned:			
(Heinz)	8¾-oz. can	196	35.6
(Nalley's)	4 oz.	85	32.4
(Van Camp)	½ cup (3.9 oz.)	96	18.2
RICE, SPANISH, SEASONING MIX (Lawry's)	1½-oz. pkg.	125	20.7
RIESLING WINE, Alsatian:			
(Willm) 11–14% alcohol	3 fl. oz.	66	3.6
(Willm) Grand Reserve Exceptionelle, 11–14% alcohol	3 fl. oz.	66	3.6
RIPPLE WINE (Gallo):			
Red, 11% alcohol	3 fl. oz.	56	3.4
White, 11% alcohol	3 fl. oz.	55	3.2

(USDA): United States Department of Agriculture
DNA: Data Not Available
* Prepared as Package Directs

Food and Description	Measure or Quantity	Calories	Carbo-hydrates (grams)
ROCKFISH (USDA):			
Raw, meat only	1 lb.	440	0.
Oven-steamed, with onions	4 oz.	121	2.2
ROCK & RYE LIQUEUR:			
(Garnier) 60 proof	1 fl. oz.	70	6.2
(Hiram Walker) 60 proof	1 fl. oz.	87	9.5
(Leroux) 60 proof	1 fl. oz.	74	8.3
(Leroux) Irish Moss, 70 proof	1 fl. oz.	110	13.0
(Old Mr. Boston) 48 proof	1 fl. oz.	72	6.0
(Old Mr. Boston) 60 proof	1 fl. oz.	94	5.8
ROE (USDA):			
Raw, carp, cod, haddock, herring, pike or shad	4 oz.	147	1.7
Raw, salmon, sturgeon, turbot	4 oz.	235	1.6
Baked or broiled, cod & shad	4 oz.	143	2.2
Canned, cod, haddock or herring, solids & liq.	4 oz.	134	.3
ROLAIDS (Warner-Lambert)	1 piece	4	1.4
ROLL & BUN:			
Barbeque (Arnold)	1 bun (1.6 oz.)	132	22.6
Brown & serve:			
Unbrowned (USDA)	1 oz.	85	14.3
Browned (USDA)	1 oz.	93	15.5
(Wonder)	1 roll (1 oz.)	79	13.9
Cinnamon nut (Pepperidge Farm)	1 roll (1 oz.)	92	12.1
Club, brown & serve (Pepperidge Farm)	1 roll (1.6 oz.)	120	23.3
Deli Twists (Arnold)	1 roll (1.2 oz.)	115	17.4
Dinner (Arnold)	1 roll (¾ oz.)	71	10.5
Dinner, fully baked (Pepperidge Farm)	1 roll (.7 oz.)	80	9.9
Dutch Egg sandwich buns (Arnold)	1 bun (1.7 oz.)	143	22.4
Finger (Arnold)	1 roll (.7 oz.)	61	9.6
Finger	1 roll (1 oz.)	84	12.0
Frankfurter or hot dog:			
(USDA)	1 roll (1.4 oz.)	119	21.2
(Arnold)	1 bun (1.4 oz.)	121	20.6
New England (Arnold)	1 roll (1.6 oz.)	130	22.0

Food and Description	Measure or Quantity	Calories	Carbo-hydrates (grams)
French, brown & serve:			
Twin (Pepperidge Farm)	1 roll (5.2 oz.)	389	75.7
Triple (Pepperidge Farm)	1 roll (3.5 oz.)	264	51.4
Giraffe sandwich buns (Arnold)	1 bun (1.6 oz.)	135	22.7
Golden Twist, brown & serve (Pepperidge Farm)	1 roll (1.2 oz.)	123	13.2
Hamburger (USDA)	1 roll (1.4 oz.)	119	21.2
Hard (USDA)	1 roll (1.8 oz.)	156	29.8
Hard (Levy's)	1 roll (2.5 oz.)	130	37.4
Hearth, brown & serve (Pepperidge Farm)	1 roll (.8 oz.)	64	11.6
Hot Cross bun (Van de Kamp's)	1 bun (1.1 oz.)	63	D.N.A.
Parker (Arnold)	1 roll (.7 oz.)	63	9.8
Plain (USDA)	1 roll (1.3 oz.)	84	15.0
Poppy finger (Arnold)	1 roll (.6 oz.)	61	9.4
Raisin (USDA)	1 bun (1 oz.)	78	16.0
Sesame crisp, brown & serve (Pepperidge Farm)	1 roll (.9 oz.)	78	13.1
Sourdough, French (Van de Kamp's)	1 roll (1.5 oz.)	130	D.N.A.
Sweet (USDA)	1 bun (1.5 oz.)	136	21.2
Tea (Arnold)	1 roll (.4 oz.)	36	5.7
Whole-wheat (USDA)	1 roll (1.3 oz.)	98	19.9
ROLL DOUGH:			
Frozen, unraised (USDA)	1 oz.	76	13.4
Frozen, baked (USDA)	1 oz.	88	15.9
Refrigerated:			
Cinnamon with icing (Pillsbury)	1 oz.	100	14.0
Dinner (Pillsbury):			
Butterflake	1 oz.	80	11.9
Crescent	1 oz.	94	10.8
Parkerhouse	1 oz.	76	12.6
Snowflake	1 oz.	84	11.9
ROLL MIX:			
Dry (USDA)	1 oz.	111	20.5

(USDA): United States Department of Agriculture
DNA: Data Not Available
* Prepared as Package Directs

Food and Description	Measure or Quantity	Calories	Carbo-hydrates (grams)
*Prepared with water			
(USDA)	1 oz.	85	15.5
(Pillsbury)	1 oz.	113	19.2
***ROMAN MEAL CEREAL**	¾ cup (1.3 oz., dry)	130	25.0
***ROOT BEER DRINK MIX**			
(Wyler's)	6 fl. oz.	69	17.2
ROOT BEER SOFT DRINK:			
Sweetened:			
(Canada Dry) *Rooti*	6 fl. oz.	76	19.6
(Clicquot Club)	6 fl. oz.	85	21.0
(Cott)	6 fl. oz.	85	21.0
(Dad's)	6 fl. oz.	79	19.6
(Dr. Brown's)	6 fl. oz.	77	19.4
(Fanta)	6 fl. oz.	77	19.8
(Hires)	6 fl. oz.	75	18.8
(Hoffman)	6 fl. oz.	77	19.4
(Key Food)	6 fl. oz.	77	19.4
(Kirsch)	6 fl. oz.	71	17.7
(Mason's)	6 fl. oz.	60	15.0
(Mission)	6 fl. oz.	85	21.0
Draft (Shasta)	6 fl. oz.	84	21.3
(Waldbaum)	6 fl. oz.	77	19.4
(Yukon Club)	6 fl. oz.	81	20.1
Low calorie:			
(Dad's)	6 fl. oz.	<1	.2
(Hoffman)	6 fl. oz.	<1	.2
(No-Cal)	6 fl. oz.	<1	<.1
Draft (Shasta)	6 fl. oz.	<1	<.1
ROSE APPLE, raw (USDA):			
Whole	1 lb. (weighed with caps & seeds)	170	43.2
Flesh only	4 oz.	64	16.1
ROSE WINE:			
(Antinori) 12% alcohol	3 fl. oz.	84	6.3
Chateau Ste. Roseline, 11–14% alcohol	3 fl. oz.	84	6.3
(Chanson) *Rose des Anges,* 12% alcohol	3 fl. oz.	84	6.3
(Cruse) 12% alcohol	3 fl. oz.	72	D.N.A.

Food and Description	Measure or Quantity	Calories	Carbohydrates (grams)
(Gallo) 13% alcohol	3 fl. oz.	55	1.8
(Gallo) *Gypsy,* 20% alcohol	3 fl. oz.	112	12.0
(Great Western) 12% alcohol	3 fl. oz.	88	4.7
(Great Western) Isabella, 12% alcohol	3 fl. oz.	84	3.8
(Italian Swiss Colony-Gold Medal) Grenache, 12.4% alcohol	3 fl. oz.	69	2.2
(Italian Swiss Colony-Private Stock) Grenache, 12% alcohol	3 fl. oz.	61	.5
(Italian Swiss Colony-Gold Medal) Napa-Sonoma-Mendocino, 12% alcohol	3 fl. oz.	67	2.2
(Louis M. Martini) Gamay, 12½% alcohol	3 fl. oz.	90	.2
(Mogen David) 12% alcohol	3 fl. oz.	75	8.9
Nectarosé, vin rosé d'Anjou, 12% alcohol	3 fl. oz.	70	2.6
(Taylor) 12.5% alcohol	3 fl. oz.	69	Tr.
ROSE WINE, SPARKLING (Chanson)	3 fl. oz.	72	3.6
RUDESHEIMER SCHLOSSBERG, German Rhine wine (Deinhard) 11% alcohol	3 fl. oz.	72	4.5
RUM (See DISTILLED LIQUOR)			
RUSK:			
(USDA)	.5 oz.	59	10.1
Dutch (Hekman's)	1 piece	55	D.N.A.
Dutch (Sunshine)	1 piece (.5 oz.)	61	10.5
Holland (Nabisco)	1 piece (.4 oz.)	49	9.0
RUTABAGA:			
Raw, without tops (USDA)	1 lb. (weighed with skin)	177	42.4

(USDA): United States Department of Agriculture
DNA: Data Not Available
* Prepared as Package Directs

Food and Description	Measure or Quantity	Calories	Carbo-hydrates (grams)
Raw, diced (USDA)	½ cup (2.5 oz.)	32	7.7
Boiled, drained, diced (USDA)	½ cup (3 oz.)	30	7.1
Boiled, drained, mashed (USDA)	½ cup (4.3 oz.)	43	10.0
Canned (King Pharr)	½ cup	52	D.N.A.
RYE, whole grain (USDA)	1 oz.	95	20.8
RYE FLOUR (See **FLOUR**)			
RYE WAFER, whole grain:			
(USDA)	1 oz.	98	21.6
(USDA)	2 wafers (1⅛″ x 3½″)	45	9.9
RYE WHISKEY (See **DISTILLED LIQUOR**)			
RYE WHISKEY EXTRACT			
(Ehlers)	1 tsp.	14	D.N.A.
RYE-KRISP:			
Pizza	1 small cracker	8	D.N.A.
Seasoned	1 cracker (1⅛″ x 3½″)	25	4.5
Traditional	1 cracker (1⅛″ x 3½″)	21	4.8
RY-KING (Wasa):			
Brown rye	1 slice (12 grams)	43	8.4
Golden rye	1 slice (10 grams)	33	6.8
Lite rye	1 slice (8 grams)	30	6.2
Seasoned rye	1 slice (9 grams)	39	6.8

Food and Description	Measure or Quantity	Calories	Carbohydrates (grams)

S

SABLEFISH, raw (USDA):
Whole	1 lb. (weighed whole)	362	0.
Meat only	4 oz.	215	0.

SABRA, Israeli liqueur (Leroux) 60 proof | 1 fl. oz. | 91 | 10.4 |

SACCHARIN (Dia-Mel) | 1 tablet | 0 | 0. |

SAFFLOWER SEED KERNELS, dry (USDA) | 1 oz. | 174 | 3.5 |

SAINT-EMILION WINE, French Bordeaux:
(Barton & Guestier) 12% alcohol	3 fl. oz.	63	.7
(Cruse) 11.5% alcohol	3 fl. oz.	69	D.N.A.

SAINT JOHN'S-BREAD FLOUR (See FLOUR, Carob)

SAINT-JULIEN WINE (Cruse) 11.5% alcohol | 3 fl. oz. | 69 | D.N.A. |

SALAD DRESSING (See also **SALAD DRESSING, LOW CALORIE**):
All purpose (Lawry's)	1 T.	59	1.5
Bleu or blue cheese:			
(USDA)	1 oz.	143	2.1
(USDA)	1 T. (.5 oz.)	76	1.1
(Kraft) Imperial	1 T. (.5 oz.)	68	.9
(Lawry's)	1 T. (.5 oz.)	57	.8
Roka (Kraft)	1 T. (.5 oz.)	55	.8
French (Wish-Bone)	1 T. (.6 oz.)	62	1.5

(USDA): United States Department of Agriculture
DNA: Data Not Available
* Prepared as Package Directs

Food and Description	Measure or Quantity	Calories	Carbohydrates (grams)
Boiled, home recipe (USDA)	1 T. (.6 oz.)	26	2.4
Caesar (Lawry's)	1 T. (.5 oz.)	70	.5
Canadian (Lawry's)	1 T. (.5 oz.)	72	.6
Cheese (Wish-Bone)	1 T.	67	1.2
Chef style, *Salad Bowl* (Kraft)	1 oz.	102	5.3
Coleslaw (Kraft)	1 T. (.5 oz.)	62	3.4
Cuisine (Kraft)	1 oz.	98	4.7
French:			
Home recipe (USDA)	1 T. (.6 oz.)	101	.6
Commercial (USDA)	1 T. (.6 oz.)	66	2.8
Commercial (USDA)	1 T. (.6 oz.)	66	2.8
(Hellmann's-Best Foods) Family	1 T. (.6 oz.)	65	2.9
(Heinz)	1 T.	78	2.0
(Kraft)	1 T. (.5 oz.)	65	1.9
(Kraft) Casino	1 T. (.5 oz.)	60	3.0
(Kraft) Catalina	1 T. (.5 oz.)	60	3.5
(Kraft) *Miracle*	1 T. (.5 oz.)	57	2.5
(Lawry's) San Francisco	1 T. (.5 oz.)	53	.8
(Marzetti's) blue	1 T. (.5 oz.)	70	3.4
(Nalley's)	1 oz.	104	3.7
(Wish-Bone) Deluxe	1 T. (.6 oz.)	60	2.3
(Wish-Bone) Garlic	1 T. (.6 oz.)	68	3.5
Garlic:			
(Hellmann's-Best Foods) *Old Homestead*	1 T. (.6 oz.)	68	3.3
(Kraft) Salad Bowl	1 oz.	105	3.9
(Lawry's) San Francisco	1 T.	53	.8
(Wish-Bone) Monaco	1 T.	84	3.6
Green Goddess:			
(Kraft)	1 T. (.5 oz.)	75	.7
(Lawry's)	1 T. (.5 oz.)	59	.7
(Wish-Bone)	1 T. (.5 oz.)	69	1.3
Hawaiian (Lawry's)	1 T. (.6 oz.)	77	5.8
Heinz Salad Dressing	1 T.	63	2.0
Herb & garlic (Kraft)	1 oz.	176	.9
Hickory Bits (Wish-Bone)	1 T.	78	.6
Italian:			
(USDA)	1 T. (.5 oz.)	83	1.0
(Hellmann's) True	1 T. (.5 oz.)	84	.8
(Kraft)	1 T. (.5 oz.)	88	.7
(Kraft) *Salad Bowl*	1 oz.	155	1.4
(Lawry's)	1 T. (.5 oz.)	80	.9

Food and Description	Measure or Quantity	Calories	Carbo-hydrates (grams)
(Lawry's) with cheese	1 T. (.5 oz.)	60	4.7
(Marzetti's) creamy	1 T. (.5 oz.)	73	1.8
(Wish-Bone)	1 T. (.6 oz.)	79	.8
(Wish-Bone) low oil	1 T.	80	.9
(Wish-Bone) Rosé	1 T. (.6 oz.)	63	.4
Mayonnaise (See **MAYONNAISE**)			
Mayonnaise-type salad dressing (USDA)	1 T. (.5 oz.)	65	2.2
Miracle Whip (Kraft)	1 T. (.5 oz.)	69	1.8
Oil & vinegar (Kraft)	1 T. (.5 oz.)	65	.6
Onion, California (Wish-Bone)	1 T. (.5 oz.)	76	1.0
Onion, creamy (Wish-Bone)	1 T. (.5 oz.)	70	.8
Roquefort (USDA)	1 T. (.5 oz.)	76	1.1
Roquefort (Kraft) refrigerated	1 T. (.5 oz.)	56	.8
Russian:			
(USDA)	1 T. (.5 oz.)	74	1.6
(Kraft) pourable	1 T. (.5 oz.)	55	4.3
(Wish-Bone)	1 T. (.6 oz.)	56	7.2
Salad Bowl (Kraft)	1 T. (.5 oz.)	53	2.2
Salad Secret (Kraft)	1 T. (.5 oz.)	56	1.8
Sherry (Lawry's)	1 T. (.5 oz.)	55	1.6
Slaw (Marzetti's)	1 T. (.5 oz.)	73	3.2
Spin Blend (Hellmann's)	1 T. (.5 oz.)	56	2.6
Sweet & Sour (Kraft)	1 T. (.5 oz.)	28	6.5
Tang (Nalley's)	1 oz.	102	4.8
Thousand Island:			
(USDA)	1 T. (.6 oz.)	80	2.5
(Best Foods) pourable	1 T. (.5 oz.)	60	2.8
(Kraft)	1 T. (.5 oz.)	71	1.9
(Kraft) pourable	1 T. (.5 oz.)	56	2.3
(Kraft) refrigerated	1 T. (.5 oz.)	73	2.1
(Kraft) *Salad Bowl*	1 oz.	128	2.4
(Lawry's)	1 T. (.5 oz.)	69	2.3
(Wish-Bone)	1 T. (.6 oz.)	73	2.6
Wine vinegar & oil (James H. Black)	1 T.	19	1.9

(USDA): United States Department of Agriculture
DNA: Data Not Available
* Prepared as Package Directs

Food and Description	Measure or Quantity	Calories	Carbo-hydrates (grams)
SALAD DRESSING, DIETETIC or LOW CALORIE:			
Bleu or blue:			
Low fat, 6% fat (USDA)	1 T. (.6 oz.)	12	.7
Low fat, 1% fat (USDA)	1 T. (.5 oz.)	3	.2
(Dia-Mel)	1 T.	12	.4
(Frenchette) chunky	1 T. (.5 oz.)	22	1.7
(Kraft)	1 T. (.5 oz.)	13	.5
(Tillie Lewis)	1 T.	12	.2
Caesar (Tillie Lewis)	1 T.	12	.2
Catalina (Kraft)	1 T. (.5 oz.)	15	2.6
Chef style (Kraft)	1 T. (.5 oz.)	16	2.6
Chefs (Tillie Lewis)	1 T. (.5 oz.)	2	.4
Cole slaw (Kraft)	1 T. (.5 oz.)	28	3.4
Diet Whip (Dia-Mel)	1 T.	10	Tr.
Diet-Aise (Slim-ette)	1 T.	15	D.N.A.
French:			
Low fat, 6% fat (USDA)	1 T. (.6 oz.)	15	2.5
Low fat, 1% fat, with artificial sweetener (USDA)	1 T. (.5 oz.)	2	.3
Medium fat, with artificial sweetener (USDA)	1 T. (.5 oz.)	23	.2
(Dia-Mel)	1 T.	15	.2
(Dia-Mel) Green Garlic	1 T.	9	Tr.
(Frenchette)	1 T. (.5 oz.)	10	2.6
(Kraft)	1 T. (.5 oz.)	21	2.0
(Marzetti's)	1 T.	24	3.6
(Tillie Lewis)	1 T. (.5 oz.)	3	.8
(Wish-Bone)	1 T. (.6 oz.)	23	3.3
(Wish-Bone) Garlic	1 T.	16	2.7
Italian:			
(USDA)	1 T. (.5 oz.)	8	.4
(Dia-Mel)	1 T.	9	.4
Italianette (Frenchette)	1 T. (.5 oz.)	7	1.5
(Kraft)	1 T. (.5 oz.)	10	.7
(Marzetti's)	1 T. (.5 oz.)	8	1.5
(Tillie Lewis)	1 T. (.5 oz.)	1	.3
(Wish-Bone)	1 T. (.6 oz.)	7	1.1
May-Lo-Naise (Tillie Lewis)	1 T. (.5 oz.)	9	.1
Mayonnaise, imitation (USDA)	1 T. (.6 oz.)	22	.8
Russian (Dia-Mel)	1 T.	24	1.4

Food and Description	Measure or Quantity	Calories	Carbohydrates (grams)
Russian (Wish-Bone)	1 T. (.6 oz.)	24	4.7
Slaw (Marzetti's)	1 T. (.5 oz.)	27	2.8
Supreme (McCormick)	1 oz.	80	2.0
Thousand Island:			
(USDA)	1 T. (.5 oz.)	27	2.3
(Kraft)	1 T. (.5 oz.)	28	2.3
(Marzetti's)	1 T. (.5 oz.)	20	2.7
(Tillie Lewis)	1 T.	10	.4
(Wish-Bone)	1 T. (.6 oz.)	27	2.9
Whipped (Tillie Lewis)	1 T. (.5 oz.)	10	.2
SALAD DRESSING MIX,			
regular & low calorie:			
Bacon (Lawry's)	1 pkg. (.8 oz.)	69	11.9
Bleu or blue cheese:			
*(Good Seasons)	1 T. (.5 oz.)	89	1.3
*(Good Seasons) thick, creamy	1 T. (.5 oz.)	96	.9
(Lawry's)	1 pkg. (.7 oz.)	79	4.5
Caesar garlic cheese (Lawry's)	1 pkg. (.8 oz.)	71	8.7
*Cheese garlic (Good Seasons)	1 T. (.5 oz.)	84	.8
*Coleslaw (Good Seasons) thick, creamy	1 T.	91	1.9
*French, old fashioned (Good Seasons)	1 T. (.5 oz.)	83	.5
French, old fashioned (Lawry's)	1 pkg. (.8 oz.)	72	16.8
*French, Riviera (Good Seasons)	1 T. (.6 oz.)	90	2.4
*Garlic (Good Seasons)	1 T. (.5 oz.)	84	.8
*Green Goddess (Good Seasons) thick, creamy	1 T.	87	.8
Green Goddess (Lawry's)	1 pkg. (.8 oz.)	69	12.7
Italian:			
*(Good Seasons)	1 T. (.5 oz.)	84	.8
*Low calorie (Good Seasons)	1 tsp.	3	.7
(Lawry's)	1 pkg. (.6 oz.)	44	9.6

(USDA): United States Department of Agriculture
DNA: Data Not Available
* Prepared as Package Directs

Food and Description	Measure or Quantity	Calories	Carbo-hydrates (grams)
(Lawry's) with cheese	1 pkg. (.8 oz.)	69	9.4
*Onion (Good Seasons)	1 T. (.5 oz.)	84	.8
*Parmesan (Good Seasons)	1 T.	87	.8
SALAD FRUIT, unsweetened, unseasoned (S and W)			
Nutradiet	4 oz.	43	9.8
SALAD SEASONING:			
(Durkee)	1 tsp.	4	.7
With cheese (Durkee)	1 tsp.	10	.4
SALAMI:			
Dry (USDA)	1 oz.	128	.3
Cooked (USDA)	1 oz.	88	.4
Cooked (Eckrich)	1 oz.	58	D.N.A.
(Vienna)	1 oz.	74	.5
Beef (Sugardale)	1-oz. slice	76	Tr.
Cotto (Oscar Mayer)	1 slice (.8 oz.)	55	.4
Cotto (Wilson)	1 oz.	84	.4
Hard (Oscar Mayer)	1 slice (.4 oz.)	41	<.1
SALISBURY STEAK:			
Canned, with mushrooms (Morton House)	12¾-oz. can	835	D.N.A.
Frozen:			
(Banquet) buffet	2-lb. pkg.	1524	46.5
(Banquet) cookin' bag	5 oz.	239	7.2
(Holloway House)	1 steak (7. oz.)	320	18.9
(Swanson) with potato	6-oz. pkg.	360	30.5
Dinner, frozen:			
(Banquet)	11-oz. dinner	335	21.5
(Morton)	11-oz. dinner	384	24.7
(Swanson) 3-course	16-oz. dinner	517	46.9
SALMON:			
Atlantic (USDA):			
Raw, whole	1 lb. (weighed whole)	640	0.
Raw, meat only	4 oz.	246	0.
Canned, solids & liq., including bones	4 oz.	230	0.
Chinook or King:			
Raw, steak (USDA)	1 lb. (weighed with bones)	886	0.

Food and Description	Measure or Quantity	Calories	Carbo-hydrates (grams)
Raw, meat only (USDA)	4 oz.	252	0.
Canned, solids & liq.:			
Including bones (USDA)	4 oz.	238	0.
(Icy Point)	7¾-oz. can	460	0.
(Pillar Rock)	7¾-oz. can	460	0.
Chum, canned, solids & liq., including bones (USDA)	4 oz.	158	0.
Coho, canned, solids & liq., including bones (USDA)	4 oz.	174	0.
Coho, canned, dietetic (Silver Beauty)	4 oz.	187	0.
Pink or Humpback:			
Raw, steak (USDA)	1 lb. (weighed with bones)	475	0.
Raw, meat only (USDA)	4 oz.	135	0.
Canned, solids & liq.:			
Including bones (USDA)	4 oz.	160	0.
(Del Monte)	7¾-oz. can	268	0.
(Icy Point)	7¾-oz. can	310	0.
(Pink Beauty)	7¾-oz. can	310	0.
Sockeye or Red or Blueback, canned, solids & liq.:			
Including bones (USDA)	4 oz.	194	0.
(Icy Point)	3¾-oz. can	181	0.
(Pillar Rock)	3¾-oz. can	181	0.
Unseasoned (S and W) *Nutradiet*	3¾-oz. can	190	1.6
Unspecified kind of salmon, baked or broiled (USDA)	4.2-oz. steak (approx. 4" x 3" x ½")	218	0.
SALMON RICE LOAF, home recipe (USDA)	4 oz.	138	8.3
SALMON, SMOKED:			
(USDA)	4 oz.	200	0.
Lox, drained (Vita)	4-oz. jar	136	.2

(USDA): United States Department of Agriculture
DNA: Data Not Available
* Prepared as Package Directs

Food and Description	Measure or Quantity	Calories	Carbohydrates (grams)
SALSIFY (USDA):			
Raw, without tops, freshly harvested	1 lb. (weighed untrimmed)	51	71.0
Raw, without tops, after storage	1 lb. (weighed untrimmed)	324	71.0
Boiled, drained solids, freshly harvested	4 oz.	14	17.1
Boiled, drained solids, after storage	4 oz.	79	17.1
SALT:			
Table (USDA)	1 tsp. (6 grams)	0	0.
Garlic (Lawry's)	1 pkg. (2.9 oz.)	116	22.9
Garlic (Lawry's)	1 tsp. (4 grams)	5	1.0
Imitation, butter flavored (Durkee)	1 tsp. (4 grams)	3	.2
Seasoned (Lawry's)	1 pkg. (3 oz.)	21	2.3
Seasoned (Lawry's)	1 tsp. (5 grams)	1	.1
Substitute (Adolph's)	1 tsp. (4 grams)	Neg.	0.
Substitute, seasoned (Adolph's)	1 tsp. (4 grams)	4	.9
SALT PORK, raw (USDA):			
With skin	1 lb. (weighed with skin)	3410	0.
Without skin	1 oz.	222	0.
SALT STICK (See BREAD STICK)			
SANCERRE WINE, French white, Loire Valley:			
(Barton & Guestier) 12% alcohol	3 fl. oz.	61	.3
(Chanson) 12½% alcohol	3 fl. oz.	87	6.3
SAND DAB, raw (USDA):			
Whole	1 lb. (weighed whole)	118	0.
Meat only	4 oz.	90	0.
SANDWICH SPREAD:			
(USDA)	1 cup (8.7 oz.)	932	39.1
(USDA)	1 T. (.5 oz.)	57	2.4

Food and Description	Measure or Quantity	Calories	Carbo-hydrates (grams)
(USDA) low calorie	1 T. (.5 oz.)	17	1.2
(Hellmann's-Best Foods)	1 T. (.5 oz.)	62	2.4
(Kraft)	1 oz.	105	5.6
(Nalley's)	1 oz.	100	7.0
(Tillie Lewis) dietetic	1 T.	9	.2
SAPODILLA, fresh (USDA):			
Whole	1 lb. (weighed whole)	323	79.1
Flesh only	4 oz.	101	24.7
SAPOTES or MARMALADE PLUM raw (USDA):			
Whole	1 lb. (weighed whole)	431	108.9
Flesh only	4 oz.	142	35.8
SARDINE:			
Atlantic, canned in oil (USDA):			
Solids & liq.	4 oz.	353	.7
Drained solids	3 oz.	173	D.N.A.
Moroccan, skinless & boneless, canned (Cresca):			
In olive oil	3¾-oz. can.	341	D.N.A.
In water	3½-oz. can	165	D.N.A.
Norwegian, canned (Underwood):			
In mustard sauce	3 oz. sardines & 1 oz. sauce	134	1.6
In oil, drained solids	3 oz.	167	.7
In tomato sauce	3 oz. sardines & 1 oz. sauce	124	1.7
Pacific (USDA):			
Raw	4 oz.	181	0.
Canned in brine or mustard, solids & liq.	4 oz.	222	1.9
Canned in tomato sauce, solids & liq.	4 oz.	223	1.9

(USDA): United States Department of Agriculture
DNA: Data Not Available
* Prepared as Package Directs

Food and Description	Measure or Quantity	Calories	Carbo-hydrates (grams)
SARSAPARILLA SOFT DRINK:			
(Hoffman)	6 fl. oz.	83	22.2
(Yukon Club)	6 fl. oz.	89	22.2
SAUCE, regular and dietetic:			
Barbecue:			
(USDA)	½ cup (4.4 oz.)	114	10.0
(Good Seasons) original *Open Pit*	1 T. (.6 oz.)	27	6.5
(Heinz) with onion	1 T.	19	4.2
(Kraft)	1 oz.	34	7.9
(Kraft) garlic	1 oz.	32	7.6
(Kraft) hot	1 oz.	31	7.0
(Kraft) smoked	1 oz.	34	7.9
Bolognaise (Crosse & Blackwell)	1 T.	24	1.4
Bordelaise (Crosse & Blackwell)	1 T.	18	1.4
Champignon (Crosse & Blackwell)	1 T.	12	1.4
Cheese (Kraft) *Deluxe Dinner*	1 oz.	77	2.0
Chili (See **CHILI SAUCE**)			
Cocktail, refrigerated (Kraft)	1 oz.	31	7.5
Enchilada (Rosarita)	1 oz.	8	1.2
Famous (Durkee)	1 T. (.6 oz.)	69	2.2
57 (Heinz)	1 T.	14	2.6
Hard (Crosse & Blackwell)	1 T.	64	8.3
Hollandaise (Cresca)	1 oz.	39	D.N.A.
Horseradish (Kraft)	1 oz.	100	3.3
Hot tomato (Rosarita)	1 oz.	7	1.2
H.P. (Lea & Perrins)	1 T. (1. oz.)	20	4.8
Marinara (Buitoni)	4 oz.	67	8.0
Marinara (Chef Boy-Ar-Dee)	3¾ oz. (¼ of 15-oz. can)	68	10.9
Mint (Crosse & Blackwell)	1 T. (.5 oz.)	16	4.0
Mushroom (Contadina)	1 fl. oz.	22	2.4
Newburg (Crosse & Blackwell)	1 T.	22	1.3
Polynesian (Crosse & Blackwell)	1 T.	16	3.6
Remoulade, dietetic (Tillie Lewis)	1 T.	11	.6

Food and Description	Measure or Quantity	Calories	Carbo- hydrates (grams)
Savory (Heinz)	1 T.	20	4.5
Seafood cocktail (Crosse & Blackwell)	1 T. (.6 oz.)	22	4.9
Shrimp cocktail (Crosse & Blackwell)	1 T.	22	5.1
Soy (USDA)	1 oz.	19	2.7
Spaghetti (See **SPAGHETTI SAUCE**)			
Steak (Crosse & Blackwell)	1 T. (.7 oz.)	21	4.8
Sweet & sour (Kraft)	1 oz.	55	13.0
Tabasco (See individual listing)			
Tartar:			
(USDA)	1 T. (.5 oz.)	74	.6
(USDA) low calorie	1 T. (.5 oz.)	31	.9
(Hellmann's-Best Foods)	1 T. (.5 oz.)	73	.3
(Kraft)	1 oz.	145	1.4
(Kraft) spice blend	1 oz.	151	.9
White:			
Home recipe:			
Thin (USDA)	1 cup (8.8 oz.)	302	18.0
Medium (USDA)	1 cup (9 oz.)	413	22.4
Thick (USDA)	1 cup (8.7 oz.)	489	27.2
Worcestershire:			
(Crosse & Blackwell)	1 T.	15	3.6
(Heinz)	1 T.	11	2.5
(Lea & Perrins)	1 T. (.6 oz.)	12	3.0
SAUCE MIX:			
*a la King, without chicken (Durkee)	1 cup (1.5 oz. dry pkg.)	273	25.5
*Barbecue (Kraft)	1 oz.	32	7.9
Cheese:			
*(Durkee)	1 cup (1¼-oz. dry pkg.)	523	31.0
(French's)	1¼-oz. pkg.	165	11.2
*(Kraft) cheddar	1 oz.	52	1.9
(McCormick)	1¼-oz. pkg.	170	4.8
*(McCormick)	1 oz.	40	2.0

(USDA): United States Department of Agriculture
DNA: Data Not Available
* Prepared as Package Directs

Food and Description	Measure or Quantity	Calories	Carbohydrates (grams)
*Chicken (Kraft)	1 oz.	15	2.3
*Cream (Kraft)	1 oz.	44	2.5
Enchilada (Lawry's)	1.6-oz. pkg.	144	27.3
Hollandaise:			
*(Durkee)	⅔ cup (1¼-oz. dry pkg.)	213	11.0
(French's)	1⅛-oz. pkg.	192	6.8
*(Kraft)	1 oz.	54	2.0
*(McCormick)	1 oz.	36	2.0
Newburg (French's)	1½-oz. pkg.	200	11.8
Seafood cocktail (Lawry's)	.6-oz. pkg.	43	9.7
Sloppy Joe (See **SLOPPY JOE MIX**)			
Sour cream:			
(French's)	1¼-oz. pkg.	192	12.7
*(Kraft)	1 oz.	61	4.1
*(McCormick)	1 oz.	20	1.2
*With skim milk (Durkee)	⅔ cup (1½-oz. dry pkg.)	186	12.0
*With whole milk (Durkee)	⅔ cup (1½-oz. dry pkg.)	216	11.4
Stroganoff (French's)	1¾-oz. pkg.	192	21.0
Tartar (Lawry's)	.6-oz. pkg.	64	9.8
*White sauce supreme (McCormick)	.6-oz. pkg.	11	2.0
SAUERKRAUT, canned:			
Solids & liq. (USDA)	1 cup (8.3 oz.)	42	9.4
Drained solids (USDA)	1 cup (5 oz.)	31	6.2
Solids & liq. (Del Monte)	1 cup (5.3 oz.)	27	6.0
Drained solids (Steinfield's)	1 cup	33	6.6
SAUERKRAUT JUICE, canned (USDA)	½ cup (4.3 oz.)	12	2.8
SAUGER, raw (USDA):			
Whole	1 lb. (weighed whole)	133	0.
Meat only	4 oz.	95	0.
SAUSAGE (See also individual kinds):			
Breakfast (Hormel)	8-oz. can	838	.7

Food and Description	Measure or Quantity	Calories	Carbo-hydrates (grams)
Brown & serve, before browning (USDA)	1 oz.	111	.8
Brown & serve, after browning (USDA)	1 oz.	120	.8
Brown & serve, canned (Hormel)	8 oz.	925	2.3
Cocktail (Cresca)	1 oz.	71	D.N.A.
New England Brand (Wilson)	2 oz.	105	.5
In sauce (Prince)	1 can (3.7 oz.)	187	4.2

SAUTERNES:

(Barton & Guestier) French white Bordeaux, 13% alcohol	3 fl. oz.	95	7.6
(Barton & Guestier) haut, French white Bordeaux, 13% alcohol	3 fl. oz.	99	8.7
(Gallo) 12% alcohol	3 fl. oz.	50	.9
(Gallo) haut, 12% alcohol	3 fl. oz.	67	2.1
(Gold Seal) dry, 12% alcohol	3 fl. oz.	82	.4
(Gold Seal) semi-soft, 12% alcohol	3 fl. oz.	87	2.6
(Great Western) Aurora, 12% alcohol	3 fl. oz.	88	4.7
(Italian Swiss Colony-Gold Medal) 11.6% alcohol	3 fl. oz.	59	.6
(Louis M. Martini) dry, 12.5% alcohol	3 fl. oz.	90	.2
(Mogen David) cream, 12% alcohol	3 fl. oz.	45	6.2
(Mogen David) dry, American, 12% alcohol	3 fl. oz.	30	1.8
(Taylor) 12.5% alcohol	3 fl. oz.	81	2.9

SCALLION (See **ONION, GREEN**)

SCALLOP:

Raw, muscle only (USDA)	4 oz.	92	3.7
Steamed (USDA)	4 oz.	127	D.N.A.

(USDA): United States Department of Agriculture
DNA: Data Not Available
* Prepared as Package Directs

Food and Description	Measure or Quantity	Calories	Carbo- hydrates (grams)
Frozen:			
Breaded, fried, reheated (USDA)	4 oz.	220	11.9
Breaded, fried, reheated (Booth)	4 oz.	220	11.9
Breaded, fried (Mrs. Paul's)	7-oz. pkg.	412	45.5
SCHAV SOUP (Manischewitz)	8 oz. (by wt.)	11	2.1
SCHNAPPS, PEPPERMINT:			
(Garnier) 60 proof	1 fl. oz.	83	8.4
(Hiram Walker) 60 proof	1 fl. oz.	78	7.2
(Leroux) 60 proof	1 fl. oz.	87	9.2
(Old Mr. Boston) 42 proof	1 fl. oz.	60	4.5
(Old Mr. Boston) 60 proof	1 fl. oz.	78	4.2
SCONE (Hostess)	1 pkg.	180	33.9
*SCOTCH BROTH (Campbell)	1 cup	84	9.8
SCOTCH WHISKEY (See **DISTILLED LIQUOR**)			
SCRAPPLE (USDA)	4 oz.	244	16.6
SCREWDRIVER MIX (Bar-Tender's)	1 serving (⅝ oz.)	70	17.4
SCREWDRIVER MIXTURE, soft drink (Canada Dry)	6 fl. oz.	75	19.3
SCUP (See **PORGY**)			
SEABASS, WHITE, raw, meat only (USDA)	4 oz.	109	0.
SEGO, diet food:			
*Instant mix with whole milk	1 cup	224	17.6
Liquid diet	10-oz. can	225	35.0
SEKT SPARKLING WINE (Deinhard)	3 fl. oz.	72	3.6
SENEGALESE SOUP (Crosse & Blackwell)	6½ oz. (½ can)	61	6.8

Food and Description	Measure or Quantity	Calories	Carbohydrates (grams)
SESAME SEEDS, dry (USDA):			
Whole	1 oz.	160	6.1
Hulled	1 oz.	165	5.0
SESAME TAHINI (A. Sahadi)	1 T. (8 grams)	57	.8
SEVEN-UP, soft drink	6 fl. oz.	73	18.0
SHAD (USDA):			
Raw, whole	1 lb. (weighed whole)	370	0.
Raw, meat only	4 oz.	193	0.
Cooked, home recipe:			
Baked with butter or margarine & bacon slices	4 oz.	228	0.
Creole	4 oz.	172	1.8
Canned, solids & liq.	4 oz.	172	0.
SHAD, GIZZARD, raw (USDA):			
Whole	1 lb. (weighed whole)	299	0.
Meat only	4 oz.	227	0.
SHAKE 'N BAKE, seasoned mix:			
Chicken-coating	2⅜-oz. pkg.	276	40.0
Fish-coating	2-oz. pkg.	224	33.0
Hamburger-coating	2-oz. pkg.	158	31.6
Pork-coating	2⅜-oz. pkg.	260	46.3
SHALLOT, raw (USDA):			
With skin	1 oz.	18	4.2
With skin removed	1 oz.	20	4.8
SHAPE (Drackett):			
Liquid, any flavor	1 can (8 fl. oz.)	225	33.2
Powder:			
Chocolate	2 scoops (1 oz.)	109	19.3
Strawberry or vanilla	2 scoops (1 oz.)	109	20.0

(USDA): United States Department of Agriculture
DNA: Data Not Available
* Prepared as Package Directs

Food and Description	Measure or Quantity	Calories	Carbohydrates (grams)
SHEEFISH (See **INCONNU**)			
SHEEPSHEAD, Atlantic, raw (USDA):			
Whole	1 lb. (weighed whole)	159	0.
Meat only	4 oz.	128	0.
SHERBET (See also individual brands):			
Orange (USDA)	1 cup (6.8 oz.)	259	59.4
Orange (USDA)	⅓ pint (4.6 oz.)	173	39.7
All flavors (Borden)	⅓ pint (4 oz.)	159	34.4
(Sealtest)	¼ pt. (3.1 oz.)	120	26.5
SHERBET & FRUIT ICE MIX, ORANGE (Junket)	6 serving pkg. (4 oz.)	388	108.8
SHERRY:			
(Gallo) 20% alcohol	3 fl. oz.	88	2.7
(Gallo) 16% alcohol	3 fl. oz.	76	3.3
(Gold Seal) 19% alcohol	3 fl. oz.	139	4.6
(Great Western) Solera, 19% alcohol	3 fl. oz.	143	8.5
Cocktail (Gold Seal) 19% alcohol	3 fl. oz.	122	1.6
Cocktail (Petri)	3 fl. oz.	102	D.N.A.
Cream:			
(Gallo) 20% alcohol	3 fl. oz.	111	8.4
(Gallo) Old Decanter, Livingston, 20% alcohol	3 fl. oz.	117	12.8
(Gold Seal) 19% alcohol	3 fl. oz.	158	9.4
(Great Western) Solera, 19% alcohol	3 fl. oz.	154	11.6
(Italian Swiss Colony-Private Stock) 19.7% alcohol	3 fl. oz.	129	8.5
(Louis M. Martini) 19.5% alcohol	3 fl. oz.	138	1.2
(Taylor) 19.5% alcohol	3 fl. oz.	150	11.3
(Williams & Humbert) Canasta, 20½% alcohol	3 fl. oz.	150	5.4
Dry:			
(Gallo) 20% alcohol	3 fl. oz.	84	1.8

Food and Description	Measure or Quantity	Calories	Carbohydrates (grams)
(Gallo) Old Decanter, very dry, 20% alcohol	3 fl. oz.	87	2.1
(Great Western) Solera, 19% alcohol	3 fl. oz.	128	4.2
(Italian Swiss Colony-Gold Medal) 19.7% alcohol	3 fl. oz.	104	1.7
(Italian Swiss Colony-Private Stock) 19.8% alcohol	3 fl. oz.	104	1.7
(Louis M. Martini) 19.5% alcohol	3 fl. oz.	138	1.2
(Williams & Humbert) Carlito Amontillado, 20½% alcohol	3 fl. oz.	120	4.5
(Williams & Humbert) Cedro, 20½% alcohol	3 fl. oz.	120	4.5
(Williams & Humbert) Dos Cortados, 20½% alcohol	3 fl. oz.	120	4.5
(Williams & Humbert) Pando, 17% alcohol	3 fl. oz.	120	4.5
Dry Sack (Williams & Humbert) 20½% alcohol	3 fl. oz.	120	4.5
Hartley (Italian Swiss Colony-Private Blend) 19.8% alcohol	3 fl. oz.	105	1.9
Medium:			
(Great Western) cooking, 19% alcohol	3 fl. oz.	135	6.4
(Italian Swiss Colony-Gold Medal) 19.7% alcohol	3 fl. oz.	106	2.6
(Italian Swiss Colony-Private Stock) 19.8% alcohol	3 fl. oz.	108	2.8
(Taylor) 19½% alcohol	3 fl. oz.	132	7.1

SHORTENING (See **FATS**)

SHREDDED OATS, cereal (USDA)	1 oz.	107	20.4

(USDA): United States Department of Agriculture
DNA: Data Not Available
* Prepared as Package Directs

Food and Description	Measure or Quantity	Calories	Carbo-hydrates (grams)
SHREDDED WHEAT, cereal:			
(USDA) plain	1 cup (1.2 oz.)	124	28.0
(Kellogg's)	4 biscuits (1 oz.)	108	23.6
(Nabisco)	1 biscuit (.9 oz.)	86	18.7
(Nabisco) *Spoon Size*	1 biscuit (1 gram)	4	.9
(Quaker)	2 biscuits (1.3 oz.)	135	28.7
(Sunshine)	1 biscuit (1 oz.)	104	22.3
SHRIMP:			
Raw:			
Whole (USDA)	1 lb. (weighed in shell)	285	4.7
Meat only (USDA)	4 oz.	103	1.7
Canned:			
Wet pack, solids & liq. (USDA)	4 oz.	91	.9
Dry pack or drained (USDA)	4 oz.	132	.8
North Pacific, tiny, drained (Icy Point)	4½-oz.-can	148	.8
North Pacific, tiny, drained (Pink Beauty)	4½-oz.-can	148	.8
Cooked, french-fried (USDA)	4 oz.	255	11.3
Frozen:			
Raw:			
Breaded, not more than 50% breading (USDA)	4 oz.	158	22.6
Breaded (Booth)	4 oz.	158	22.6
Breaded (Chicken of the Sea)	4 oz.	158	22.6
Unbreaded (Chicken of the Sea)	4 oz.	103	D.N.A.
Fried (Chicken of the Sea)	4 oz.	255	D.N.A.
Fried (Mrs. Paul's)	4 oz.	258	D.N.A.
SHRIMP COCKTAIL:			
(Sau-Sea)	4 oz.	80	18.0
(Sea Snack)	4 oz.	110	14.8
SHRIMP DINNER, frozen:			
(Morton)	7¾-oz. dinner	379	37.3
(Swanson)	8-oz. dinner	358	41.5

Food and Description	Measure or Quantity	Calories	Carbohydrates (grams)
SHRIMP PASTE, canned (USDA)	1 oz.	51	.4
SHRIMP PUFF, frozen (Durkee)	1 piece (.5 oz.)	44	3.0
SHRIMP ROLL, frozen (Temple)	2½-oz. roll	117	20.7
SHRIMP SOUP, Cream of:			
Canned (Crosse & Blackwell)	½ can (6½ oz.)	92	6.5
Frozen:			
Condensed (USDA)	8 oz. (by wt.)	302	16.3
*Prepared with equal volume water (USDA)	1 cup (8.5 oz.)	158	8.4
*Prepared with equal volume milk (USDA)	1 cup (8.6 oz.)	243	15.2
SILVER SATIN WINE (Italian Swiss Colony-Gold Medal):			
19.7% alcohol	3 fl. oz.	130	8.9
With bitter lemon, 19.7% alcohol	3 fl. oz.	130	8.9
SIMBA, soft drink	6 fl. oz.	77	19.7
SKATE, raw, meat only (USDA)	4 oz.	111	0.
SLENDER, coffee (Carnation)	1 envelope (1 oz.)	104	16.1
SLOE GIN (See **GIN, SLOE**)			
SLOPPY JOE:			
Canned, with beef (Morton House)	15-oz. can	860	D.N.A.
Frozen (Banquet) cookin' bag	5 oz.	251	36.0

(USDA): United States Department of Agriculture
DNA: Data Not Available
* Prepared as Package Directs

Food and Description	Measure or Quantity	Calories	Carbo-hydrates (grams)
SLOPPY JOE SEASONING MIX:			
(French's)	1½-oz. pkg.	117	26.0
*With meat & tomato paste (Durkee)	3 cups (½-oz. dry pkg.)	1432	50.3
(Lawry's)	1½-oz. pkg.	139	27.7
(McCormick)	1⁵⁄₁₆-oz. pkg.	112	D.N.A,
*(Wyler's)	6 fl. oz.	25	4.3
SMELT, Atlantic, jack & bay (USDA):			
Raw, whole	1 lb. (weighed whole)	244	0.
Raw, meat only	4 oz.	111	0.
Canned, solids & liq.	4 oz.	227	0.
SMOKIE SAUSAGE:			
(Eckrich):			
Smoked, not bulk	4-oz. piece	344	D.N.A.
Smokee, from 1-lb. pkg.	1 link	115	D.N.A.
Smokee, from 12-oz. pkg.	1 link	150	D.N.A.
Smokette	1 piece	75	D.N.A.
Smok-Y-Links	1 piece	75	D.N.A.
(Oscar Mayer) 8 per ¾ lb.	1 link (1.5 oz.)	131	1.0
Little Smokies (Oscar Mayer)	1 link (9 grams)	29	.2
(Wilson)	1 oz.	84	.5
SNACK (See CRACKER, POPCORN, POTATO CHIPS, etc.)			
SNAIL, raw:			
(USDA)	4 oz.	102	2.3
Giant African (USDA)	4 oz.	83	5.0
SNAPPER (See RED SNAPPER)			
SNO BALL (Hostess) 2 to pkg.	1 cake (1.5 oz.)	135	25.8
SOAVE WINE, Italian white (Antinori) 12% alcohol	3 fl. oz.	84	6.3

Food and Description	Measure or Quantity	Calories	Carbo-hydrates (grams)
SODA or SOFT DRINK (See individual kinds listed by flavor or brand name)			
SOFT SWIRL (Jell-O):			
All flavors except chocolate	½ cup (3.8 oz.)	168	25.8
Chocolate	½ cup (4 oz.)	190	27.4
SOLE, raw (USDA):			
Whole	1 lb. (weighed whole)	118	0.
Meat only	4 oz.	90	0.
SORGHUM (USDA):			
Grain	1 oz.	94	20.7
Syrup	1 T. (.7 oz.)	54	12.2
SORREL (See **DOCK**)			
SOUP (See individual listing by kind)			
SOUR MIXER, soft drink (Canada Dry)	6 fl. oz.	71	18.4
SOURSOP, raw (USDA):			
Whole	1 lb. (weighed with skin & seeds)	200	50.3
Flesh only	4 oz.	74	18.5
SOUSE (USDA)	1 oz.	51	.3
SOUTHERN COMFORT, 100 proof	1 oz.	120	3.5
SOYBEAN (USDA):			
Young seeds:			
Raw	1 lb. (weighed in pods)	322	31.7
Boiled, drained	4 oz.	134	11.5

(USDA): United States Department of Agriculture
DNA: Data Not Available
* Prepared as Package Directs

Food and Description	Measure or Quantity	Calories	Carbohydrates (grams)
Canned, solids & liq.	4 oz.	85	7.1
Canned, drained solids	4 oz.	117	8.4
Mature seeds, dry:			
Raw	1 lb.	1828	152.0
Raw	1 cup (7.4 oz.)	846	70.4
Cooked	4 oz.	147	12.2
Roasted, *Soy Town*	1 oz.	152	5.1
SOYBEAN CURD or TORFU:			
(USDA)	4 oz.	82	2.7
(USDA)	4.2-oz. cake (2¾" x 2½" x 1")	86	2.9
SOYBEAN FLOUR (See FLOUR)			
SOYBEAN GRITS, high fat			
(USDA)	1 cup (4.9 oz.)	524	46.0
SOYBEAN MILK (USDA):			
Fluid	4 oz.	37	2.5
Powder	1 oz.	122	7.9
SOYBEAN PROTEIN			
(USDA)	1 oz.	91	4.3
SOYBEAN PROTEINATE			
(USDA)	1 oz.	88	2.2
SOYBEAN SPROUT (See BEAN SPROUT)			
SOY SAUCE (See SAUCE)			
SPACE FOOD:			
*Applesauce mix (Epicure)	1.5 oz.	191	40.5
*Banana pudding powder (Epicure)	2.5 oz.	299	49.7
*Beef bites (Epicure)	.6 oz.	73	.1
*Beef pot roast bars (Epicure)	1 oz.	121	0.
*Beef sandwich bites (Epicure)	.8 oz.	95	7.8
*Beef & vegetable bar (Epicure)	.9 oz.	170	5.8
*Brownie bites (Epicure)	1.1 oz.	184	23.6

Food and Description	Measure or Quantity	Calories	Carbo-hydrates (grams)
*Butterscotch pudding powder (Epicure)	2.5 oz.	299	49.7
Caramel stick (Pillsbury)	1 oz.	118	19.8
*Caramel stick (Pillsbury)	1 piece	41	6.7
*Cheese sandwich bites (Epicure)	.8 oz.	168	3.0
*Chicken bites (Epicure)	.8 oz.	103	0.
*Chicken sandwich bites (Epicure)	.8 oz.	101	7.5
*Chicken & vegetable bar (Epicure)	.8 oz.	60	6.8
Chocolate malt stick (Epicure)	1 oz.	118	19.8
*Chocolate pudding powder (Epicure)	2.5 oz.	299	49.4
Chocolate stick (Pillsbury)	1 oz.	118	19.8
*Chocolate stick (Pillsbury)	1 piece	41	6.7
*Cinnamon toast bites (Epicure)	.8 oz.	117	14.9
*Cocoa beverage powder (Epicure)	1.5 oz.	180	27.4
*Corn bar (Epicure)	1 oz.	107	22.8
*Corn flake mix (Epicure)	1.3 oz.	143	31.0
*Fruit cocktail bar (Epicure)	.8 oz.	88	21.3
*Mushroom soup powder (Epicure)	1.1 oz.	184	12.2
*Orange beverage powder (Epicure)	.6 oz.	65	15.2
*Pea bar (Epicure)	.7 oz.	73	13.6
*Peach bar (Epicure)	.8 oz.	75	17.4
*Peanut butter sandwich bite (Epicure)	1.1 oz.	153	12.7
Peanut butter stick (Pillsbury)	1 oz.	118	19.8
Peanut butter stick (Pillsbury)	1 piece	41	6.7
*Pea soup powder (Epicure)	1.7 oz.	186	30.8
*Pineapple beverage powder (Epicure)	.6 oz.	60	15.0
*Potato salad bar (Epicure)	.9 oz.	113	10.0

(USDA): United States Department of Agriculture
DNA: Data Not Available
* Prepared as Package Directs

Food and Description	Measure or Quantity	Calories	Carbo-hydrates (grams)
*Shrimp cocktail bar (Epicure)	1.1 oz.	140	13.9
*Spaghetti & sauce (Epicure)	.7 oz.	96	7.3
*Toast bites (Epicure)	.6 oz.	76	8.2
SPAGHETTI. Plain spaghetti products are essentially the same in caloric value and carbohydrate content on the same weight basis. The longer the cooking, the more water is absorbed and this affects the nutritive value (USDA):			
Dry	1 oz.	105	21.3
Dry, broken	1 cup (2.5 oz.)	262	53.4
Cooked:			
8–10 minutes, "al dente"	1 cup (5.1 oz.)	216	43.9
8–10 minutes, "al dente"	4 oz.	168	34.1
14–20 minutes, tender	1 cup (4.9 oz.)	155	32.2
14–20 minutes, tender	4 oz.	126	26.1
SPAGHETTI DINNER:			
With meat balls:			
*(Chef Boy-Ar-Dee)	8¾-oz. pkg.	362	62.0
*With meat sauce (Chef Boy-Ar-Dee)	7-oz. pkg.	251	50.3
*With meat sauce (Kraft) *Deluxe Dinner*	4 oz.	151	23.1
*With mushroom sauce (Chef Boy-Ar-Dee)	7-oz. pkg.	229	51.5
Frozen:			
(Banquet)	11½-oz. dinner	423	57.2
(Morton)	11-oz. dinner	368	55.9
(Swanson)	11½-oz. dinner	323	44.4
SPAGHETTI & FRANKFURTERS in TOMATO SAUCE, canned:			
SpaghettiOs (Franco-American)	1 cup	253	25.7
(Heinz)	8½-oz. can	308	28.2

Food and Description	Measure or Quantity	Calories	Carbo-hydrates (grams)
SPAGHETTI & GROUND BEEF in TOMATO SAUCE, canned:			
Buitoni	8 oz.	266	23.6
(Chef Boy-Ar-Dee)	7½ oz. (½ of 15-oz. can)	192	26.4
(Franco-American)	1 cup	272	25.5
(Nalley's)	8 oz.	204	28.6
SPAGHETTI & MEATBALLS in TOMATO SAUCE:			
Home recipe (USDA)	1 cup (8.7 oz.)	332	38.7
Canned:			
(USDA)	1 cup (8.8 oz.)	258	28.5
(Austex)	15½-oz. can	437	48.5
(Buitoni)	8 oz.	258	21.1
(Chef Boy-Ar-Dee)	8 oz. (⅛ of 40-oz. can)	213	27.2
(Franco-American)	1 cup	264	24.3
SpaghettiOs (Franco-American)	1 cup	215	23.0
(Hormel)	15-oz. can	348	20.0
(Morton House)	4 oz.	288	D.N.A.
Frozen (Buitoni)	8 oz.	262	31.2
Frozen (Buitoni)	4 oz.	131	15.6
SPAGHETTI with MEAT SAUCE:			
Canned (Heinz)	8½-oz. can	207	26.3
Frozen:			
(Banquet) cookin' bag	8 oz.	323	33.8
(Kraft)	12½-oz. pkg.	343	48.9
(Morton)	8-oz. casserole	289	28.9
(Swanson)	8-oz. pkg.	233	28.5
SPAGHETTI MIX:			
*American style (Kraft)	4 oz.	121	22.2
*Italian style (Kraft)	4 oz.	119	20.1
SPAGHETTI SAUCE:			
Clam, red (Buitoni)	4 oz.	106	1.4

(USDA): United States Department of Agriculture
DNA: Data Not Available
* Prepared as Package Directs

Food and Description	Measure or Quantity	Calories	Carbo-hydrates (grams)
Clam, white (Buitoni)	4 oz.	140	2.2
Marinara (See **SAUCE, Marinara**)			
Meat:			
(Buitoni)	4 oz.	111	5.0
(Chef Boy-Ar-Dee)	3¾ oz. (¼ of 15-oz. can)	93	10.1
With ground meat (Chef Boy-Ar-Dee)	4⅐ oz. (⅐ of 29-oz. jar)	136	10.2
(Heinz)	1 cup	220	30.8
(Prince)	½ cup (4.9 oz.)	144	11.0
Meatball (Chef Boy-Ar-Dee)	5 oz. (⅓ of 15-oz. can)	170	21.2
Meatless or plain:			
(Buitoni)	4 oz.	76	9.5
(Chef Boy-Ar-Dee)	4 oz. (¼ of 16-oz. jar)	73	12.4
(Heinz)	½ cup	98	15.4
(Prince)	½ cup (4.6 oz.)	88	13.0
(Ronzoni)	4 oz.	110	D.N.A.
Mushroom:			
(Buitoni)	4 oz.	69	7.6
(Chef Boy-Ar-Dee)	3¾ oz. (¼ of 15-oz. can)	68	11.4
With meat (Heinz)	½ cup	106	14.0
(Franco-American)	4 oz.	87	12.4
Arturo (Naas)	8-oz. can	132	D.N.A.
SPAGHETTI SAUCE MIX:			
*(Kraft)	4 oz.	60	9.0
(McCormick)	1½-oz. pkg.	147	D.N.A.
*(McCormick)	4 oz.	80	13.0
(Wyler's)	1½-oz. pkg.	D.N.A.	25.0
Italian (French's)	1½-oz. pkg.	108	22.6
*Prepared without oil (Spatini)	½ cup (4.2 oz.)	26	9.0
*Prepared with oil (Spatini)	½ cup (4.2 oz.)	52	9.0
With mushrooms (French's)	1⅜-oz. pkg.	122	17.6
With mushrooms (Lawry's)	1½-oz. pkg.	147	22.6
*With mushrooms, tomato paste (Durkee)	2⅔ cups (1.2-oz. pkg.)	209	48.1

Food and Description	Measure or Quantity	Calories	Carbohydrates (grams)
*Without meat (Durkee)	2 cups (2.1-oz. pkg.)	167	38.8
SPAGHETTI with TOMATO SAUCE:			
Twists (Buitoni)	8 oz.	142	24.1
(Van Camp)	½ cup (3.9 oz.)	84	16.9
SPAGHETTI in TOMATO SAUCE with CHEESE:			
Home recipe (USDA)	1 cup (8.8 oz.)	260	37.0
Canned:			
(USDA)	1 cup (8.8 oz.)	190	38.5
(Chef Boy-Ar-Dee)	8 oz. (⅕ of 40-oz. can)	156	31.8
Italian style (Franco-American)	1 cup	174	30.9
(Heinz)	8½-oz. can	178	31.1
SPAM (Hormel) canned:			
Regular	12-oz. can	1180	4.8
Spread	3-oz. can	217	.8
SPANISH MACKEREL, raw (USDA):			
Whole	1 lb. (weighed whole)	490	0.
Meat only	4 oz.	201	0.
SPANISH-STYLE VEGETABLES, frozen (Birds Eye)	⅓ pkg. (3⅓ oz.)	85	7.1
SPEARMINT EXTRACT (Ehlers)	1 tsp.	12	D.N.A.
SPECIAL K, cereal (Kellogg's)	1¼ cups (1 oz.)	109	20.9
SPICE CAKE MIX:			
*(Duncan Hines)	¹⁄₁₂ of cake (2.7 oz.)	199	35.0

(USDA): United States Department of Agriculture
DNA: Data Not Available
* Prepared as Package Directs

Food and Description	Measure or Quantity	Calories	Carbohydrates (grams)
*& apple with raisins (Betty Crocker)	½₂ of cake	206	37.7
Honey: (USDA)	1 oz.	126	21.6
*Prepared with caramel icing (USDA)	2 oz.	200	34.5
*Layer (Betty Crocker)	½₂ of cake	202	36.1

SPICES. Most spices, such as cinnamon, saffron and allspice, are used in such small quantities that the contribution of calories and carbohydrates can be disregarded in dieting for weight control.

SPINACH:

Food and Description	Measure or Quantity	Calories	Carbohydrates (grams)
Raw (USDA):			
Untrimmed	1 lb. (weighed with large stems & roots)	85	14.0
Trimmed or packaged	1 lb.	118	19.5
Trimmed, whole leaves	1 cup (1.2 oz.)	9	1.4
Trimmed, chopped	1 cup (1.8 oz.)	14	2.2
Boiled, drained whole leaves (USDA)	1 cup (5.5 oz.)	36	5.6
Canned, regular pack:			
Solids & liq. (USDA)	½ cup (4.1 oz.)	22	3.5
Drained solids (USDA)	½ cup (4 oz.)	27	4.0
Drained liq. (USDA)	4 oz.	7	1.5
Drained solids (Del Monte)	½ cup (4 oz.)	28	4.0
Canned, dietetic pack:			
Solids & liq. (USDA)	4 oz.	24	3.7
Drained solids (USDA)	4 oz.	29	4.5
Drained liq. (USDA)	4 oz.	9	2.3
Solids & liq. (Blue Boy)	4 oz.	22	2.4
Frozen:			
Chopped:			
Not thawed (USDA)	4 oz.	27	4.3
Boiled, drained (USDA)	4 oz.	26	4.2
(Birds Eye)	⅓ pkg. (3.3 oz.)	23	2.7
Deviled, with cheddar cheese, casserole (Green Giant)	⅓ of 10-oz. pkg.	67	5.2

Food and Description	Measure or Quantity	Calories	Carbo-hydrates (grams)
Leaf:			
Not thawed (USDA)	4 oz.	28	4.8
Boiled, drained (USDA)	4 oz.	27	4.4
(Birds Eye)	⅓ pkg. (3.3 oz.)	23	3.1
In butter sauce (Green Giant)	⅓ of 10-oz. pkg.	44	3.4

SPINACH, NEW ZEALAND (See **NEW ZEALAND SPINACH**)

SPINACH SOUFFLE, frozen:

(Stouffer's)	12-oz. pkg.	484	29.0
(Swanson)	7½-oz. pkg.	260	15.9

SPINY LOBSTER (See **CRAYFISH**)

SPLEEN, raw (USDA):

Beef & calf	4 oz.	118	0.
Hog	4 oz.	121	0.
Lamb	4 oz.	130	0.

SPONGE CAKE, home recipe (USDA)

	1/12 of 10″ cake (2.3 oz.)	196	35.7

SPORT COLA, soft drink (Canada Dry)

	6 fl. oz.	77	20.0

SPOT, fillets (USDA):

Raw	1 lb.	993	0.
Baked	4 oz.	335	0.

SPRITE, soft drink

	6 fl. oz.	70	18.1

SQUAB, pigeon, raw (USDA):

Dressed	1 lb. (weighed with feet, inedible viscera & bones)	569	0.

(USDA): United States Department of Agriculture
DNA: Data Not Available
* Prepared as Package Directs

Food and Description	Measure or Quantity	Calories	Carbo-hydrates (grams)
Meat & skin	4 oz.	333	0.
Meat only	4 oz.	161	0.
Giblets	1 oz.	44	.3
SQUASH SEEDS, dry (USDA):			
In hull	4 oz.	464	12.6
Hulled	1 oz.	157	4.3
SQUASH, SUMMER:			
Fresh (USDA):			
Crookneck & Straightneck, yellow:			
Whole	1 lb. (weighed untrimmed)	89	19.1
Boiled, drained, diced	½ cup (3.6 oz.)	15	3.2
Boiled, drained, slices	½ cup (3.1 oz.)	13	2.7
Scallop, white & pale green:			
Whole	1 lb. (weighed untrimmed)	93	22.7
Boiled, drained, mashed	½ cup (4.2 oz.)	19	4.5
Zucchini & Cocozelle, green:			
Whole	1 lb. (weighed untrimmed)	73	15.5
Boiled, drained, slices	½ cup (2.7 oz.)	9	1.9
Canned, zucchini (Del Monte)	½ cup (4.1 oz.)	25	5.6
Frozen:			
Not thawed (USDA)	4 oz.	24	5.3
Boiled, drained (USDA)	4 oz.	24	5.3
Parmesan (Mrs. Paul's)	12-oz. pkg.	259	16.0
Zucchini, slices (Birds Eye)	½ cup (3.3 oz.)	20	3.8
SQUASH, WINTER:			
Fresh (USDA):			
Acorn:			
Whole	1 lb. (weighed with skin & seeds)	152	38.6
Baked, flesh only, mashed	½ cup (3.6 oz.)	56	14.3
Boiled, flesh only, mashed	½ cup (4.1 oz.)	39	9.7
Butternut:			
Whole	1 lb. (weighed with skin & seeds)	171	44.4

Food and Description	Measure or Quantity	Calories	Carbo-hydrates (grams)
Baked, flesh only	4 oz.	77	19.8
Boiled, flesh only	4 oz.	46	11.8
Hubbard:			
Whole	1 lb. (weighed with skin & seeds)	117	28.1
Baked, flesh only	4 oz.	57	13.3
Baked, flesh only, mashed	½ cup (3.6 oz.)	51	11.9
Boiled, flesh only, diced	½ cup (4.2 oz.)	35	8.1
Frozen:			
Not thawed (USDA)	4 oz.	43	10.4
Heated (USDA)	½ cup (4.2 oz.)	46	11.0
SQUID, raw, meat only (USDA)	4 oz.	95	1.7
STARCH (See **CORNSTARCH**)			
***START,** instant breakfast drink	½ cup (4.7 oz.)	60	14.9
STEINWEIN REBENGOLD, Franconia wine (Deinhard) 11% alcohol	3 fl. oz.	60	1.0
STOMACH, PORK, scalded (USDA)	4 oz.	172	0.
STRAINED FOOD (See **BABY FOOD**)			
STRAWBERRY:			
Fresh, whole (USDA)	1 lb. (weighed with caps & stems)	161	36.6
Fresh, capped (USDA)	1 cup (5.1 oz.)	53	12.1
Canned, unsweetened or low calorie:			
Water pack, solids & liq. (USDA)	4 oz.	25	6.4
Solids & liq. (Blue Boy)	4 oz.	16	7.8

(USDA): United States Department of Agriculture
DNA: Data Not Available
* Prepared as Package Directs

Food and Description	Measure or Quantity	Calories	Carbo-hydrates (grams)
(White Rose)	4 oz.	26	5.8
Frozen, sweetened:			
Whole (USDA)	16-oz. can	418	106.7
Slices (USDA)	10-oz. pkg.	310	79.0
Whole (Birds Eye)	¼ pkg. (4 oz.)	101	26.6
Halves (Birds Eye)	½ cup (5 oz.)	162	39.9
Quick thaw (Birds Eye)	½ cup (5 oz.)	122	30.7
STRAWBERRY CRISPS, dehydrated snack (Epicure)	1 oz.	85	19.2
***STRAWBERRY DANISH DESSERT** (Junket)	½ cup	138	33.8
***STRAWBERRY DRINK MIX:**			
Quik	2 heaping tsp. (.6 oz.)	62	15.9
*(Wyler's)	6 fl. oz.	64	15.8
STRAWBERRY FLAVORING, imitation:			
(Ehlers)	1 tsp.	12	D.N.A.
(No-Cal)	1 tsp.	<1	Tr.
STRAWBERRY ICE CREAM (Sealtest)	¼ pt. (2.3 oz.)	133	19.5
STRAWBERRY ICE CREAM MIX (Junket)	6 serving pkg. (4 oz.)	388	110.0
STRAWBERRY LIQUEUR (Leroux) 50 proof	1 fl. oz.	74	8.3
STRAWBERRY PIE:			
Home recipe (USDA)	⅛ of 9" pie (5.6 oz.)	313	48.8
Creme (Tastykake)	4-oz. pie	356	50.7
Frozen:			
(Morton)	⅙ of 20-oz. pie	253	36.8
Cream (Banquet)	2½ oz.	187	27.5
Cream (Morton)	¼ of 14.4-oz. pie	247	32.4

Food and Description	Measure or Quantity	Calories	Carbo-hydrates (grams)
Cream (Mrs. Smith's)	⅛ of 8" pie (2.3 oz.)	204	23.6
STRAWBERRY PIE FILLING, (Lucky Leaf)	8 oz.	248	60.0
STRAWBERRY PRESERVE or JAM, dietetic or low calorie:			
(Dia-Mel)	1 T.	22	5.4
(Diet Delight)	1 T. (.6 oz.)	23	5.7
(Slenderella)	1 T. (.6 oz.)	22	5.6
(Smucker's)	1 T. (.5 oz.)	3	.8
(Tillie Lewis)	1 T. (.5 oz.)	10	2.4
STRAWBERRY RENNET CUSTARD MIX:			
Powder:			
(Junket)	1 oz.	115	27.9
*(Junket)	4 oz.	108	14.7
Tablet:			
(Junket)	1 tablet	1	.2
*With sugar (Junket)	4 oz.	101	13.5
STRAWBERRY-RHUBARB PIE:			
(Tastykake)	4-oz. pie	399	63.5
Frozen (Mrs. Smith's)	⅛ of 8" pie (4.2 oz.)	312	45.8
STRAWBERRY-RHUBARD PIE FILLING (Lucky Leaf)	8 oz.	258	62.8
STRAWBERRY SOFT DRINK:			
Sweetened:			
(Canada Dry)	6 fl. oz.	85	22.2
(Fanta)	6 fl. oz.	88	22.7
(Shasta)	6 fl. oz.	80	20.3
(Yoo-Hoo)	6 fl. oz.	90	18.0

(USDA): United States Department of Agriculture
DNA: Data Not Available
* Prepared as Package Directs

Food and Description	Measure or Quantity	Calories	Carbohydrates (grams)
High-protein (Yoo-Hoo)	6 fl. oz.	114	24.6
Low calorie (Shasta)	6 fl. oz.	<1	<.1
STRAWBERRY SYRUP, dietetic:			
(Dia-Mel)	1 T.	22	5.5
(No-Cal)	1 tsp.	<1	0.
STRAWBERRY TURNOVER, frozen (Pepperidge Farm)	1 turnover (3.3 oz.)	326	34.5
STROGANOFF, BEEF:			
Canned (Hormel)	1-lb. can	645	9.5
Frozen (Swanson)	6.5-oz. pkg.	213	5.8
Mix (Chef Boy-Ar-Dee)	6⅔-oz. pkg.	232	30.6
Mix (Lipton)	6¼-oz. pkg.	380	48.5
*Mix (Noodle-Roni)	4 oz.	126	18.6
Seasoning mix (Lawry's)	1½-oz. pkg.	118	23.4
Skillet (Hunt's)	1-lb. 2-oz. pkg.	817	94.0
STRUDEL, frozen (Pepperidge Farm):			
Apple	⅛ of strudel (2.5 oz.)	202	26.0
Blueberry	⅛ of strudel (2.5 oz.)	240	28.4
Cherry	⅛ of strudel (2.5 oz.)	204	26.8
Pineapple-cheese	⅛ of strudel (2.3 oz.)	209	21.2
STURGEON (USDA):			
Raw, section	1 lb. (weighed with bones & skin)	362	0.
Raw, meat only	4 oz.	107	0.
Smoked	4 oz.	169	0.
Steamed	4 oz.	181	0.
SUCCOTASH, frozen:			
Not thawed (USDA)	4 oz.	110	24.4
Boiled, drained (USDA)	½ cup (3.4 oz.)	89	19.7
(Birds Eye)	½ cup (3.3 oz.)	87	19.4

Food and Description	Measure or Quantity	Calories	Carbohydrates (grams)
SUCKER, CARP, raw (USDA):			
Whole	1 lb. (weighed whole)	196	0.
Meat only	4 oz.	126	0.
SUCKER, including **WHITE** and **MULLET,** raw:			
Whole (USDA)	1 lb. (weighed whole)	203	0.
Meat only (USDA)	4 oz.	118	0.
SUET (USDA)	1 oz.	242	0.
SUGAR, beet or cane (There is no difference in calories and carbohydrates among brands):			
Brown:			
(USDA)	1 lb.	1692	437.3
Firm-packed (USDA)	1 cup (7.5 oz.)	791	204.4
Firm-packed (USDA)	1 T. (.5 oz.)	48	12.5
Confectioners':			
(USDA)	1 lb.	1746	451.3
Sifted (USDA)	1 cup (3.4 oz.)	366	94.5
Sifted (USDA)	1 T. (6 grams)	23	5.9
Granulated:			
(USDA)	1 lb.	1746	451.3
(USDA)	1 cup (6.9 oz.)	751	194.0
(USDA)	1 T. (.4 oz.)	46	11.9
Lump (USDA)	1⅛″ x ¾″ x ⅜″ piece (6 grams)	23	6.0
Maple (USDA)	1 lb.	1579	408.0
Maple (USDA)	1¾″ x 1¼″ x ½″ piece (1.2 oz.)	104	27.0
SUGAR APPLE, raw (USDA):			
Whole	1 lb. (weighed with skin & seeds)	192	48.4
Flesh only	4 oz.	107	26.9

(USDA): United States Department of Agriculture
DNA: Data Not Available
* Prepared as Package Directs

Food and Description	Measure or Quantity	Calories	Carbohydrates (grams)
SUGAR FROSTED FLAKES, cereal	¾ cup (1 oz.)	109	25.2
SUGAR JETS, cereal	1 cup (1 oz.)	111	23.7
SUGAR POPS, cereal	1 cup (1 oz.)	112	25.6
SUGAR SMACKS, cereal	1 cup (1 oz.)	112	25.3
SUGAR SUBSTITUTE:			
(Adolph's)	1 tsp. (1 gram)	Neg.	Neg.
Sweetness & Light	1 tsp. (1 gram)	4	.9
Sweetnin (Tillie Lewis)	1 tsp. (5 grams)	0	0.
Sweet'n It, liquid (Dia-Mel)	1 tsp.	0	0.
Sweet'n It, powdered (Dia-Mel)	1 packet (1 gram)	3	.8
(Weight Watchers)	1 packet (1 gram)	4	.9
SUNFLOWER SEED (USDA):			
In hulls	4 oz. (weighed in hull)	343	12.2
Hulled	1 oz.	159	5.6
SUNFLOWER SEED FLOUR (See **FLOUR**)			
SURINAM CHERRY (See **PITANAGA**)			
SUZY Q (Hostess)	1 cake (2¼ oz.)	141	23.1
SWAMP CABBAGE (USDA):			
Raw, whole	1 lb. (weighed untrimmed)	107	19.8
Boiled, trimmed, drained	4 oz.	24	4.4
SWEETBREADS (USDA):			
Beef, raw	1 lb.	939	0.
Beef, braised	4 oz.	363	0.
Calf, raw	1 lb.	426	0.
Calf, braised	4 oz.	191	0.
Hog (See **PANCREAS**)			
Lamb, raw	1 lb.	426	0.
Lamb, braised	4 oz.	198	0.

Food and Description	Measure or Quantity	Calories	Carbohydrates (grams)
SWEET POTATO:			
Raw (USDA):			
All kinds, unpared	1 lb. (weighed whole)	419	96.6
Jersey types, pared	4 oz.	116	25.5
Puerto Rico variety, pared	4 oz.	133	31.0
Baked, peeled after baking (USDA)	3.9-oz. sweet potato (5″ x 2″)	155	35.8
Boiled, peeled after boiling (USDA)	5-oz. sweet potato (5″ x 2″)	168	38.7
Candied, home recipe (USDA)	1 sweet potato (3½″ x 2¼″)	294	59.8
Canned, regular pack:			
In syrup, solids & liq. (USDA)	4 oz.	129	31.2
Vacuum or solid pack (USDA)	½ cup (3.8 oz.)	118	27.1
In syrup, solids & liq. (Del Monte)	½ cup (4.2 oz.)	138	33.7
(King Pharr)	½ cup	118	22.5
Yam (King Pharr)	½ cup	114	27.0
Vacuum pack (Taylor's)	½ cup	135	32.0
Canned, dietetic pack, without added sugar & salt (USDA)	4 oz.	52	12.2
Dehydrated flakes, dry (USDA)	½ cup (2 oz.)	220	52.2
*Dehydrated flakes, prepared with water (USDA)	½ cup (4.4 oz.)	120	28.5
Frozen, candied (Mrs. Paul's)	12-oz. pkg.	557	135.0
Frozen, candied, yams (Birds Eye)	½ cup (4 oz.)	215	53.3
SWEET POTATO PIE:			
Home recipe (USDA)	⅛ of 9″ pie (5.4 oz.)	324	36.0
(Tastykake)	4-oz. pie	359	50.0

(USDA): United States Department of Agriculture
DNA: Data Not Available
* Prepared as Package Directs

Food and Description	Measure or Quantity	Calories	Carbo-hydrates (grams)
SWEETSOP (See **SUGAR APPLE**)			
SWING (Shasta):			
Sweetened	6 fl. oz.	80	20.3
Low calorie	6 fl. oz.	<1	<.1
SWISS STEAK, frozen:			
(Stouffer's)	10-oz. pkg.	569	14.0
Dinner (Swanson)	10-oz. dinner	361	35.0
With gravy (Holloway House)	1 steak (7 oz.)	236	5.6
SWISS UP WINE (Italian Swiss Colony-Gold Medal) 19.7% alcohol	3 fl. oz.	132	9.3
SWORDFISH (USDA):			
Raw, meat only	1 lb.	535	0.
Broiled with butter or margarine	3″ x 3″ x ½″ steak (4.4 oz.)	218	0.
Canned, solids & liq.	4 oz.	116	0.
SYLVANER WINE (Louis M. Martini) 12.5% alcohol	3 fl. oz.	90	.2
SYRUP. (See also individual listings by kind, such as **PANCAKE & WAFFLE SYRUP** or by brand name, such as **LOG CABIN**):			
Cane and maple blend (USDA)	1 T.	50	13.0
All fruit flavors (Smucker's)	1 T.	50	12.5

Food and Description	Measure or Quantity	Calories	Carbo-hydrates (grams)

I

| *TABASCO* (McIlhenny) | ¼ tsp. (1 gram) | <1 | <.1 |

TACO, beef, frozen:
Regular size:

(Banquet)	1 taco	101	14.0
(Patio)	1 taco (2¼ oz.)	179	15.1
(Rosarita)	1 taco (2 oz.)	138	D.N.A.
Cocktail (Patio)	1 taco (½ oz.)	39	4.8
Cocktail (Rosarita)	1 taco (½ oz.)	30	D.N.A.

TACO FILLING, beef, canned

(Rosarita)	1 oz.	61	D.N.A.

TACO SEASONING MIX

(Lawry's)	1¼-oz. pkg.	120	21.8

TAHITIAN TREAT, soft

drink (Canada Dry)	6 fl. oz.	95	23.9

TAMALE:
Canned:

(Hormel)	15-oz. can	582	41.2
(Rutherford)	6 oz.	242	D.N.A.
(Wilson)	15½-oz. can	601	63.3
Frozen:			
(Banquet) cookin' bag	2 tamales with sauce (3 oz. each)	279	26.0
(Rosarita)	3⅓-oz. tamale	256	D.N.A.
Hot, with gravy (Patio)	1 pkg.	1011	D.N.A.
With chili gravy (Patio)	1 piece	175	6.3

TAMARIND, fresh (USDA):

Whole	1 lb. (weighed with pods & seeds)	520	136.1
Flesh only	4 oz.	271	70.9

(USDA): United States Department of Agriculture
DNA: Data Not Available
* Prepared as Package Directs

Food and Description	Measure or Quantity	Calories	Carbo-hydrates (grams)
TANDY TAKE (Tastykake):			
Chocolate	1 cake (⅔ oz.)	147	21.0
Choc-o-mint	1 cake (.6 oz.)	102	13.0
Dandy Kake	1 cake (.6 oz.)	102	13.0
Karamel	1 cake (⅔ oz.)	100	12.2
Orange	1 cake (.6 oz.)	103	13.6
Peanut butter	1 cake (⅔ oz.)	194	32.1
***TANG**, instant breakfast drink	½ cup (4 oz.)	61	15.8
TANGELO, fresh (USDA):			
Juice from whole fruit	1 lb. (weighed with peel, membrane & seeds)	104	24.6
Juice	½ cup (4.4 oz.)	51	12.0
TANGERINE or MANDARIN ORANGE, fresh:			
Whole (USDA)	1 lb. (weighed with skin & seeds)	154	38.9
Whole (USDA)	4.1-oz. tangerine (2⅜" dia.)	39	10.0
Peeled (Sunkist)	1 large tangerine	39	10.0
Sections, without membranes (USDA)	1 cup (6.8 oz.)	89	22.4
TANGERINE JUICE:			
Fresh (USDA)	½ cup (4.4 oz.)	53	12.5
Canned, unsweetened (USDA)	½ cup (4.4 oz.)	53	12.6
Canned, sweetened (USDA)	½ cup (4.4 oz.)	62	14.9
Frozen, concentrate, unsweetened:			
Undiluted (USDA)	6-oz. can	340	80.4
*Diluted with 3 parts water by volume (USDA)	½ cup (4.4 oz.)	57	13.4
*(Minute Maid)	½ cup (4.2 oz.)	57	13.9
*(Snow Crop)	½ cup (4.2 oz.)	57	13.9
TAPIOCA, dry, quick-cooking granulated: (USDA)	1 cup (5.4 oz.)	535	131.3

Food and Description	Measure or Quantity	Calories	Carbohydrates (grams)
(USDA)	1 T. (10 grams)	35	8.6
(Minute Tapioca)	1 T.	40	10.0
TAPIOCA PUDDING:			
Apple, home recipe (USDA)	½ cup (4.4 oz.)	146	36.8
Cream, home recipe (USDA)	½ cup (2.9 oz.)	110	14.0
Canned (Aunt's)	5-oz. can	166	25.6
Mix:			
*All flavors (Jell-O)	½ cup (5.1 oz.)	166	27.6
*Fluffy recipe (Minute Tapioca)	½ cup (5.8 oz.)	150	20.1
*Chocolate (Royal)	½ cup (5.1 oz.)	184	29.0
*Vanilla (My-T-Fine)	½ cup (5 oz.)	144	25.2
*Vanilla (Royal)	½ cup (5.1 oz.)	175	29.1
TARO, raw:			
Tubers, whole (USDA)	1 lb. (weighed with skin)	373	90.3
Tubers, skin removed (USDA)	4 oz.	111	26.9
Leaves & stems (USDA)	1 lb.	181	33.6
TAUTOG or BLACKFISH, raw:			
Whole (USDA)	1 lb. (weighed whole)	149	0.
Meat only (USDA)	4 oz.	101	0.
TEA:			
Bag (Tender Leaf)	1 bag	1	Tr.
Canned (Lipton)	12 fl. oz.	138	34.6
Instant:			
(USDA)	1 tsp.	1	.4
(Tender Leaf)	1 rounded tsp.	1	Tr.
*Lemon flavored (Lipton)	8 fl. oz.	3	.8
TEAM, cereal (Nabisco)	1⅓ cup (1 oz.)	107	24.2
TEA MIX, iced:			
All flavors _Nestea_	3 tsp. (.6 oz.)	58	15.1

(USDA): United States Department of Agriculture
DNA: Data Not Available
* Prepared as Package Directs

Food and Description	Measure or Quantity	Calories	Carbo- hydrates (grams)
*All flavors (Salada)	1 cup	57	13.6
*(Tender Leaf)	1 cup	57	14.2
(*Wyler's)	1 cup	56	14.0
Lemon flavored:			
*(Lipton)	1 cup	102	25.5
*Low calorie (Lipton)	1 cup	4	1.2
*Low calorie (Tender Leaf)	1 cup	12	3.1
TEE UP, soft drink (Kirsch)	6 fl. oz.	64	16.1
TEMPTYS (Tastykake):			
Butter creme	1 cake (⅔ oz.)	94	12.9
Chocolate	1 cake (⅔ oz.)	95	17.1
Lemon	1 cake (⅔ oz.)	95	17.3
TENDERGREEN (See MUSTARD SPINACH)			
TENDER MADE MAIN MEAL MEAT, canned (Wilson):			
Beef roast	3 oz.	100	0.
Corned beef brisket	3 oz.	135	.8
Ham	3 oz.	129	.8
Picnic	3 oz.	137	.8
Pork roast	3 oz.	133	0.
Pork loin, smoked	3 oz.	114	.8
Turkey & dressing	3 oz.	159	8.5
Turkey roast	3 oz.	87	0.
TEQUILA (See DISTILLED LIQUOR)			
TEQUILA SOUR (Calvert) 55 proof	3 fl. oz.	185	11.4
TERRAPIN, DIAMOND BACK, raw (USDA):			
In shell	1 lb. (weighed in shell)	106	0.
Meat only	4 oz.	126	0.
THICK & FROSTY (General Foods)	1 cup (8.3 oz.)	314	37.7

Food and Description	Measure or Quantity	Calories	Carbohydrates (grams)
THUNDERBIRD WINE (Gallo):			
14% alcohol	3 fl. oz.	86	8.1
20% alcohol	3 fl. oz.	106	7.5
THURINGER, sausage (USDA)	1 oz.	87	.5
TIA MARIA, liqueur (Hiram Walker) 63 proof	1 fl. oz.	92	10.0
TIKI, soft drink (Shasta):			
Regular	6 fl. oz.	84	21.3
Diet	6 fl. oz.	<1	<.1
TILEFISH (USDA):			
Raw, whole	1 lb. (weighed whole)	183	0.
Baked, meat only	4 oz.	156	0.
TOASTER BAKED PRODUCTS:			
Toast 'Em (General Foods):			
Danka, Danish	1 piece (1½ oz.)	210	24.5
Pop-ups, fruit flavors	1 piece (1.8 oz.)	191	34.1
Toastette (Nabisco):			
Apple	1 piece (1⅔ oz.)	184	32.3
Blueberry	1 piece (1⅔ oz.)	184	33.0
Brown sugar, cinnamon	1 piece (1⅔ oz.)	189	31.9
Cherry	1 piece (1⅔ oz.)	182	32.7
Strawberry	1 piece (1⅔ oz.)	184	32.7
Toast-r-Cake, bran (Thomas')	1 piece (1.2 oz.)	116	19.6
Toast-r-Cake, corn (Thomas')	1 piece (1.2 oz.)	118	18.1
Toaster-r-Cake, orange (Thomas')	1 piece (1.2 oz.)	117	17.9
TODDLER FOOD (See **BABY FOOD**)			
TOKAY WINE:			
(Gallo)	3 fl. oz.	107	7.5
(Gallo) 14% alcohol	3 fl. oz.	86	8.1

(USDA): United States Department of Agriculture
DNA: Data Not Available
* Prepared as Package Directs

Food and Description	Measure or Quantity	Calories	Carbo-hydrates (grams)
(Italian Swiss Colony-Gold Medal) 19.7% alcohol	3 fl. oz.	128	8.1
(Taylor) white, 18.5% alcohol	3 fl. oz.	144	11.3
TOMATO:			
Fresh, green, whole, untrimmed (USDA)	1 lb. (weighed with core & stem)	99	21.1
Fresh, ripe (USDA):			
Whole, eaten with skin	1 lb.	100	21.3
Whole, eaten without skin	1 small (1¾" x 2¼", 3.9 oz.)	24	5.2
Whole, eaten without skin	1 med. (2" x 2½", 15.3 oz.)	33	7.0
Peeled	1 lb. (weighed with skin, stem ends & hard core)	88	18.8
Sliced, peeled	½ cup (3.2 oz.)	20	4.2
Boiled (USDA)	½ cup (4.3 oz.)	31	6.7
Canned, regular pack:			
Whole, solids & liq. (USDA)	½ cup (4.2 oz.)	25	5.1
(Contadina)	½ cup	28	5.6
Diced, in purée (Contadina)	½ cup	44	9.2
Sliced (Contadina)	½ cup	36	8.4
Stewed (Contadina)	½ cup	36	8.0
Stewed (Del Monte)	½ cup (4.2 oz.)	31	7.1
Whole, peeled (Hunt's)	½ cup (4.2 oz.)	24	5.6
Canned, dietetic pack:			
Solids & liq. (USDA)	4 oz.	23	4.8
Solids & liq. (Blue Boy)	4 oz.	25	4.8
Whole, peeled (Diet Delight)	½ cup (4.3 oz.)	39	5.4
Whole, unseasoned (S and W) *Nutradiet*	4 oz.	24	5.2
Solids & liq. (Tillie Lewis)	½ cup (4.3 oz.)	25	4.6
TOMATO JUICE:			
Canned, regular pack:			
(USDA)	6 fl. oz.	35	7.8
(USDA)	½ cup (4.3 oz.)	23	5.2
(Campbell)	6 fl. oz.	33	6.6

Food and Description	Measure or Quantity	Calories	Carbo-hydrates (grams)
(Del Monte)	½ cup (4.3 oz.)	22	4.9
(Heinz)	5½ fl.-oz. can	34	6.6
(Hunt's)	5½ fl.-oz. can	30	7.2
Canned, dietetic pack:			
(USDA)	4 oz. (by wt.)	22	4.9
(Blue Boy)	4 oz. (by wt.)	24	4.5
(Diet Delight)	½ cup (4.2 oz.)	24	4.9
Unseasoned (S and W) *Nutradiet*	4 oz. (by wt.)	25	5.0
Concentrate, canned (USDA)	4 oz. (by wt.)	86	19.4
*Concentrate, canned, diluted with 3 parts water by volume (USDA)	4 oz. (by wt.)	23	5.1
Dehydrated (USDA)	1 oz.	86	19.3
*Dehydrated (USDA)	½ cup (4.3 oz.)	24	5.4
TOMATO JUICE COCKTAIL:			
(USDA)	4 oz. (by wt.)	24	5.7
(College Inn)	4 oz.	29	6.3
TOMATO PASTE, canned:			
(USDA)	6 oz.	139	31.6
(Contadina)	6-oz. can	143	30.1
(Hunt's)	1 T. (.6 oz.)	14	3.2
TOMATO PUREE:			
Canned, regular pack:			
(USDA)	1 cup (8.8 oz.)	98	22.2
(Contadina)	1 cup	96	20.
(Hunt's)	1 cup (8.8 oz.)	104	2.2
Canned, dietetic pack (USDA)	1 oz.	11	2.5
TOMATO SALAD, jellied (Contadina)	½ cup	60	13.6
TOMATO SAUCE:			
(Contadina)	1 cup	80	16.8
(Del Monte)	1 cup (8.8 oz.)	60	14.0

(USDA): United States Department of Agriculture
DNA: Data Not Available
* Prepared as Package Directs

Food and Description	Measure or Quantity	Calories	Carbo-hydrates (grams)
(Hunt's) plain	1 cup (8.7 oz.)	78	18.7
(Hunt's) with bits	1 cup (8.7 oz.)	82	19.4
(Hunt's) with cheese	1 cup (8.8 oz.)	107	20.6
TOMATO SOUP:			
Canned, regular pack:			
Condensed (USDA)	8 oz. (by wt.)	163	28.8
*Prepared with equal volume water (USDA)	1 cup (8.6 oz.)	88	15.7
*Prepared with equal volume milk (USDA)	1 cup (8.6 oz.)	172	22.5
*(Campbell)	1 cup	79	14.0
*(Heinz) California	1 cup (8½ oz.)	87	18.3
*(Manischewitz)	8 oz. (by wt.)	60	9.1
*Beef (Campbell) Noodle-O's	1 cup	109	15.5
*Bisque (Campbell)	1 cup	115	20.9
*Rice, old fashioned (Campbell)	1 cup	99	16.7
*Rice (Manischewitz)	8 oz. (by wt.)	78	12.8
With vegetables (Heinz) Great American	1 cup (8¾ oz.)	126	17.6
Canned, dietetic pack:			
Low sodium (Campbell)	7¼-oz. can	97	16.9
*With rice (Claybourne)	8 oz.	73	14.6
(Tillie Lewis)	1 cup	70	11.8
TOMATO VEGETABLE SOUP MIX:			
With noodles (USDA)	1 oz.	98	17.8
*With noodles (USDA)	1 cup (8 oz.)	62	11.6
*(Golden Grain)	1 cup	80	13.3
*(Lipton) with noodles	1 cup	69	12.0
TOMCOD, ATLANTIC, raw (USDA):			
Whole	1 lb. (weighed whole)	136	0.
Meat only	4 oz.	87	0.
TOM COLLINS or COLLINS MIXER SOFT DRINK:			
(Dr. Brown's)	6 fl. oz.	64	16.1
(Hoffman)	6 fl. oz.	64	16.1

Food and Description	Measure or Quantity	Calories	Carbo-hydrates (grams)
(Key Food)	6 fl. oz.	66	16.5
(Kirsch)	6 fl. oz.	60	15.1
(Waldbaum)	6 fl. oz.	66	16.5
(Yukon Club)	6 fl. oz.	60	15.0
TONGUE (USDA):			
Beef, medium fat, raw, untrimmed	1 lb.	714	1.4
Beef, medium fat, braised	4 oz.	277	.5
Calf, raw, untrimmed	1 lb.	454	3.1
Calf, braised	4 oz.	181	1.1
Hog, raw, untrimmed	1 lb.	741	1.7
Hog, braised	4 oz.	287	.6
Lamb, raw, untrimmed	1 lb.	659	1.7
Lamb, braised	4 oz.	288	.6
Sheep, raw, untrimmed	1 lb.	877	7.9
Sheep, braised	4 oz.	366	2.7
TONGUE, CANNED:			
Pickled (USDA)	1 oz.	76	<.1
Potted or deviled (USDA)	1 oz.	82	.2
(Hormel)	12-oz. can	802	.7
TONIC WATER (See **QUININE SOFT DRINK**)			
TOPPING (See also **CHOCOLATE SYRUP**)			
Sweetened:			
Butterscotch:			
(Kraft)	1 oz.	84	18.9
(Smucker's)	1 T. (.7 oz.)	63	15.3
Caramel:			
(Smucker's)	1 T. (.7 oz.)	61	15.3
Chocolate (Kraft)	1 oz.	84	18.7
Vanilla (Kraft)	1 oz.	84	19.2
Chocolate or chocolate-flavored:			
(Kraft)	1 oz.	73	18.0
Fudge (Hershey's)	1 oz.	96	15.8

(USDA): United States Department of Agriculture
DNA: Data Not Available
* Prepared as Package Directs

Food and Description	Measure or Quantity	Calories	Carbohydrates (grams)
Fudge (Smucker's)	1 T. (.7 oz.)	53	12.6
Marshmallow creme (Kraft)	1 oz.	90	22.9
Pecan in syrup (Smucker's)	1 T. (.7 oz.)	86	8.9
Pineapple (Kraft)	1 oz.	80	19.7
Spoonmallow (Kraft)	1 oz.	83	21.9
Strawberry (Kraft)	1 oz.	80	19.7
Walnut (Kraft)	1 oz.	113	14.3
Dietetic, chocolate (Diet Delight)	1 T. (.6 oz.)	20	4.7
TOPPING, WHIPPED:			
(Birds Eye) *Cool Whip*	1 T. (4 grams)	16	1.1
(Kraft)	1 oz.	79	4.3
(Lucky Whip)	1 T. (4 grams)	12	.5
(Sealtest) *Big Top*	1½ fl. oz.	15	.7
TOPPING, WHIPPED, MIX:			
*(D-Zerta)	1 T.	7	.3
*(Dream Whip)	1 T.	14	1.2
*(Lucky Whip)	1 T. (4 grams)	10	1.0
TORTILLA:			
(USDA)	.7-oz. tortilla (5″)	42	9.7
Corn, frozen (Patio)	1 tortilla	64	D.N.A.
TOTAL, cereal (General Mills)	1¼ cups (1 oz.)	100	23.0
TOWEL GOURD, raw (USDA):			
Unpared	1 lb. (weighed with skin)	69	15.8
Pared	4 oz.	20	4.6
TREET (Armour)	1 oz.	84	.3
TRIPE, beef (USDA):			
Commercial	4 oz.	113	0.
Pickled	4 oz.	70	0.
TRIPLE JACK WINE (Gallo) 20% alcohol	3 fl. oz.	102	6.5

Food and Description	Measure or Quantity	Calories	Carbo-hydrates (grams)
TRIPLE SEC LIQUEUR:			
(Bols) 78 proof	1 fl. oz.	101	8.8
(Garnier) 60 proof	1 fl. oz.	83	8.5
(Hiram Walker) 80 proof	1 fl. oz.	105	9.8
(Leroux) 80 proof	1 fl. oz.	102	8.9
(Old Mr. Boston) 42 proof	1 fl. oz.	97	10.1
(Old Mr. Boston) 60 proof	1 fl. oz.	105	10.1
TRIX, cereal (General Mills)	1 cup (1 oz.)	110	25.2
TROPICAL PUNCH SOFT DRINK (Yukon Club)	6 fl. oz.	90	22.5
TROUT:			
Brook, fresh, whole (USDA)	1 lb. (weighed whole)	224	0.
Brook, fresh, meat only (USDA)	4 oz.	115	0.
Lake (See **LAKE TROUT**)			
Rainbow (USDA):			
Fresh, meat with skin	4 oz.	221	0.
Canned	4 oz.	237	0.
Frozen (1000 Springs):			
Dressed	5-oz. trout	164	3.2
Boned	5-oz. trout	135	2.7
Boned & breaded	5-oz. trout	245	D.N.A.
TUNA:			
Raw, bluefin, meat only (USDA)	4 oz.	164	0.
Raw, yellowfin, meat only (USDA)	4 oz.	151	0.
Canned in oil:			
Solids & liq.:			
(USDA)	4 oz.	327	0.
(Breast O'Chicken)	6½-oz. can	540	0.
(Star-Kist)	7-oz. can	577	0.
Chunk (Star-Kist)	6½-oz. can	535	0.
Chunk (Star-Kist)	3¼-oz. can	268	0.
Chunk, light (Chicken of the Sea)	6½-oz. can	405	0.

(USDA): United States Department of Agriculture
DNA: Data Not Available
* Prepared as Package Directs

Food and Description	Measure or Quantity	Calories	Carbo-hydrates (grams)
Chunk, light (Icy Point)	6½-oz. can	530	0.
Chunk, light (Pillar Rock)	6½-oz. can	530	0.
Solid (Star-Kist)	7-oz. can	577	0.
White Albacore (Del Monte)	6½-oz. can	543	0.
Drained solids:			
(USDA)	4 oz.	223	0.
(Del Monte)	1 cup (5.6 oz.)	306	0.
Chunk, light (Chicken of the Sea)	6½-oz. can	294	0.
Chunk, light (Del Monte)	1 cup (5.6 oz.)	374	0.
Solid, white (Icy Point)	7-oz. can	286	0.
Solid, white (Pillar Rock)	7-oz. can	286	0.
Canned in water:			
Solids & liq. (USDA)	4 oz.	144	0.
(Breast O'Chicken)	6½-oz. can	230	0.
(Deep Blue)	7-oz. can	215	0.
Solids & liq. (Star-Kist)	7-oz. can	210	0.
Canned, dietetic:			
Drained, chunk, light (Chicken of the Sea)	6½-oz. can	200	0.
Solids & liq. (Star-Kist)	6½-oz. can	207	0.
Solids & liq. (Star-Kist)	3¼-oz. can	112	0.
TUNA & NOODLE DINNER (Star-Kist)	15-oz. can	364	D.N.A.
TUNA PIE, frozen:			
(Banquet)	8-oz. pie	479	40.2
(Morton)	8-oz. pie	385	35.8
(Star-Kist)	8-oz. pie	450	D.N.A.
TUNA SALAD, home recipe (USDA)	4 oz.	193	4.0
TUNA SOUP, Creole, canned (Crosse & Blackwell)	6½ oz. (½ can)	57	6.6
TURBOT Greenland (USDA):			
Raw, whole	1 lb. (weighed whole)	344	0.
Raw, meat only	4 oz.	166	0.

Food and Description	Measure or Quantity	Calories	Carbo-hydrates (grams)
TURKEY:			
Raw, ready-to-cook (USDA)	1 lb. (weighed with bones)	722	0.
Roasted (USDA):			
Flesh & skin	4 oz.	253	0.
Meat only:			
Chopped	1 cup (5 oz.)	268	0.
Diced	1 cup (4.8 oz.)	257	0.
Light	4 oz.	200	0.
Dark	4 oz.	230	0.
Skin only	1 oz.	128	0.
Canned, boned (USDA)	4 oz.	229	0.
Canned, boned, solids & liq. (Lynden)	5-oz. jar	239	0.
TURKEY DINNER, frozen:			
Sliced turkey, mashed potato, peas (USDA)	12 oz.	381	43.2
(Banquet)	11½-oz. dinner	280	28.2
(Morton) 3-course	1-lb. 1-oz. dinner	634	79.4
(Swanson)	11½-oz. dinner	401	43.7
(Swanson) 3-course	16-oz. dinner	501	54.5
(Weight Watchers)	16-oz. dinner	320	23.4
TURKEY GIZZARD (USDA):			
Raw	4 oz.	178	1.2
Simmered	4 oz.	222	1.2
TURKEY PIE:			
Home recipe, baked (USDA)	⅓ of 9″ pie (8.2 oz.)	550	42.2
Frozen:			
Commercial, unheated (USDA)	8 oz.	447	45.6
(Banquet)	8-oz. pie	398	38.0
(Morton)	8-oz. pie	411	35.7
(Swanson)	8-oz. pie	422	37.5
(Swanson) deep dish	1-lb. pie	746	63.8

(USDA): United States Department of Agriculture
DNA: Data Not Available
* Prepared as Package Directs

Food and Description	Measure or Quantity	Calories	Carbo- hydrates (grams)
TURKEY SOUP:			
Noodle:			
Condensed (USDA)	8 oz. (by wt.)	147	15.9
*Prepared with equal			
volume water (USDA)	1 cup (8.8 oz.)	82	8.8
*(Campbell)	1 cup	72	7.5
*(Heinz)	1 cup (8½ oz.)	83	10.0
(Heinz) *Great American*	1 cup (8¾ oz.)	97	12.1
Low sodium (Campbell)	7½-oz. can	78	9.2
*Vegetable (Campbell)	1 cup	73	8.0
TURKEY TETRAZZINI,			
frozen:			
(Morton) casserole	9-oz. pkg.	429	29.8
(Stouffer's)	12-oz. pkg.	694	68.7
TURNIP (USDA):			
Fresh, without tops	1 lb. (weighed with skins)	117	25.7
Boiled, drained, diced	½ cup (2.8 oz.)	18	3.8
Boiled, drained, mashed	½ cup (4 oz.)	26	5.6
TURNIP GREENS, leaves &			
stems:			
Fresh (USDA)	1 lb. (weighed untrimmed)	107	19.0
Boiled, in small amount water, short time, drained (USDA)	½ cup (2.6 oz.)	14	2.6
Boiled, in large amount water, long time, drained solids (USDA)	½ cup (2.6 oz.)	14	2.4
Canned, solids & liq. (USDA)	½ cup (4 oz.)	21	3.7
Frozen:			
Not thawed (USDA)	4 oz.	26	4.5
Boiled, drained (USDA)	4 oz.	26	4.4
Boiled, drained (USDA)	½ cup (2.9 oz.)	19	3.2
Chopped (Birds Eye)	½ cup (3.3 oz.)	22	2.7
TURNOVER (See individual kinds)			

Food and Description	Measure or Quantity	Calories	Carbohydrates (grams)
TURTLE, GREEN (USDA):			
Raw, in shell	1 lb. (weighed in shell)	97	0.
Raw, meat only	4 oz.	101	0.
Canned	4 oz.	120	0.
TV DINNER (See individual listing such as: **BEEF DINNER, CHICKEN DINNER, CHINESE DINNER, ENCHILADA DINNER,** etc.			
20-20 WINE (Mogen David) 20% alcohol	3 fl. oz.	105	9.8
TWINKIE (Hostess) 2 to pkg.	1 cake (1.5 oz.)	144	25.0
TWISTER, wine (Gallo) 20% alcohol	3 fl. oz.	109	8.4

(USDA): United States Department of Agriculture
DNA: Data Not Available
* Prepared as Package Directs

Food and Description	Measure or Quantity	Calories	Carbo-hydrates (grams)

U

UPPER-10, soft drink	6 fl. oz. (6.5 oz.)	78	18.5

V

VALPOLICELLA WINE, Italian red (Antinori)	3 fl. oz.	84	6.3
VANDERMINT, Dutch liqueur, (Leroux) 60 proof	1 fl. oz.	90	10.2
VANILLA CAKE, frozen (Pepperidge Farm)	⅛ of cake (3.1 oz.)	332	47.3
VANILLA CAKE MIX, French (Betty Crocker)	1-lb. 2.5-oz. pkg.	2202	423.6
VANILLA DRINK MIX, *Quik*	2 heaping tsp	60	15.6
VANILLA EXTRACT (Ehlers)	1 tsp.	8	D.N.A.
VANILLA ICE CREAM (See also individual brand names):			
(Borden's) 10.5% fat	¼ pt. (2.3 oz.)	132	15.8
Lady Borden, 14% fat	¼ pt. (2.5 oz.)	162	17.0
(Sealtest) *Party Slice*	1 slice (¼ pt., 2.3 oz.)	133	15.8
(Sealtest) 10.2% fat	¼ pt. (2.3 oz.)	133	15.8
(Sealtest) 12.1% fat	¼ pt. (2.3 oz.)	144	16.1
French (Prestige)	¼ pt. (2.3 oz.)	183	15.8
Fudge royale (Sealtest)	¼ pt. (2.3 oz.)	132	18.2
VANILLA ICE CREAM MIX (Junket)	6 serving pkg. (4 oz.)	388	110.0
VANILLA ICE MILK (Borden)	½ pt.	216	34.3
VANILLA PIE FILLING MIX: (See **VANILLA PUDDING MIX**)			

Food and Description	Measure or Quantity	Calories	Carbo-hydrates (grams)
VANILLA PUDDING:			
Blancmange, home recipe, with starch base (USDA)	½ cup (4.5 oz.)	142	20.4
(Betty Crocker)	½ cup	170	29.5
Canned (Del Monte)	5-oz. can	190	32.8
Canned (Hunt's)	5-oz. can	238	30.2
Canned (Thank You)	½ cup	169	29.2
Chilled (Sealtest)	4 oz.	125	20.9
VANILLA PUDDING or PIE FILLING MIX:			
Sweetened:			
*Regular (Jell-O)	½ cup (5.3 oz.)	173	29.3
*Instant (Jell-O)	½ cup (5.3 oz.)	178	30.5
*French, instant (Jell-O)	½ cup (5.3 oz.)	173	29.3
*Regular (My-T-Fine)	½ cup (5 oz.)	176	32.7
*Regular (Royal)	½ cup (5.1 oz.)	171	27.5
*Instant (Royal)	½ cup (5.1 oz.)	179	30.3
*Shake-A-Pudd'n (Royal)	½ cup (5.6 oz.)	165	32.3
Low calorie:			
*With whole milk (Dia-Mel)	4 oz.	90	8.1
*With nonfat milk (Dia-Mel)	4 oz.	53	8.2
*With whole milk (D-Zerta)	½ cup (4.6 oz.)	107	12.2
*With nonfat milk (D-Zerta)	½ cup (4.6 oz.)	72	12.7
VANILLA RENNET CUSTARD MIX:			
Powder:			
(Junket)	1 oz.	116	28.0
*(Junket)	4 oz.	108	14.7
Tablet:			
(Junket)	1 tablet	1	.2
*With sugar (Junket)	4 oz.	101	13.5
VANILLA SOFT DRINK:			
(Yoo-Hoo)	6 fl. oz.	90	18.0
High-protein (Yoo-Hoo)	6 fl. oz.	114	24.6

(USDA): United States Department of Agriculture
DNA: Data Not Available
* Prepared as Package Directs

Food and Description	Measure or Quantity	Calories	Carbohydrates (grams)
VEAL, medium fat (USDA):			
Chuck, raw	1 lb. (weighed with bone)	628	0.
Chuck, braised, lean & fat	4 oz.	266	0.
Flank, raw	1 lb. (weighed with bone)	1410	0.
Flank, stewed, lean & fat	4 oz.	442	0.
Foreshank, raw	1 lb. (weighed with bone)	368	0.
Foreshank, stewed, lean & fat	4 oz.	245	0.
Loin, raw	1 lb. (weighed with bone)	681	0.
Loin, broiled, medium done, chop, lean & fat	4 oz.	265	0.
Plate, raw	1 lb. (weighed with bone)	828	0.
Plate, stewed, lean & fat	4 oz.	344	0.
Rib, raw, lean & fat	1 lb. (weighed with bone)	723	0.
Rib, roasted, medium done, lean & fat	4 oz.	305	0.
Round & rump, raw	1 lb. (weighed with bone)	573	0.
Round & rump, broiled, steak or cutlet, lean & fat	4 oz.	245	0.
VEAL PARMIGIANA DINNER, frozen (Swanson)	12¼-oz. dinner	492	47.7
VEGETABLE BOUILLON CUBE:			
(Herb-Ox)	1 cube (4 grams)	6	.5
(Wyler's)	1 cube (4 grams)	7	.3
VEGETABLE FAT (See **FAT**)			
VEGETABLE JUICE COCKTAIL, canned:			
(USDA)	4 oz. (by wt.)	19	4.1
Unseasoned (S and W) Nutradiet	4 oz. (by wt.)	24	5.1
V-8 (Campbell)	¾ cup	31	6.0
Vegemato (College Inn)	4 oz.	22	4.7
VEGETABLE, MIXED:			
Canned (Veg-All)	4 oz.	39	7.8

Food and Description	Measure or Quantity	Calories	Carbo-hydrates (grams)
Frozen:			
Not thawed (USDA)	4 oz.	74	15.5
Boiled, drained (USDA)	½ cup (3.2 oz.)	58	12.2
(Birds Eye)	½ cup (3.3 oz.)	50	12.4
Jubilee (Birds Eye)	½ cup (3.3 oz.)	138	18.9
(Blue Goose)	4 oz.	60	12.8
In butter sauce (Green Giant)	⅓ of 10-oz. pkg.	59	8.7
With onion sauce (Birds Eye)	½ cup (2.7 oz.)	117	13.6
VEGETABLE OYSTER (See SALSIFY)			
VEGETABLE SOUP:			
Canned, regular pack:			
(Campbell) *Chunky*	1 cup	105	16.5
Beef, condensed (USDA)	8 oz. (by wt.)	147	17.9
*Beef, prepared with equal volume water (USDA)	1 cup (8.6 oz.)	78	9.6
With beef broth, condensed (USDA)	8 oz. (by wt.)	145	24.9
*With beef broth, prepared with equal volume water (USDA)	1 cup (8.8 oz.)	80	13.8
*(Campbell)	1 cup	77	12.6
*(Campbell) old fashioned	1 cup	70	8.9
*Beef (Campbell)	1 cup	75	7.3
*(Campbell) *Noodle-O's*	1 cup	71	9.7
*Beef (Heinz)	1 cup (8½ oz.)	66	9.6
Beef (Heinz) *Great American*	1 cup (8¾ oz.)	126	12.2
With beef broth (Heinz) *Great American*	1 cup (8¾ oz.)	144	18.4
*With beef stock (Heinz)	1 cup (8½ oz.)	83	13.4
With ground beef (Heinz) *Great American*	1 cup (8¾ oz.)	139	12.1
Vegetarian:			
Condensed (USDA)	8 oz. (by wt.)	145	24.0
*Prepared with equal volume water (USDA)	1 cup (8.6 oz.)	78	13.2
*(Campbell)	1 cup	71	11.8

(USDA): United States Department of Agriculture
DNA: Data Not Available
* Prepared as Package Directs

Food and Description	Measure or Quantity	Calories	Carbo- hydrates (grams)
*(Heinz)	1 cup (8¾ oz.)	83	14.2
(Heinz) *Great American*	1 cup (8½ oz.)	125	18.1
*(Manischewitz)	8 oz. (by wt.)	63	10.2
Canned, dietetic pack:			
Low sodium (Campbell)	7½-oz. can	83	14.4
Beef, low sodium			
(Campbell)	7½-oz. can	78	8.8
*(Claybourne)	1 cup	104	21.0
(Tillie Lewis)	1 cup	62	11.1
Frozen:			
With beef, condensed			
(USDA)	8 oz. (by wt.)	159	15.9
*With beef, prepared with equal volume water			
(USDA)	8 oz. (by wt.)	79	7.7
VEGETABLE SOUP MIX:			
*(Wyler's)	6 fl. oz.	42	7.0
Beef (Lipton)	1 cup	53	7.3
*& noodle (Lipton)	1 cup	73	13.3
VENISON, raw, lean meat only (USDA)	4 oz.	143	0.
VERMOUTH:			
Dry & extra dry:			
(C & P) 19% alcohol	3 fl. oz.	90	3.0
(Gallo) 18% alcohol	3 fl. oz.	75	1.7
(Gancia) 21% alcohol	3 fl. oz.	126	D.N.A.
(Lejon) 18.5% alcohol	3 fl. oz.	99	2.2
(Noilly Pratt) 19% alcohol	3 fl. oz.	101	1.6
(Taylor) 17% alcohol	3 fl. oz.	102	.9
Rosso, (Gancia) 21% alcohol	3 fl. oz.	153	6.9
Sweet:			
(C & P) 16% alcohol	3 fl. oz.	120	14.4
(Gallo) 18% alcohol	3 fl. oz.	118	2.3
(Lejon) 18.5% alcohol	3 fl. oz.	134	11.4
(Noilly Pratt) 16% alcohol	3 fl. oz.	128	12.1
(Taylor) 17% alcohol	3 fl. oz.	132	10.4
White (Gancia) 16.8% alcohol	3 fl. oz.	132	7.8
White (Lejon) 18.5% alcohol	3 fl. oz.	101	2.6
VERNORS, soft drink:			
Regular	6 fl. oz. (6.2 oz.)	70	16.8
Low calorie	6 fl. oz.	1	<.1

Food and Description	Measure or Quantity	Calories	Carbo-hydrates (grams)
VICHYSSOISE SOUP			
(Crosse & Blackwell)	6½ oz. (½ can)	94	9.4
VIENNA SAUSAGE, canned:			
(USDA)	1 oz.	68	<.1
(Armour Star)	5-oz. can	393	0.
(Armour Star)	1 sausage (.6 oz.)	45	0.
(Hormel)	4-oz. can	323	.6
(Wilson)	1 oz.	85	<.1
VILLA ANTINORI, Italian white wine, 12½% alcohol	3 fl. oz.	87	6.3
VINEGAR:			
Cider:			
(USDA)	1 T. (.5 oz.)	2	.9
(USDA)	½ cup (4.2 oz.)	17	7.1
(Hunt's)	1 oz.	4	1.7
Distilled:			
(USDA)	1 T. (.5 oz.)	2	.8
(USDA)	½ cup (4.2 oz.)	14	6.0
(Hunt's)	1 oz.	3	1.4
VINESPINACH or BASELLA, raw (USDA)	4 oz.	22	3.9
VINO PRIMO WINE (Italian Swiss Colony Gold Medal) 12% alcohol	3 fl. oz.	66	1.6
VIN ROSE (See **ROSE WINE**)			
VODKA, unflavored (See **DISTILLED LIQUOR**)			
VODKA COCKTAIL:			
Martini (Calvert) 75 proof	3 fl. oz.	188	Tr.
Screwdriver (Old Mr. Boston) 25 proof	3 fl. oz.	117	10.5
VODKA, FLAVORED (Old Mr. Boston):			
Wild cherry, grape, lemon, lime or orange, 70 proof	1 fl. oz.	100	8.0
Peppermint, 70 proof	1 fl. oz.	90	5.0
VOIGNY WINE (Chanson) 13% alcohol	3 fl. oz.	96	7.5

(USDA): United States Department of Agriculture
DNA: Data Not Available
* Prepared as Package Directs

Food and Description	Measure or Quantity	Calories	Carbohydrates (grams)

W

WAFER (See **COOKIE** or **CRACKER**)

WAFFLE:

Food and Description	Measure or Quantity	Calories	Carbohydrates (grams)
Home recipe (USDA)	2.6-oz. waffle (½″ x 4½″ x 5½″)	209	28.1
Frozen:			
(USDA)	1 waffle (8 in 13-oz. pkg.)	116	19.3
(USDA)	1 waffle (6 in 5-oz. pkg.)	61	10.1
Original (Aunt Jemima)	2 sections (1.5 oz.)	117	16.2

WAFFLE MIX (USDA) (See also **PANCAKE & WAFFLE MIX**):

Food and Description	Measure or Quantity	Calories	Carbohydrates (grams)
Dry	1 oz.	130	18.5
*Prepared with water	2.6-oz. waffle (½″ x 4½″ x 5½″)	229	30.2

WAFFLE SYRUP (See **SYRUP**)

WALNUT:

Food and Description	Measure or Quantity	Calories	Carbohydrates (grams)
Black:			
In shell, whole (USDA)	1 lb. (weighed in shell)	627	14.8
Shelled, whole (USDA)	4 oz.	712	16.8
Chopped (USDA)	½ cup (2.1 oz.)	377	8.9
Kernel (Hammons)	1 lb.	2985	46.3
English or Persian:			
In shell, whole (USDA)	1 lb. (weighed in shell)	1329	32.2
Shelled, whole (USDA)	4 oz.	738	17.9
Chopped (USDA)	½ cup (2.1 oz.)	391	9.5
Chopped (USDA)	1 T. (8 grams)	49	1.2
Chopped (Diamond)	1 T.	49	1.2
Halves (USDA)	½ cup (1.8 oz.)	326	7.9

Food and Description	Measure or Quantity	Calories	Carbo-hydrates (grams)
Halves (Diamond)	½ cup	327	7.8
Halves (Diamond)	8–15 halves	98	2.3
WALNUT, BLACK, EXTRACT (Ehlers)	1 tsp.	4	D.N.A.
***WALNUT CAKE MIX, BLACK** (Betty Crocker)	¹⁄₁₂ of cake	202	36.3
WATER CHESTNUT, CHINESE, raw (USDA):			
Whole	1 lb. (weighed unpeeled)	272	66.4
Peeled	4 oz.	90	21.5
WATERCRESS, raw (USDA):			
Whole	½ lb. (weighed untrimmed)	40	6.2
Trimmed	½ cup (.6 oz.)	3	.5
WATERMELON, fresh (USDA):			
Whole	1 lb. (weighed with rind)	54	13.4
Wedge	2-lb. wedge (4″ x 8″ measured with rind)	111	27.3
Diced (USDA)	1 cup (5.6 oz.)	42	10.2
WATERMELON RIND (Crosse & Blackwell)	1 T.	38	9.3
WAX GOURD, raw (USDA):			
Whole	1 lb. (weighed with skin & cavity contents)	41	9.4
Flesh only	4 oz.	15	3.4
WEAKFISH (USDA):			
Raw, whole	1 lb. (weighed whole)	263	0.
Broiled, meat only	4 oz.	236	0.

(USDA): United States Department of Agriculture
DNA: Data Not Available
* Prepared as Package Directs

Food and Description	Measure or Quantity	Calories	Carbo-hydrates (grams)
WELSH RAREBIT, home recipe (USDA)	1 cup (8.2 oz.)	415	14.6
WEST INDIAN CHERRY (See **ACEROLA**)			
WHALE MEAT, raw (USDA)	4 oz.	177	0.
WHEAT CHEX, cereal (Ralston)	½ cup (1 oz.)	108	23.0
*WHEATENA, cereal	½ cup (.9 oz., dry)	88	18.1
WHEAT FLAKES, cereal:			
Crushed (USDA)	1 cup (2.5 oz.)	248	56.4
Dietetic (Van Brode)	1 oz.	109	23.0
WHEAT GERM, crude, commercially milled (USDA)	1 oz.	103	13.2
WHEAT GERM, CEREAL:			
(USDA)	¼ cup (1 oz.)	110	14.0
(Kretschmer)	¼ cup (1 oz.)	106	12.6
With sugar & honey (Kretschmer)	¼ cup (1 oz.)	107	26.9
WHEAT HONEYS, cereal	1 cup (1⅛ oz.)	152	32.7
WHEATIES, cereal	1 cup (1 oz.)	101	23.1
WHEAT OATA, cereal, dry	¼ cup (1 oz.)	109	19.6
WHEAT, PUFFED, cereal:			
(USDA)	1 cup (.4 oz.)	44	9.4
Frosted (USDA)	1 cup (.4 oz.)	45	10.6
(Checker)	½-oz. serving	51	11.0
(Quaker)	1⅛ cups (.5 oz.)	51	11.2
WHEAT, SHREDDED, cereal (See **SHREDDED WHEAT**)			
*WHIP'N CHILL (Jell-O):			
*All flavors except chocolate	½ cup (3 oz.)	135	19.3
*Chocolate	½ cup (3 oz.)	144	22.0

Food and Description	Measure or Quantity	Calories	Carbo-hydrates (grams)
WHISKEY or WHISKY (See **DISTILLED LIQUOR**)			
WHISKEY SOUR:			
(Calvert) 60 proof	3 fl. oz.	190	9.5
(Hiram Walker) 52.5 proof	3 fl. oz.	177	12.0
WHISKEY SOUR MIX:			
(Bar-Tender's)	1 serving (⅝ oz.)	70	17.2
Low calorie, *Sip 'n Slim*	1 serving (¾ oz.)	2	.5
WHISKEY SOUR SOFT DRINK:			
(Canada Dry)	6 fl. oz.	71	18.4
(Shasta)	6 fl. oz.	65	16.5
WHITEFISH, LAKE (USDA):			
Raw, whole	1 lb. (weighed whole)	330	0.
Raw, meat only	4 oz.	176	0.
Baked, stuffed, home recipe	4 oz.	244	6.6
Smoked	4 oz.	176	0.
WHOOPEE PIE (Berwick)	1 pie	300	45.0
WIENER (Oscar Mayer):			
Regular	1 link	161	D.N.A.
Little	1 link	30	D.N.A.
WILD BERRY, fruit drink (Hi-C)	6 fl. oz.	92	22.7
WILD RICE, raw:			
(USDA)	4 oz.	400	85.4
(USDA)	½ cup (2.9 oz.)	289	61.7
WINE (Most wines are listed by kind, brand, vineyard, region or grape name): Dessert (USDA) 18.8% alcohol	3 fl. oz.	122	6.9
Dessert (Petri)	3 fl. oz.	124	D.N.A.
Flavored (Petri)	3 fl. oz.	124	D.N.A.

(USDA): United States Department of Agriculture
DNA: Data Not Available
* Prepared as Package Directs

Food and Description	Measure or Quantity	Calories	Carbo-hydrates (grams)
Red (Great Western) *Pleasant Valley*, 12% alcohol	3 fl. oz.	88	4.7
Table:			
(USDA) 12.2% alcohol	3 fl. oz.	75	3.7
(Petri)	3 fl. oz.	59	D.N.A.
White (Great Western) *Pleasant Valley*, 12% alcohol	3 fl. oz.	88	4.7
WINK, soft drink (Canada Dry)	6 fl. oz.	85	22.0
WINTERGREEN EXTRACT (Ehlers)	1 tsp.	11	D.N.A.
WONTON SOUP, canned (Mow Sang)	10-oz. can	134	21.0
WORCESTERSHIRE SAUCE (See **SAUCE,** Worcestershire)			
WRECKFISH, raw, meat only (USDA)	4 oz.	129	0.

Y

YAM (USDA):			
Raw, whole	1 lb. (weighed with skin)	394	90.5
Raw, flesh only	4 oz.	115	26.3
Canned and frozen (See **SWEET POTATO)**			
YAM BEAN, raw (USDA):			
Unpared	1 lb. (weighed unpared)	225	52.2
Pared	4 oz.	62	14.5
YANKEE DOODLES (Drake's)	1 cake (1 oz.)	120	18.0

Food and Description	Measure or Quantity	Calories	Carbo-hydrates (grams)
YEAST:			
Baker's:			
Compressed (USDA)	1 oz.	24	3.1
Compressed (Fleischmann's)	⅜-oz. cake	19	1.9
Dry (USDA)	1 oz.	80	11.0
Dry (USDA)	1 pkg. (7 grams)	20	2.7
Dry (Fleischmann's)	¼ oz. (pkg. or jar)	24	2.9
Brewer's dry, debittered (USDA)	1 oz.	80	10.9
Brewer's dry, debittered (USDA)	1 T. (8 grams)	23	3.1
YELLOWTAIL, raw, meat only (USDA)	4 oz.	156	0.
YOGURT:			
Made from whole milk (USDA)	½ cup (4.3 oz.)	76	6.0
Made from partially skimmed milk, plain or vanilla:			
(USDA)	½ cup (4.3 oz.)	61	6.3
(USDA)	8-oz. container	113	11.8
Plain:			
(Borden) Swiss style	5-oz. container	82	9.9
(Borden) Swiss style	8-oz. container	131	15.9
(Breakstone)	8-oz. container	141	12.7
(Breakstone)	1 T. (.5 oz.)	10	.8
(Dannon)	8-oz. container	136	14.1
Apple, Dutch (Dannon)	8-oz. container	258	51.1
Apricot:			
(Breakstone)	8-oz. container	220	37.4
(Breakstone) *Swiss Parfait*	8-oz. container	249	42.9
(Dannon)	8-oz. container	258	51.1
Black cherry (Breakstone) *Swiss Parfait*	8-oz. container	256	44.9
Blueberry:			
(Breakstone)	8-oz. container	252	46.3
(Breakstone) *Swiss Parfait*	8-oz. container	286	53.1
(Dannon)	8-oz. container	258	51.1

(USDA): United States Department of Agriculture
DNA: Data Not Available
* Prepared as Package Directs

Food and Description	Measure or Quantity	Calories	Carbo-hydrates (grams)
(Meadow Gold)	8-oz. container	249	54.0
(Meadow Gold) Swiss style	8-oz. container	245	49.0
(Sanna) *Swiss Miss*	4-oz. container	125	19.0
(Sealtest) *Light n' Lively*	8-oz. container	257	50.6
(SugarLo)	8-oz. container	117	14.6
Boysenberry:			
(Dannon)	8-oz. container	258	51.1
(Meadow Gold)	8-oz. container	249	54.0
Cherry:			
(Dannon)	8-oz. container	258	51.1
(Meadow Gold)	8-oz. container	249	54.0
Dark (SugarLo)	8-oz. container	117	14.6
Cinnamon apple (Breakstone)	8-oz. container	229	39.9
Coffee (Dannon)	8-oz. container	198	33.3
Danny (Dannon):			
Cuplet, any flavor	4-oz. container	129	25.5
Frozen pop	2½-oz. pop	127	18.0
Honey (Breakstone) *Swiss Parfait*	8-oz. container	277	51.5
Lemon:			
(Breakstone) *Swiss Parfait*	8-oz. container	254	44.9
(Sealtest) *Light n' Lively*	8-oz. container	229	43.4
Lime (Breakstone) *Swiss Parfait*	8-oz. container	243	40.1
Mandarin orange:			
(Borden) Swiss style	5-oz. container	142	28.7
(Borden) Swiss style	8-oz. container	227	45.9
(Breakstone) *Swiss Parfait*	8-oz. container	263	48.3
Peach:			
(Borden) Swiss style	5-oz. container	138	27.8
(Borden) Swiss style	8-oz. container	221	44.5
(Breakstone) *Swiss Parfait*	8-oz. container	254	47.4
Melba (Breakstone) *Swiss Parfait*	8-oz. container	268	49.4
(Meadow Gold)	8-oz. container	249	54.0
(Sealtest) *Light n' Lively*	8-oz. container	252	49.3
(SugarLo)	8-oz. container	117	14.6
Pineapple:			
(Breakstone)	8-oz. container	220	37.9
(Meadow Gold)	8-oz. container	249	54.0
(Sealtest) *Light n' Lively*	8-oz. container	241	47.2
(SugarLo)	8-oz. container	117	14.8
Pineapple-orange (Dannon)	8-oz. container	258	51.1

Food and Description	Measure or Quantity	Calories	Carbo-hydrates (grams)
Prune whip (Breakstone)	8-oz. container	231	41.1
Prune whip (Dannon)	8-oz. container	258	51.1
Raspberry:			
(Borden) Swiss style	5-oz. container	147	29.5
(Borden) Swiss style	8-oz. container	236	47.2
(Breakstone)	8-oz. container	249	45.8
(Dannon)	8-oz. container	258	51.1
Red (Breakstone) *Swiss Parfait*	8-oz. container	263	46.5
(Meadow Gold) Swiss style	8-oz. container	245	49.0
(Sanna) *Swiss Miss*	4-oz. container	125	19.0
Red (Sealtest) *Light n' Lively*	8-oz. container	225	41.8
(SugarLo)	8-oz. container	118	14.8
Strawberry:			
(Borden) Swiss style	5-oz. container	142	27.8
(Borden) Swiss style	8-oz. container	227	44.5
(Breakstone)	8-oz. container	225	43.5
(Breakstone) *Swiss Parfait*	8-oz. container	259	50.6
(Dannon)	8-oz. container	258	51.1
(Meadow Gold)	8-oz. container	249	54.0
(Meadow Gold) Swiss style	8-oz. container	245	49.0
(Sanna) *Swiss Miss*	4-oz. container	125	19.0
(Sealtest) *Light n' Lively*	8-oz. container	234	44.3
(SugarLo)	8-oz. container	111	13.2
Vanilla:			
(Borden) Swiss style	5-oz. container	148	28.4
(Borden) Swiss style	8-oz. container	235	45.4
(Breakstone)	8-oz. container	195	29.5
(Dannon)	8-oz. container	198	33.3

YOUNGBERRY, fresh (See **BLACKBERRY,** fresh)

(USDA): United States Department of Agriculture
DNA: Data Not Available
* Prepared as Package Directs

Food and Description	Measure or Quantity	Calories	Carbo- hydrates (grams)

Z

ZELTINGER ANGLERWEIN,
German Moselle wine

| (Deinhard) 11% alcohol | 3 fl. oz. | 60 | 1.0 |

ZINFANDEL WINE:
(Italian Swiss Colony-Gold

| Medal) 12.3% alcohol | 3 fl. oz. | 63 | .7 |

(Louis M. Martini) 12.5%

| alcohol | 3 fl. oz. | 90 | .2 |

| **ZITI,** baked, frozen (Buitoni) | 4 oz. | 128 | 21.4 |

ZUCCHINI (See **SQUASH, SUMMER**)

ZWIEBACK:

| (USDA) | 1 oz. | 120 | 21.1 |
| (Nabisco) | 1 piece (7 grams) | 31 | 5.4 |

BIBLIOGRAPHY

Dawson, Elsie H., Gilpin, Gladys L., and Fulton, Lois H., *Average weight of a measured cup of various foods.* U.S.D.A. ARS 61–6, February 1969. 19 pp.

Merrill, A. L. and Watt, B. K., *Energy value of foods—basis and derivation.* U.S.D.A. Handb. 74, 105 pp. 1955.

Pecot, Rebecca K., Jaeger, Carol M., and Watt, Bernice K., *Proximate composition of beef from carcass to cooked meat: Method of derivation and tables of values.* U.S.D.A. Home Economics Research Report 31, 32 pp. 1965.

Pecot, Rebecca K. and Watt, Bernice K., *Food yields: Summarized by different stages of preparation.* U.S.D.A. Handb. 102, 93 pp. 1956.

U.S.D.A. Nutritive value of foods. Home and Garden Bul. 72, 36 pp. 1964 and revised edition, 1970. 41 pp.

U.S.D.A. Unpubl. Data 1969.

Watt, Bernice K., Merrill, Annabel L., et al., *Composition of foods: Raw, processed, prepared.* U.S.D.A. Agriculture Handb. 8, 190 pp. 1963.